T0316726

Medicine and the Workhouse

Rochester Studies in Medical History

Senior Editor: Theodore M. Brown
Professor of History and Preventive Medicine
University of Rochester

ISSN 1526-2715

Additional Titles of Interest

A complete list of titles in the Rochester Studies in Medical History series
may be found on our website, www.urpress.com.

Medicine and
the Workhouse

EDITED BY
JONATHAN REINARZ AND LEONARD SCHWARZ

UNIVERSITY OF ROCHESTER PRESS

First published 2013

University of Rochester Press
668 Mt. Hope Avenue, Rochester, NY 14620, USA
www.urpress.com
and Boydell & Brewer Limited
PO Box 9, Woodbridge, Suffolk IP12 3DF, UK
www.boydellandbrewer.com

ISBN-13: 978-1-58046-448-2
ISSN: 1526-2715

Library of Congress Cataloging-in-Publication Data

Medicine and the workhouse / edited by Jonathan Reinarz and Leonard Schwarz.
    pages cm. — (Rochester studies in medical history, ISSN 1526-2715 ; volume 27)
    Includes bibliographical references and index.
    ISBN 978-1-58046-448-2 (hardcover : alk. paper) 1. Poor—Medical care—History.
2. Workhouses—History. I. Reinarz, Jonathan. II. Schwarz, Leonard.
    RA418.5.P6M433   2013
    362.1086'942—dc23

                                                              2013011382

A catalogue record for this title is available from the British Library.

This publication is printed on acid-free paper.
Printed in the United States of America.

Contents

Preface

This book had its origins in a two-day conference on "Medicine and the Workhouse" in November 2008, sponsored by the University of Birmingham and the Wellcome Trust. It drew together scholars whose current work directly addresses the issue of medicine and the workhouse. It also included a number of historians who have investigated the subject of health, illness, and the workhouse and whose names frequently appear in the references of the selection of papers that were chosen to present in this volume. The first day of the event was devoted to the Old Poor Law, while the papers presented on the second day concentrated on the New Poor Law. This structure was retained for the organization of this volume to demonstrate change and particular themes that emerged during the conference. The afterword was initially a keynote delivered at the outset of the event but has been situated at the end of the volume, given that it serves as a bridge between the two periods and offers a fitting conclusion to the subject as a whole, outlining both achievements in this area of research and some future challenges.

We wish to thank the conference sponsors, particularly the Wellcome Trust, for making this event possible and all the presenters for their stimulating papers and discussions. We are especially grateful to Steven King, Alistair Ritch, and Kevin Siena for reading through the introductory section of the volume and their many helpful comments. We also wish to thank Kiran Hallan for assisting with the organization of the event and Frances Worrall for aiding with the footnotes and tables.

—The Editors

Introduction

JONATHAN REINARZ AND LEONARD SCHWARZ

Despite a relative dearth of work on the subject, the student of workhouses is bound, within a short space of time, to be led into the field of medicine.[1] Nevertheless, one might ask why there has not been more work on this subject, given that emotional responses to suffering within the workhouse led the institution to figure so prominently in popular literature of the nineteenth century, the most well-known case being Charles Dickens's *Oliver Twist* (1838). In any case, what is becoming ever clearer is that workhouses were not established simply to warehouse the destitute, but they had their own, often specialist, sick wards, and sickness was a common cause of poverty, as well as a common route into the workhouse. However, the stories of inmates, where they have been collected and compiled, present some common, but also very diverse, experiences. The records, when they do go into sufficient detail, present a host of diseases and afflictions, at least as broad as recorded in the earliest voluntary hospital records.[2] They also offer concentrations of particular cases, as illustrated in a number of the chapters in this volume, encouraging what at times might be described as an early period of specialization at some institutions. Nevertheless, few medical practitioners, let alone inmates, were eager to enter workhouses, usually spending short periods there before securing more prestigious posts at voluntary and endowed hospitals. As late as the second half of the twentieth century, medical schools in England continued to refuse to recognize the sheer variety of medical conditions in a workhouse, as the chapter by Jonathan Reinarz and Alistair Ritch in this volume makes clear. Within the voluminous medical history literature for England, these institutions have been equally sidelined.

The historian of workhouses is confronted with many potential themes for research, nearly as diverse and numerous as the cases that presented themselves to medical staff in these institutions in the past. As a result, it is a rich seam for future historical research. If not immediately evident in subsequent chapters, many of these strands are clearly outlined in Steven King's afterword. The scope of this volume was, however, restricted by the papers that were presented at an original conference and, of these, the editors have decided to concentrate on a handful that dominated discussion over the two-day event and recurred in papers across periods. The papers chosen for this volume, as the title declares, all very clearly focus on medical aspects of workhouse care. They also concentrate on both medical staff, primarily doctors and surgeons, less often the nursing staff, as well as the sick inmates. In terms of the medical staff, some effort has been made to trace a selection of medical careers and medical activity in the workhouse in greater detail than has been the case previously; relations between medical staff and lay governors and authorities are also explored, as are the roles of both groups as advocates, and opponents, of change. In the process, there is an attempt to chart the gradual professionalization of workhouse medical officers as a group. Often, these arguments are made by way of case studies. Among other matters, these regional studies are meant to reflect workhouse medicine's profound geographic diversity, between metropolis and province, as well as colony, but also between relatively proximate provincial towns. Together, they demonstrate the variety of practice encompassed by workhouse medicine, as well as some very real challenges of research in this area.

Some subjects are noticeably absent. The chapters do not, for example, consider in any depth the history of workhouse architecture, which clearly impacted on the types of patients seen at institutions and determined their experiences at the workhouse, as this has been attempted elsewhere.[3] Nor do they consider Scotland, for which there is, as yet, no detailed analysis of the situation before 1834, though some new work has recently built on Stephanie Blackden's research on Glasgow and is ongoing.[4] There is also a great deal of scope for additional research into the poor law in Wales. This volume, however, does look beyond England, to later nineteenth-century Ireland and even attempts a comparison with the Caribbean workhouse, whose penal and medical functions are highlighted in Rita Pemberton's chapter.[5] Also, they consider workhouse patients. Most authors have attempted to break down the sick workhouse population in the traditional way, namely by classifying them into identifiable "types," including young women, syphilitics and other venereal cases, patients suffering from fevers, the very young and older inmates. While some offer only rare snapshots of the sick poor in a particular year or region, as in Alannah Tomkins's contribution, others, such as Susannah Ottaway, map distinct groups, like the elderly, and make a case for gradual change in their representation and care over several decades. In general, the organization of the volume in two parts encourages these and other reflections, but comparisons often extend beyond the Old and New Poor Laws. Occasionally, comparisons may appear problematic, as they did when draft papers were first presented at our conference, and, at these points, authors focus instead on the methodological and practical issues that will challenge and frustrate future scholars who engage with the records of workhouses, their infirmaries, and the medical staff and patients who spent time there. As other biographies of workhouse inmates emerge, scholars will undoubtedly grapple with issues raised by Tomkins; for example, even the most depressing of workhouse cases appear to have had some kind words for the treatment they received in poor law establishments.

Many of the problems faced by the researchers who have confronted this subject stem directly from terminology. Though perhaps less complicated when first read in the title of this book, the term "workhouse" does not always appear in poor law records dealing with institutional care, or adequately describe the work undertaken in the buildings originally established as workhouses in name. Or, as Kevin Siena helpfully suggests, the workhouse was not only about "work." This theme recurs throughout this volume. As King suggests in his concluding section, whether described as "workhouses," "hospitals for the poor," or "poor houses," these institutions were regularly reinvented, if not modified, to deal with the problems and concerns that parish and union authorities faced during the eighteenth and nineteenth centuries. Workhouses were often described as "prisons," especially in their early years, although their roles contrasted significantly among communities. Whether in England or America, they could function as refuge or prison, shelter or even a basic hospital.[6]

Those who visited distant institutions usually perceived these differences the quickest. The difference between English and Caribbean workhouses was, not surprisingly, noted by English observers in the early nineteenth century, as recounted by Pemberton. Irish workhouses, following a tour of the country's institutions in 1895, were described by Catherine Wood to be dirtier and smaller than English ones, but also overcrowded. This sort of variation between institutions internationally, however, also characterized workhouses in London, where some, including those investigated by Jeremy Boulton, Romola Davenport, and Leonard Schwarz; Ottaway, and Siena, could more appropriately have been renamed hospices, which might go some of the way toward solving the problem of workhouse definition that existed at least under the Old Poor Law. In cases where the functions of the institution may have appeared less medical, such as those that operated as prisons, the intended outcomes were perhaps not that different when considered more fully. Most of these institutions, whether taking on predominantly prisoners, the destitute, or sick poor, aimed primarily at bringing about some sort of transformation; as argued elsewhere, they refashioned incarcerated and troublesome bodies, returning healthy and productive members of the poor to the community.[7] In the case of the workhouse and prison, two seemingly different institutions were even linked by the treadmill, which promised "salvation through hard work." Both were equally renowned for their restrictive diets. Virginia Crossman is also one of the few contributors to remind us that visiting at workhouses was similarly restricted, especially when compared with voluntary hospitals and asylums.[8] In nearly every case explored here, workhouses, regardless of geographic distribution, retained both their medical and punitive functions.

With so few public institutions in existence at the time, it should perhaps not surprise historians that eighteenth-century workhouses themselves did occasionally transform, at times resembling prisons, hospices, hospitals, or even homes for the elderly, depending on the needs, values, or simply the wishes of influential staff and authorities. In the case of eighteenth-century London, whose workhouses have attracted much attention from scholars in the past decade, this variation has become apparent. For the eighteenth century, Siena presents the sheer extent of illness among the poor, while attempting to demonstrate how London workhouses rapidly became "medicalized" after their foundation, usually in the 1720s. Interestingly, he also argues that it was users' needs that led the way in which workhouses altered and evolved. Ottaway points to the growing importance of the elderly in the late eighteenth century to explain the simultaneous medicalization of old age that took place in this period. Though troubled to a certain extent by its use as a home for the elderly, contemporaries who supported these institutions gradually transformed large parts of them into hospitals or at least added medical wings. In their case study, Boulton, Davenport, and Schwarz show how one large London workhouse, that of St. Martin in the Fields, became medicalized during the earlier eighteenth century. The intention was usually to manage a large workhouse and a small infirmary; the outcome might reverse the process. The same was constantly true under the New Poor Law, at least in London, as the commissioners found to their cost.[9] Nevertheless, in English provincial workhouses, as outlined by Leonard Smith, a space for the least dangerous poor lunatics often developed into multiple wards, which, nevertheless, also occasionally housed very dangerous inmates. While this was perhaps intended as a temporary measure that would be remedied through the construction of English county asylums, overcrowding prevented the transfer of all those deemed unsuitable for the workhouse wards and, as a result, poor law regulations were gradually modified. Many of these wards also began to house significant numbers of epileptics, as was the case in Birmingham and Leicester, eventually leading these spaces to be renamed "epileptic wards" in the former city, even if not entirely suited to their new functions.

For what was a workhouse? As a number of contributors point out, at least under the Old Poor Law, and quite possibly under the New, a workhouse evolved as a *complex* of different buildings that had sometimes been constructed to take care of a particular situation. In the Caribbean, they were often formerly prisons put to new uses. As in the British context, the workhouse was partly designed to drive poor or work-shy members of society back to work; in part it served as a hospital. For those hitherto active, but now ill, the workhouse's rate of "cure" (that is, of symptom prevention) may not have been so different from that of the hospital. For the aged poor, it was sometimes a port of call—often the last port of call—before death. For all the very poor, it was a place of last resort, and that is unlikely to have changed very much into the nineteenth century and under the New Poor Law.

Medical history can often provide an entry to urban history, more particularly the lives of the poor. So as with John Landers's book, Boulton, Davenport, and Schwarz's chapter on the one hand, and Siena's on the other, can both be read as detailed studies of London.[10] For instance, London is supposed to have had an unusual number of people with settlements elsewhere. Siena has found a number of references to charities stating that they cared only for nonsettled Londoners; it is not generally appreciated how rare such references are. The overwhelming majority of dispensaries, most of which were founded in the 1770s and beyond, made no reference to the Settlement Acts at all.[11] It is as though they were under an obligation not to mention poor relief. Yet the more is known about parish provision of medicine, the more likely it becomes that dispensaries catered to the nonsettled poor. This, in turn, means that immigration figures based on dispensaries are too high. For instance, it has become customary to quote Robert Bland's records for the Westminster General Dispensary from 1774 to 1781, which state that three-quarters of patients were born outside London.[12] But, if we accept Edward Anthony Wrigley's estimate of some 8,000 migrants to London a year between 1650 and 1750 and make the exaggerated assumption that all the immigrants stayed in London for thirty years, that comes to only 240,000 in 1750, or 36 percent of a population of 675,000.[13] Incidentally, Bland's sample refers only to married women.[14]

While such research demonstrates how resourceful historians of the metropolis have been in accessing the records that allow them to reconstruct the lives of the poor, it is a mistake to draw too broad conclusions from London: first, London had more people on relief than the rest of England, and, of those, far more were in its fifty-four workhouses;[15] second, London workhouses were exceptionally large, at least by the standards of most provincial workhouses;[16] and, third, a greater proportion of the poor were relieved inside the workhouse.[17] The Commissioners' Report, dominated by the commissioners' panic about able-bodied adult poor, hardly discussed illness and old age, although these were two of the most common causes of poverty.[18] In 1803 a parliamentary report gave aged and infirm adults as 16 percent of the whole. In 1851 they were 42.1 percent, with the insane another 1.7 percent.[19] In 1896 Birmingham's workhouse had 1,123 inmates, compared with 917 at the workhouse infirmary at Dudley Road, Birmingham. In the case of Ireland, such calculations are complicated by

the existence of a national dispensary system from 1851 and an expansion
in out-relief from the 1860s. Crossman also reminds us that infirmaries there
were opened to paying patients around this time. In the Caribbean even less
is known about the sick inmates of the workhouse, given the poor survival
rates of doctors' journals.

Despite such difficulties, most chapters in this volume attempt to break
down some general statistics into regional and key diagnostic subgroups.
In their chapter Boulton, Davenport, and Schwarz, for example, come
near arguing that sickness can be divided into three categories: that of
children, for whom the death rate might be high, even omitting the infant
year; that of old people (sixty plus), also with a high death rate; and those
between. Ottaway does not disagree with this, at least as far as the elderly
are concerned. For his purposes, Siena has concentrated on the fever, itch,
and venereal cases. He also highlights that workhouse populations were
disproportionately female, although a more sustained consideration of
gender, despite its significant role in the workhouse, is not a feature of this
particular volume.[20] Reinarz and Ritch identify four specific categories:
children, venereal cases, epileptics, and the elderly. Angela Negrine, in
her examination of another provincial workhouse, charts a complex range
of patients in Leicester but also identifies the imbecile patient as composing a significant constituency. Smith examines this same, ubiquitous
category in additional detail and suggests that workhouses were an important, neglected element in the institutional provision for the insane, nine
thousand having been recorded among the English workhouse population
in 1847. Additionally, he attempts to differentiate between the mentally
ill and those who were potentially dangerous to staff and other inmates.
Ottaway, in turn, focuses on the elderly, who regularly appear in lists of
workhouse inmates for an earlier period. By the late nineteenth century, Irish workhouses also housed many elderly sick and infirm inmates.
Crossman further distinguishes extensive maternity departments and great
numbers of venereal cases. While percentages and concentrations of particular cases might easily vary as a result of time and place, Pemberton
usefully reminds us that this list could change dramatically internationally,
the Caribbean workhouse having regularly hosted the leper, a less common diagnostic category in the English context. Though such cases look
less familiar than the fever and ulcerous cases housed in London workhouses, these, too, appeared among the inmates in Caribbean workhouse,
but less apparent to Pemberton are those who must have been injured as
a result of the vicious punishments meted out by the cruelest members of
the workhouse staff.

Regardless of the diagnostic labels workhouse inmates carried, many of
those who entered these institutions quite soon sickened and died there.
It follows that the workhouse doctor had an important role to play. Who

were these doctors? Surprisingly, workhouse doctors have remained almost as unfamiliar to eighteenth-century historians as the patients treated in workhouses and their infirmaries. Unlike the successful medical careers charted in anniversary histories of voluntary hospitals, the names, let alone the careers, of workhouse doctors are less often documented in the medical history literature. In eighteenth-century London these medical practitioners seem to have sprung primarily from the ranks of apothecaries. In nineteenth-century Ireland, on the other hand, the poor law service was well stocked with members of the Catholic community. Until the nineteenth century in England, apothecaries were the doctors of the poor. A glance at the *Old Bailey Online* confirms this for London. When faced with a medical emergency, people often visited the nearest apothecary, their collective position having been revised recently as a consequence by Penelope Corfield: "Growing numbers of medical practitioners described themselves as surgeon-apothecaries or as surgeons and apothecaries, providing the bedrock of working doctors."[21] And, just as workhouses underwent medicalization, staff steadily medicalized and professionalized. Gradually, apothecaries elevated themselves to "surgeon-apothecaries," and, on occasion, they were called doctors, and this was long before the Apothecaries Act of 1815.[22] However, apothecaries rose a great deal in status in the eighteenth century, as the chapter by Boulton, Davenport, and Schwarz shows, particularly in its discussion of the parish apothecaries. St. Martin in the Fields's medical staff performed postmortems and honed other skills that possibly delayed the death of inmates; Siena equally uncovers considerable evidence of their early forensic work.

These are developments one would expect at most nineteenth-century workhouses, and it is in the second part of this volume that we hear much more about these individuals, their work, and their growing reputations. As already suggested, Crossman alerts us to the fact that doctors in Irish workhouses were more often Catholics, given that the more prestigious professional posts in Ireland tended to go to Protestant practitioners. She also argues a case for professionalization after 1860, a process that was aided by the system's organization. This extended to the nursing staff, where Catholic nuns perhaps hastened a decline in the use of pauper nurses. Either way, this did not delay the appearance of trained nurses, many of whom acquired their skills at workhouses, some of which, including the institution at Cork, established nurse training centers. In the English case, the General Medical Order (1842), as we are reminded by Samantha Shave and Negrine, ensured that qualification, not cost, guided the appointment of poor law medical officers and their qualifications in both medicine and surgery, technically making them better qualified than most local private practitioners. In an age when cost took precedence in guardians' appointment decisions, as covered by Shave, these seem inevitably, and repeatedly, to have led to the now infamous "workhouse scandal." Even if subsequent inquiries led to changes in regulations and procedures, it sometimes took much longer to alter practice. Negrine strengthens her case for professionalization by charting in detail the work of two medical officers at the Leicester workhouse, whose work and relations with poor law guardians demonstrated their growing confidence over the second half of the nineteenth century. Similar evidence, if shorter tenures, are presented by Reinarz and Ritch. Apart from Tobago, the Caribbean workhouses also had identifiable medical personnel and better medical provision than prisons. Though medical officers' individual journals have yet to be recovered, after a perusal of the workhouse records for several Caribbean islands, Pemberton is convinced that medical staff in Trinidad, for example, professionalized early, even if the odd workhouse hospital at this time might have been described as a "shed."

One might also judge the success of workhouse medical officers by returning to a question posed by historians of voluntary hospitals some decades ago in attempts to determine whether these institutions were in fact "gateways to death," as suggested by some of their most vocal contemporary critics.[23] This issue is tackled early on by Boulton, Davenport, and Schwarz, whose research indicates that many of the poor in fact entered the workhouse to die, but did not necessarily do so. Siena also indicates that the workhouse was, at times, regarded as a fever pit, but structure and admission procedures were altered in accordance and perhaps limited or controlled contagion. There is, in fact, a major difference between Siena's contribution and the chapter by Boulton, Davenport, and Schwarz. Siena argues that workhouses were obliged to take the sick poor whether the workhouse wanted them or not and contains examples to that effect; Boulton, Davenport, and Schwarz argue that at least one London workhouse, but it was the third largest in the metropolis, could keep out some sick poor, and this exclusion was caused not only by the end of adult smallpox in St. Martin's—and thus in Westminster—during the early 1770s.[24]

Perhaps part of this difference was caused by the limited capacity of the workhouses, as well as by the decision of the poor to stay away from what they—rightly or wrongly—regarded as a death trap; either way, it seems to have mattered a lot in which parish a pauper resided when he fell ill. Adults with settlements in the parish were unlikely to be particularly vulnerable to infectious diseases after exposure at a younger age, although the cause of death given as "aged" could hide a multitude of infectious diseases. The multiplication of wards at workhouses in the late nineteenth century, in theory, allowed more efficient segregation, but, oddly, fever could as easily increase after reconstruction, as indicated by Negrine. The establishment of separate isolation hospitals, however, would have limited the numbers of fever cases entering the workhouse in some communities and perhaps finally lowered the chances of inmates contracting infection while residing there.

That said, the limited surgical work undertaken at many English and Irish provincial workhouses would also have kept death rates under control, though acute cases appear to have grown at most English institutions by the end of the nineteenth century and seem periodically to have been treated at eighteenth-century institutions. A decline in the proportion of sick inmates at Irish workhouses until the 1890s, as argued by Crossman, would also have left its impact on the institutions' mortality figures. In earlier decades the propensity for dispensaries and out-relief to impact on figures must also be considered, as would a policy that involved the release of the sick, as uncovered by Pemberton for at least one Caribbean workhouse. Although cleanliness at workhouses appears to have been as much a problem as in England, ironically, the public work undertaken by inmates—cleaning burial grounds, removing filth from neighborhoods—may have gone some way toward improving the health of those who inhabited the "blighted" zones in which these institutions were often located. In any case, though crucial to answering this question, the effectiveness of workhouse medicine, or even the experience of those who resided in these institutions, cannot be determined in isolation from the wider health of the communities in which prospective inmates dwelt, their ill health having been the result of bad diet and poor living conditions more generally. If anything, their condition was less a reflection of the attainments of workhouse medicine than a barometer of the society from which inmates stemmed.

Some may argue that the benefits of workhouse care were equally outbalanced by the stigma attached to the institution and the harsh conditions inmates often encountered during periods of residence. This argument is perhaps easiest to uphold in the case of Pemberton's workhouses, in which cross infection appears to have been less a threat than regular floggings or periods on the treadmill. So, too, might the impact of separation, punishment, poor diet, and occasionally murder, as featured in English workhouse scandals, such as Bridgwater, have undone the benefits of medical care, should one consider the psychological impact alone. It is for this reason that the contribution from Tomkins will perhaps surprise many readers. Against all the negative testimony collected following local visits and national inquiries, let alone that depicted in Victorian literature, her findings support Tim Hitchcock's suggestion that a bed in the workhouse was a hard-won resource that was both prized and appreciated.[25] The testimony she presents here demonstrates that some experiences of the workhouse were "unduly positive." Negrine also emphasizes the way in which efforts by medical staff to improve the surroundings of the workhouse had the potential to improve the care offered. Neither were such actions restricted to medical staff alone but often attributed to guardians and workhouse masters, among other poor law officers. Though such evidence is difficult to find, these examples should remind us that emotional responses to the workhouse were far more complex than hitherto suggested. Moreover, many of these chapters remind us not only that medicine and the emotions are interlinked but that workhouse historians might usefully contribute to an emerging interest in the emotions among medical historians.[26]

A more immediate concern, considering the volume's organization, would be to explore further how the introduction of the New Poor Law in 1834 changed matters. In the Irish case, this is perhaps most easily answered, if only because its system of workhouses was introduced as late as 1838. One might equally expect a disconnection from English workhouses when examining their development in the Caribbean, given that these institutions grew out of the already existing penal system. However, even here, 1834 stands out as a turning point, the Jamaican Gaols Act of that year having commenced a transfer in the control of workhouses, though the parish remained the key administrative unit. It also instigated the appointment of medical officers at these institutions, which clearly would have improved medical services. In the English context, we see less evidence of an immediate improvement of this kind. Negrine and Shave remind us that the Poor Law Amendment Act (1834) required all unions to appoint a medical officer; however, King concludes that most commentators agree "the early decades of the New Poor Law witnessed (and caused) a decline in the scale and standard of medical care." This may have resulted from the sort of medical practitioner who applied for these lowly posts. What is becoming clear is that most medical posts were filled by junior doctors and surgeons, occasionally originating from outside the communities they served; in which case they were both easily hindered in their efforts to improve services by local guardians more concerned with saving money than lives. Interestingly, this decline in services coincided with a period in which progress in the establishment of voluntary hospitals nationally also appeared to slow, as enthusiasm for direct charity waned and arguments for economic independence prevailed.[27]

What remains to be argued convincingly, however, as noted by King, is "when this situation was put into reverse." The Medical Order of 1842 may have been an important factor, for it required poor law medical officers to be "dually qualified" and restricted the size of the districts they served. Real change to practice took much longer, not least because the stipulation regarding qualification applied only to medical officers who resided in the district. Technicalities aside, one could hardly expect such rapid change nationally, or even just in Leicester, when pauper nurses were done away with by the town's guardians in 1899. In the case of Irish workhouses, Crossman is more decisive in her claim that workhouse medicine improved after 1860. Though suggesting that medical care at Caribbean workhouses improved even earlier, Pemberton indicates that prisoners and inmates continued to undertake much of the overseeing and nursing. Additionally, medical officers at English workhouses, it is well known, continued to complain of their work in the medical journals throughout the nineteenth century. Improvements in individual circumstances, as Negrine points out, appear to depend on the length of time medical officers remained in post. Following this model, those in Leicester would have enjoyed some increase in status, if not influence, while those attached to the Birmingham workhouse, by way of contrast, likely had more reason to complain, given their shorter tenures. One major difference accounting for these shorter terms of service seems to have been the requirement for medical officers at the Birmingham workhouse to be resident at the institution. Seemingly insignificant, such details remind us of the need for additional microstudies of workhouses, especially under the New Poor Law.

Despite such variations, we persist in arguing that the New Poor Law marked a break with what had gone before, a caesura—even for medicine and even for the aged—while the New Poor Law did not specifically encourage the poor to return to work. Anyway, the old and the ill (often the same people) were frequently incapable of work, or at least of prolonged work. But there were other factors at play also. First of all, the New Poor Law is much more conveniently documented. Instead of relying on the chance preservation of parish documents, the researcher is often able to go directly to the published (and now online) *Parliamentary Papers*.[28] Second, and related to this, in its way the Old Poor Law marked a high point of parochial government, a point that later commentators, from Edwin Chadwick to Sidney and Beatrice Webb, found intolerable. Certainly, we now know a great deal about the Old Poor Law and the contracts customarily signed by doctors, but despite the volumes written on the subject, we know less in detail of the earliest years of the New Poor Law. The Old Poor Law was administered by the parish and scandals tended to be confined there. Under the New Poor Law, crises, conflict, and scandals were liable eventually to burst into the open, as Shave's chapter on the Bridgwater workhouse indicates. As has been demonstrated in the case of the infamous Andover scandal, such episodes revealed a great deal of tension between officials at the local level and occasionally unleashed a period of change, if not just in the outlook of local authorities and taxpayers, among other interest groups. They also generated a great deal of documentation, which outlines the relations and decision-making process in great detail, among many other aspects of workhouse life and administration. As such, besides shedding much light on the medical services of a neglected institution and the lives of the poor, workhouses potentially open avenues for further explorations in the history of governance.

Many previous histories of the poor law have also explored the way in which the workhouse was governed, but equally the way in which it functioned as a form of government. As noted earlier, accounts have analyzed the often uneasy, and now familiar, relationship between the drive to improve institutional governance and the drive to improve the status (and income) of doctors, as well as the experience of paupers, both sick and well. Like the history of towns and cities, the early history of workhouses, or medical institutions for that matter, appears to be a struggle for sanitary reform. John Howard, for instance, believed this could be achieved through implementing good processes; a well-run prison would not suffer much from jail fever.[29] Our first chapter, however, indicates that the initial decision to transform workhouses into warehouses of the sick or unruly was less the result of such clearly articulated examples of good governance than the unintended consequence of the harsh exclusion criteria of other institutions, as well as the unwillingness or inability of families to care for all their members, whether due to difficulties brought on by age, disability, or mental illness. As such, poor law guardians, as Siena states, were oftentimes less proactive planners than "reluctant saviors." On finding themselves responsible for new inmates, workhouses might indeed implement rational improvements, including the designation of separate wards for cases deemed disruptive, diseased, or morally dangerous, though taxpayers quickly aired their views when they felt they had stumped up enough.

Yet there was an inherent tension, as Crossman notes in chapter 6 of this volume: "In far too many unions [in Ireland], poor law guardians found it impossible to reconcile their desire to keep rates low and adhere to the principle of less eligibility with the requirement to provide efficient and effective medical services." Reforms introduced with the New Poor Law only increased these tensions by augmenting the plurality of actors who, rather than pursue common goals, attempted to steer the course of local provisions. It is, therefore, not surprising that it is in the first years following the introduction of this legislation that one comes across accusations of bad governance. In fact, the workhouse system, according to some, appeared to be as sick as its inmates. Investigators or critics, such as John Bowen, as demonstrated by Shave, directed their gaze at the institution and easily identified numerous "pathologies" that impeded it from operating in an effective manner; interestingly, in the case of Bowen, his opponents already appear to have been transformed into faceless figures of authority or bureaucrats, in contrast to the colorful individuals who critiqued the system in these decades. Undoubtedly, other regions witnessed numerous examples of collaboration, if not the emergence of new networks, which not only challenged obstructive guardians where they existed but steered decisions and influenced policy implementation. Alternatively, medical officers left to their own devices also regularly appear to have been able to ensure that patients received effective treatment and were well cared for in reasonably comfortable surroundings. Neither should one forget about the pauper at the heart of this political epistemic complex, who surely exercised agency and resisted disciplinary regimes, as well as the most blatant attempts by masters and guardians to inculcate "positive" values and habits. In the Caribbean context, these tensions in workhouse governance are less evident, although they certainly extended further to colonial subject and colonizer. That said, in that particular setting, both parties bought into the workhouse project, given its reforming potential, the unsuitability of English law and concerns about public security, as individual islands, like generations of inmates, worked toward becoming independent and productive nations.

Pemberton's research on the West Indies can of course stand in its own right; however, in the context of this volume, and precisely because conditions were different, it can also be seen as a kind of extended commentary on developments in England, which had a native aristocracy but not planters and had not known slavery since anyone could remember. English doctors, particularly under the New Poor Law, though not paid particularly well, expected to be consulted—indeed the acts to which Pemberton refers make explicit reference to this—which did not necessarily happen in the West Indies. They might not succeed in this, but if they failed repeatedly, at least some time after the harsh introduction of the New Poor Law, there were the makings of a scandal. On the whole, it could not be said that "medicine practiced there buttressed, rather than relieved, the cruel impositions of prison and workhouse operations of the day on the inmates." It may have been rather different in English prisons, but under the New Poor Law, workhouses were far more widespread than prisons. Perhaps most important of all, the English, or enough of them, were accustomed to a culture of time discipline. Lunatics were exempt from this, of course, but then lunatics were usually exempt from many things and their imperviousness to time discipline was one of the signs of their lunacy. Workhouses formed one end of a spectrum that stretched from workhouses to lunatic asylums to prisons and out to barracks and ships in England, and again in its colonies, and reading Pemberton is a reminder that they have not been considered as an entity. This, or at least the colonial connection, is something that legal historians have long taken for granted. Jeremy Bentham, of course, recognized the connections.[30] The Prison Medical Service developed after the Poor Law, though individual counties might have made reforms earlier; the connections between the poor law and prisons should be further investigated.[31]

This book is divided into two parts. We begin with the Old Poor Law, with chapters by Siena; Boulton, Davenport, and Schwarz, concentrating on London; and an intervening chapter by Ottaway, who, in charting the institutionalization of the aged in workhouses, widens her perspective to encompass experiences outside the English capital, including the counties of Essex, Yorkshire, Suffolk, and Leicestershire. Tomkins's chapter noticeably shifts the focus to the Midlands and comes closest to presenting the voices of former inmates. Smith's chapter on lunacy is a transitional piece that exceeds the dates of the Old Poor Law and, like earlier chapters, explores the changing roles of workhouses in communities. Part 2 shifts the focus onto the nineteenth century and the New Poor Law. It is not "top down" history, but proceeds from somewhere around the middle—again with exceptions, beginning with Crossman's valuable survey of Irish workhouses and Reinarz and Ritch's and Negrine's detailed studies of two provincial workhouses. Shave proceeds to dissect one of the lesser known workhouse scandals, one concentrated in the southwest of England, to illuminate the way in which scandals fed into the policy process. We then make an excursion into the Caribbean with Pemberton, before concluding with a separate agenda, or afterword, sketched out by King, which, like many of the chapters collected here, will undoubtedly steer further explorations into the field of workhouse medicine.

Notes

1. If the subject of medicine is left unremarked, this is by deliberate choice, to highlight other aspects, as in David R. Green, *Pauper Capital: London and the Poor Law, 1790–1870* (Farnham, UK: Ashgate, 2010).

2. Guenter B. Risse, *Hospital Life in Enlightenment Scotland: Care and teaching at the Royal Infirmary of Edinburgh* (Cambridge: Cambridge University Press, 1986), 121–72.

3. Kathryn Morrison, *The Workhouse: A Study of Poor Law Buildings in England* (Swindon: English Heritage, 1999).

4. David A. Sutton, "The Public-Private Interface of Domiciliary Medical Care for the Poor in Scotland, c. 1875–1911" (PhD diss., University of Glasgow, 2009). See also Stephanie Blackden, "The Poor Law and Health: A Survey of Medical Aid in Glasgow, 1845–1900," in *The Search for Wealth and Stability: Essays in Economic and Social History Presented to M. W. Flinn,* ed. Thomas Christopher Smout, 263–82 (London: Macmillan, 1979); and Stephanie Blackden, "The Board of Supervision and the Scottish Parochial Medical Service," *Medical History* 30, no. 2 (1986): 145–72.

5. Other recent histories of workhouses outside the European context include Simon P. Newman, *Embodied History: The Lives of the Poor in Early Philadelphia* (Philadelphia: University of Pennsylvania Press, 2003); and Kevin Siena, "Hospitals for the Excluded or Convalescent Homes? Workhouses, Medicalization and the Poor Law in Long Eighteenth-Century London and Pre-confederation Toronto," *Canadian Bulletin of Medical History* 27, no. 1 (2010): 5–25.

6. Newman, *Embodied History,* 20, 24.

7. Ibid., 19.

8. Graham Mooney and Jonathan Reinarz, eds., *Permeable Walls: Historical Perspectives on Hospital and Asylum Visiting* (Amsterdam: Rodopi, 2009).

9. Margaret Anne Crowther, *The Workhouse System, 1834–1929: The History of an English Social Institution* (London: Methuen, 1983), 54–87.

10. John Landers, *Death and the Metropolis: Studies in the Demographic History of London, 1670–1830* (Cambridge: Cambridge University Press, 1993).

11. For instance, the usual appeal for patronage of dispensaries as set out in Bronwyn Croxson, "The Public and Private Faces of Eighteenth-Century London Dispensary Charity," *Medical History* 41 (1997): 127–49.

12. Robert Bland, *Some Calculations of the Numbers of Accidents or Deaths Which Happen in Consequence of Parturition Taken from the Midwifery Reports of the Westminster General Dispensary, London* (London: J. Nichols, 1781), 6–7.

13. Edward Anthony Wrigley, "A Simple Model of London's Importance in Changing English Society and Economy, 1650–1750," *Past and Present* 37 (1967): 46; Robert Bland, "Midwifery Reports of the Westminster General Dispensary," *Philosophical Transactions* 71 (1781): 370; also quoted in Dorothy George, *London Life in the Eighteenth Century* (London: Kegan Paul, 1925), 118.

14. This type of calculation omits Londoners with settlements in their parish, who chose to leave the capital, but it is unlikely to be very wrong.

15. This figure is from David R. Green, "Icons of the New System: Workhouse Construction and Relief Practices in London under the Old and New Poor Law," *London Journal* 34 (2009): 267.

16. Green, "Icons," 264–84; in 1803 the average capacity of a London workhouse was 257, and some were much larger than this: calculated from "Abstract of Answers and Returns under Act for Procuring Returns Relative to Expense and Maintenance of Poor in England," Parliament Papers, 1803–4, available online via subscription at: http://parlipapers.chadwyck.co.uk/marketing/index.jsp. English workhouses have also been examined by James S. Taylor, "The Unreformed Workhouse, 1776–1834," in *Comparative Development in Social Welfare*, ed. Ernest A. Martin (London: George Allen and Unwin, 1972), 57–84.

17. Green, *Pauper Capital*, 38–41.

18. Margaret Anne Crowther, "Health Care and Poor Relief in Provincial England," and David Green, "Medical Relief and the New Poor Law in London," both in *Health Care and Poor Relief in 18th and 19th Century Northern Europe*, ed. Ole P. Grell, Andrew Cunningham, and Robert Jütte (Aldershot, UK: Ashgate, 2002), 209–13 and 220–23.

19. Karel Williams, *From Pauperism to Poverty* (London: Routledge and Kegan Paul, 1981), 230–31; Lynn Hollen Lees, *The Solidarities of Strangers: The English Poor Laws and the People, 1700–1949* (Cambridge: Cambridge University Press, 1998), 192.

20. For an example of some of the work on gender and the poor law, see Marjorie Levine-Clark, "Engendering Relief: Women, Ablebodiedness, and the Poor Law in Early Victorian England," *Journal of Women's History*, 11, no. 4 (2000): 107–30, as well as her *Beyond the Reproductive Body: The Politics of Women's Health and Work in Early Victorian England* (Columbus: Ohio State University Press, 2004).

21. Penelope J. Corfield, "From Poison Peddlers to Civic Worthies: The Reputation of the Apothecaries in Georgian England," *Social History of Medicine* 22 (2009): 6.

22. Jane Austen takes the pivotal role of apothecaries for granted in *Emma*: even the valetudinarian Mr. Woodward relies on Mr. Perry, "an intelligent gentlemanlike man" (chap. 2), *Emma: A Novel* (London, John Murray, 1816). Minutes, Overseers of St. Martin's, City of Westminster Archives Centre (hereafter COWAC). For the Apothecaries Act, see Irvine Loudon, *Medical Care and the General Practitioner, 1750–1850* (Oxford: Oxford University Press, 1986), 167–88.

23. John Woodward, *To Do the Sick No Harm: A Study of the Voluntary Hospital System to 1875* (London: Routledge, 1974).

24. Romola Davenport, Leonard Schwarz, and Jeremy Boulton, 'The Decline of Adult Smallpox in Eighteenth-Century London," *Economic History Review* 64, no. 4 (2011): 1289–314.

25. Tim Hitchcock, *Down and Out in Eighteenth-Century London* (London: Hambledon and London, 2007), 139–40, 149.

26. Tom Dixon, "Patients and Passions: Languages of Medicine and Emotion, 1789–1850" and Hilary Marland, "Languages and Landscapes of Emotion: Motherhood and Puerperal Insanity in the Nineteenth Century," both in *Medicine, Emotion and Disease, 1700–1950*, ed. Fay Bound Alberti (Basingstoke, UK: Palgrave Macmillan, 2006), 22–52 and 53–78.

27. John V. Pickstone, *Medicine and Industrial Society: A History of Hospital Development in Manchester and Its Region, 1752–1946* (Manchester: Manchester University Press, 1985), 63.

28. The Parliamentary Papers are available online via subscription at:http://parlipapers.chadwyck.co.uk/marketing/index.jsp.

29. Roy Porter, "Howard's Beginning: Prisons, Disease, Hygiene," in *The Health of Prisoners: Historical Essays*, ed. Richard Creese, William F. Bynum, and Joseph Bearn (Amsterdam: Rodopi, 1995), 11.

30. For instance, see the literature on apprenticeship, for example, Marc W. Steinberg, "Unfree Labor, Apprenticeship and the Rise of the Victorian Hull Fishing Industry: An Example of the Importance of Law and the Local State in British Economic Change," *International Review of Social History* 51, no. 2 (2006): 243–76; Douglas Hay and Paul Craven, ed., *Masters, Servants, and Magistrates in Britain and the Empire, 1562–1955* (Chapel Hill: University of North Carolina Press, 2004). Jeremy Bentham's *Management of the Poor* (Dublin, James Moore, 1796) proposed panopticons for penitentiaries, prisons, houses of industry, workhouses, poor houses, manufactories, mad houses, and hospitals. Green, *Pauper Capital*, 11. Of course, Foucault drew attention to this also; see Michel Foucault, *Discipline and Punish: The Birth of the Prison* (Harmondsworth: Penguin, 1977).

31. Anne Hardy, "Development of the Prison Medical Service," and Anthony J. Standley, "Medical Treatment and Prisoners' Health in Stafford Gaol during the Eighteenth Century," both in *The Health of Prisoners: Historical Essays*, ed. Creese, Bynum, and Bearn, 59–82 and 27–43; Peter M. Higgins, *Punish or Treat? Medical Care in English Prisons, 1770–1850* (Victoria: Trafford, 2007).

Part One

The Old Poor Law

Chapter One

Contagion, Exclusion, and the Unique Medical World of the Eighteenth-Century Workhouse

London Infirmaries in Their Widest Relief

KEVIN SIENA

Georgian workhouses served many functions. Although they were nominally devoted to work, they routinely provided care and education for children and refuge for single mothers, as social historians know well. They sheltered, fed, and nursed the elderly, disabled, and mad and acted as de facto employment agents, placing young people in apprenticeships and jobs. They also provided considerable medical care. Medical historians have been slow to explore workhouses, even though simply itemizing their medical services impresses; a partial list includes obstetrical care, surgery, outpatient care, emergency medicine, doctor training, and even trials of experimental drugs and procedures. Workhouses need to be integrated into the history of eighteenth-century institutional medicine, which, for the most part, has remained a history of hospitals.[1]

However, workhouse infirmaries were not just smaller versions of existing institutions, hospitals in miniature. This chapter seeks to show how workhouse infirmaries became unique medical spaces, where particular forms of care for particular kinds of patients occurred. Workhouses' special obligations determined that, in practice, they evolved into institutions quite unlike those around them. While this chapter cannot comprehensively analyze all forms of care in workhouses, two related themes allow one to cast workhouse medicine in wide relief: contagion and exclusion. While no parish can be considered typical of so varied a city as London, the documentation related to the workhouse in St. Margaret's Westminster, when enriched with evidence from other parishes, demonstrates some of the distinctive features of

Georgian workhouse infirmaries, especially their concentration on patients excluded from other forms of care and their growing use as isolation hospitals for infectious diseases.

The 1725 foundation of St. Margaret's workhouse was hardly special. Like many parishes feeling the pressures of rising relief costs, it seized on a workhouse as a solution. Vestrymen feared that workhouses in neighboring parishes encouraged paupers to "Crowd into and shelter themselves in this Parish to avoid their being putt to Labour."[2] Lest St. Margaret's become a magnet for the idle, the vestry voted unanimously to establish a workhouse. Its debate reveals that vestrymen had absorbed the rhetoric of groups like the Society for the Promotion of Christian Knowledge (SPCK), which advocated workhouses as panaceas for idleness, immorality, unemployment, and high taxes.[3] The vestrymen again: "the poor rate will be very Considerably less and the streets cleared of Crowds of Sturdy Idle Vagrants who rather than be maintained in a Workhouse will Quit their Pensions and maintain themselves."[4] Like elsewhere, St. Margaret's established a workhouse to toughen poor relief and ease rates by scaring away applicants.[5]

Though initially built on the SPCK model, St. Margaret's workhouse transformed radically. Within twenty-four months it was a different institution. The term "medicalization" best describes the change. In early plans an infirmary was not integral. Indeed, medical space was mentioned only as one possible use of rooms in a stable that were also being considered for lodgings.[6] Yet within a year, because of repeated requests by the workhouse's surgeon, the vestry begrudgingly established a piecemeal infirmary, converting rooms originally devoted to other purposes to house the sick, venereal patients, "lunaticks," pediatrics, contagious patients, and medical supplies and appointing nursing staff for this newly medicalized space. Even this infirmary proved insufficient, as evidenced by successful requests for more medical resources and the conversion of more rooms into sick wards during the following year.[7] In less than two years, St. Margaret's went from having space atop its stable *possibly* to be used for the sick to having fourteen of its thirty-three rooms dedicated to medicine. Similar rapid medicalization occurred in workhouses in St. George's Hanover Square and St. Sepulchre's, London Division.[8]

St. Margaret's vestrymen envisioned a correctional factory, not an infirmary. They sought not a hospital but rather a house of hard labor to which only the desperate would apply. They got it half right. The less-than-desperate—like the 55 percent of pensioners who surrendered their pensions rather than accept incarceration in the new institution—stayed out of the workhouse at all costs.[9] The problem with the vestry's master plan was that the truly desperate were a very sick bunch. In early years almost 38 percent of applicants to St. Margaret's workhouse cited illness or injury as the reason they applied.[10] Again, varied though similar figures emerge in other workhouses such as St. Sepulchre's or St. Luke's Chelsea's.[11] Early reports show that medical demands were considerable. In 1734 St. Margaret's surgeon reported curing nearly two hundred people in the workhouse infirmary of more than thirty different conditions. His report indicated that parochial medical care stretched well beyond the infirmary itself, noting that his data did not include "many others cured of various Distempers in the other buildings," as well as "outpatients without number." The picture appears, then, of workhouse committees being quickly overrun with sick paupers seeking help. Officials certainly seemed surprised at the intensity of the demand for medicine. In 1734 the committee had to order that "the Board with the Inscription Surgery done Gratis, be taken down, Great Inconveniences arising by the same."[12]

Such quick, unplanned medicalization sheds important light on the history of poor law entitlement. Vestrymen probably lamented reconfiguring almost half of their workhouse away from the intended aims of discipline, work, and production. It is likely that their hands were forced due to the right to relief that settled paupers could claim. Here medical historians can contribute to the larger debate about the extent and meaning of poor law entitlement.[13] The transformation of workhouses away from founders' intentions and toward users' needs offers evidence that paupers who could prove settlement had real traction in their exchanges with parochial authorities. This suggestion finds support in evidence from workhouses in other parts of the British Atlantic world, which witnessed more advanced medicalization where poor laws were adopted (and thus where the poor could lay claim to resources based on statutory entitlement) and much weaker medicalization where the poor laws were rejected (where workhouse administrators had no legal obligation to accept the sick).[14] The story in the provinces may well be different, but in London workhouses found themselves legally obliged to care for settled paupers who were not fit workers but rather sick, weak, and broken. Workhouse admission was always a negotiation, but the force of large numbers of settled paupers demanding relief due to sickness, relief that was difficult to deny them legally, forced parochial authorities, probably begrudgingly, to reform their workhouses significantly.

This further seems the case when we consider who ended up in workhouse infirmaries, and here is where the theme of exclusion begins to emerge. We know that factors such as gender and age drove workhouse admissions in the eighteenth century, and there is no reason to think St. Margaret's was exceptional.[15] Its workhouse minutes do not record applicants' ages, but in terms of gender the pattern is typical. Three of four sick paupers cared for by the parish were women.[16]

Workhouse infirmaries such as St. Margaret's came to be a primary center of medical care for London's poorest, a demographic group that was disproportionately female. That the poor entered workhouses only as a last resort begs an important question: why did patients in workhouse infirmaries lack other medical options? Accessing the backstories of what paupers did before entering workhouses is difficult, but evidence suggests that many ended up in workhouses only because they had been excluded from other forms of medical care. Such exclusion was multifaceted. Obviously, it meant those excluded economically, unable to afford the services of private practitioners in the medical marketplace. But it also meant those excluded in other ways. Many sick paupers hoping to avoid a workhouse sought care in a hospital. However, two developments changed paupers' access to hospitals in the early eighteenth century. First, the largest hospitals in the city, the royal hospitals of St. Thomas's and St. Bartholomew's, began charging fees, pricing their beds out of reach for the absolutely destitute.[17] Second, a new type of hospital, the voluntary hospital, spread throughout the metropolis.[18] These offered free care but stipulated that paupers must first obtain a nomination by a hospital governor.[19] Here a moral litmus test determined whether paupers were "worthy" objects of charity, meaning legitimately needy but also morally sound. The networking and strategizing necessary to contact a governor and successfully lobby for a hospital bed is a topic deserving of more focused study.[20] But a letter to William Blair, surgeon and governor of the Lock Hospital, reveals that there could be many degrees of separation (in this case five) between pauper applicant and hospital governor:

> The Bearer is the servant of a friend of mine, and he unfortunately has a relation in a deplorable state. If you can take her under your care, in the Lock Hospital, you will very much oblige, Dear Sir, your faithful humble servant,
>
> James Seaton.[21]

Here an impoverished sick woman had to convince some male relative (the servant) to ask his employer to ask a friend (Seaton) to persuade Blair to nominate a woman he had never met. Getting into a voluntary hospital was fraught with uncertainty, and it was particularly hard for those with dubious reputations or no connections or those suffering from ailments like syphilis that called their character into question. Indeed, syphilitics faced greater difficulties because most voluntary hospitals excluded them.[22] In addition to the networking resources needed to contact a governor, a successful applicant required the important skill of *appearing* worthy. That some hospitals treated more men than women suggests that poor women may have fared worse in these exchanges, whether because gender prejudices created different yardsticks for male and female "worthiness" or because governors privileged the health of breadwinning men and steered resources accordingly.[23] In any case, many of the poor women who crowded into St. Margaret's infirmary had likely failed to secure a hospital bed.

Testimony in coroners' inquests captures well the stories of paupers' failed attempts to enter hospitals and their immediate turn to a workhouse. Carpenter Richard Field testified of his attempt to get his sick coworker, Richard Haywood, into the Westminster Infirmary:

> [Field] applied for an Order to get the Deced. [Haywood] into the Westmr. Hospital and when Deced went with this Dept. to the Westmr. Hospital the Gentleman there refused to take him in unless some Person would Engage to Bury him in case he might die there. Says that he went away with the Deced and walked with him as far as Chapel Street in the Parish of St. Margaret Westmr. in order to apply to Mr Loton the Church Warden.[24]

Haywood died en route, but what is important is how the two men went literally from the steps of the hospital to a parish official. Had Field lived it is likely that the churchwarden would have ordered him into St. Margaret's workhouse. That is precisely what happened to Joseph Pauley, whose story is similar, save for the different parish and hospital, St. Ann's Soho and the Middlesex Hospital, respectively. Pauley's friend, James Whitmore, testified "that he endeavored to get a Letter for [Pauley] to go to the Midsex Hospital but being Disappointed, he applied to the Overseer of the Parish, and the Deced was carried to the Poor House, where he died."[25] The very syntax of this sentence captures the immediacy of the move from hospital exclusion to workhouse admission: "Being Disappointed, he applied to the Overseer."

Some paupers faced what might be called diagnostic exclusion from hospitals, and here the issue of contagion surfaces. In addition to venereal disease, two diagnoses stand out. First, hospitals frequently refused patients with "the itch," a common skin condition that may have been scabies, but which is difficult to identify retrospectively.[26] Whether a rash or a parasite, the itch was assumed to be highly contagious. In the crowded conditions of hospitals in which patients frequently shared beds, the itch spread quickly. Thus it was that hospitals like the London Infirmary refused patients with communicable skin conditions: "no Person suspected to have the Small-pox, Itch, Scald-head or Leprosy, shall be taken under the care of this Infirmary."[27] If the itch was troublesome, "fever" was deadly. It is not coincidental that both Joseph Pauley and Richard Haywood, refused admission by the Middlesex and Westminster Infirmaries, suffered from forms of fever. Nearly every hospital refused contagious patients. The London Infirmary again: "No Persons with incurable or infectious Distempers . . . are admitted to partake of this Charity."[28] Such rules gave hospital staff latitude to refuse patients with many disorders, but patients with "malignant" or "putrid" fevers were among the most frightening. Looking again at St. Margaret's workhouse infirmary we see the effects of diagnostic exclusion and clear evidence that workhouses specialized in caring for those unable to obtain care elsewhere;

in 1734 three diagnoses—the pox, the itch, and fever—accounted for 79 percent of the infirmary's population.[29]

That three out of four of workhouse infirmary patients were women, four out of five suffered from a contagious or scandalous ailment, and that all of them were poor would have meant that these patients' chances of accessing medical care on their own were slim. They probably did not want to be in the workhouse any more than their overseers wanted them there. After all, their ailments were no less troublesome for workhouses than they were for hospitals. Indeed, the itch was the very first medical condition mentioned by St. Margaret's workhouse committee. Within three months of opening its doors the committee had to order "that such persons as are suspected to be infected with the Itch be removed into one particular Ward and that the Nurse or Nurses & other officers of the house do strictly observe the directions which shall be given by Dr. Harvey & Mr. Westbrook or either of them till this house shall be Intirely cleared of that Distemper."[30] But whereas voluntary hospitals could refuse such patients, it seems that workhouses had to accept them and make do. Workhouse provision for contagious patients offers a telling manifestation of the "dance of interlocking obligation" connecting paupers and parochial officials in the Old Poor Law system.[31]

Because paupers faced difficulties entering hospitals, workhouses often served as conduits arranging and paying for hospital beds that paupers could not secure themselves. During just two weeks in September 1727, St. Margaret's committee arranged beds in St. Bartholomew's and Guy's hospitals for Arrabella Hopkins, Lucinda Hammond, Elizabeth Valens, Elizabeth Ackley, and Mary Holman.[32] Workhouses also admitted patients needing hospitalization temporarily while overseers worked to secure them a hospital bed. Parishes like St. Sepulchre's found that such stays could become permanent because placing workhouse patients in hospitals was easier said than done.[33] Indeed, workhouses faced unique obstacles when trying to place patients in hospitals. Some voluntary hospitals openly resisted accepting parish paupers. Here we see a different kind of exclusion at work, as governors of charities refused shouldering what they saw as parochial financial obligations. The Lock Hospital, to take one example, refused patients from workhouses unless overseers paid two guineas toward their care. Parishes questioning the policy were told,

> The Gov[ernor]s present are sorry you shou'd so far misunderstand the intent of this charity, as to imagine that the nobility & gentry who support it by Voluntary Subsc[riptio]ns ever meant to receive people from parish workhouses who by the laws of the land have or ought to have very sufficient Provision[. T]he Design of the Gov[ernor]s was to relieve those who are destitute of any known Relief whats[oever] who by distance from or ignorance of their settlements must perish with[ou]t the assistance of this hospital.[34]

Looking beyond the Lock and even beyond London this seems to be a common response.[35] The relationship between voluntary hospitals and workhouses marks another issue deserving of its own study, for the voluntary charity movement was from its inception forged in dynamic relation, nay tension, with parish medicine. England's first voluntary hospital, the Westminster Infirmary, was located right in St. Margaret's, Westminster. The very first words put to paper at its inaugural meeting demonstrate that it was conceived in direct relation to the parish and that it sought to focus on those *excluded* from parish care. The preamble of its subscription roll begins, "Whereas great Numbers of sick Persons in this City languish for want of Necessaries, and too often die miserably, who are not entitled to a Parochial Relief." However, note the immediate tension: "And whereas amongst those who do receive Relief from their respective Parishes, many suffer extremely, and are sometimes lost, partly for want of Accommodations and proper Medicines in their own Houses . . . [or] by the Ignorance and Carelessness of ill Management of those about them."[36] Thus the voluntary charity movement's inaugural statement sent mixed messages, suggesting on the one hand that the hospital intended to treat those who (usually because of migration) lived a great distance from their parish of settlement, but on the other hand, also those who had a local settlement but needed better care than the parish could provide.[37] This was not inconsistent in 1719, when most London parishes had yet to build workhouses and accompanying infirmaries.

But fast-forward a decade and even the Westminster Infirmary's home parish now had a large workhouse with a sophisticated infirmary. Consequently, as sick Londoners requested relief, governors of charities began questioning whether paupers with access to workhouses were truly "destitute" and thus "worthy" of the free care their hospitals bestowed. One passage shows nicely the multiple forms of exclusion functioning at voluntary hospitals and demonstrates how, as early as 1735, the Westminster Infirmary was already moving to concentrate on the unsettled, leaving parish workhouses to look after their own. Commenting on a prospective patient named Mary Gill, the board accepted her as a proper object of its charity because "it appears that [her distemper] has not been contracted by vice, that she has no relation able to support her, [and] that the place of her legal settlement cannot be found."[38] The Westminster Infirmary was the model for later voluntary infirmaries. Indeed, its preamble emphasizing the neediness of people excluded from parochial medicine was recycled by other voluntary hospitals.[39] However, by the 1730s notable changes can be found. London's second voluntary hospital, St. George's Hospital, modeled its preamble on the Westminster Infirmary's but cut the phrase that included settled paupers among potential recipients of charity. Its preamble simply targeted the sick and indigent of Westminster "no way entitled to Parochial Relief."[40]

A survey of printed reports confirms that other London hospitals similarly steered resources toward paupers lacking access to workhouse infirmaries. John Nichols of the London Lying-in Charity thus lamented, "All this Charity can do, is . . . receive poor married Women, recommended by the Governors, Subscribers, or Contributors, not supported by their Parishes."[41] We have seen this policy at the Lock Hospital, and the Scottish Hospital established on Fleet Street in 1775 was explicit: "The Object of the Establishment was the Relief and Support of Poor Persons, natives of Scotland, *not having any parochial settlement in England.*"[42] The little known Ossulston Dispensary explained its move to Bloomsbury specifically to treat "the many foreign and other extra-parochial Poor."[43] Even on the outskirts of London, institutions such as the Kent Dispensary specified the same policy of exclusion; forbidden were "any person[s] entitled to assistance from the Infirmary at the Royal Hospital, Greenwich; or the Surgeon of Deptford or Woolwich Yards; or being in any parish workhouse."[44] Scholars must thus acknowledge the multiple, reciprocal forms of exclusion at work in eighteenth-century institutions. Workhouses and voluntary infirmaries were each in their own ways hospitals for the excluded; workhouses cared for paupers excluded from hospitals, and hospitals increasingly focused on those excluded from workhouses.

Some parishes tried to subscribe to voluntary hospitals to gain the right to nominate patients from their workhouses. The Lock Hospital's board probably surprised officials by refusing such requests.[45] Whether parishes should be allowed to subscribe to hospitals was a vexing question. Noted prison reformer George Onesiphorus Paul crystallized the tension. Subscribing was "a good bargain for the Parish," but allowing workhouses to send patients to hospitals would only "relieve the opulent," using funds donated for the poor to ease the burdens of taxpayers. Printed treatises suggest different practices in London and the provinces, although more research is needed here. Infirmaries in Gloucester, Leicester, Lincoln, and Manchester all listed parishes among their subscribers, enabling overseers to nominate patients from workhouses.[46] By contrast, London charities, including the Middlesex Hospital, St. George's Hospital, the London Hospital, and the Lock Hospital, do not.[47] However, even at provincial infirmaries that allowed parochial subscriptions there was tension, evidenced by the 1775 rules for the Hereford Infirmary, demanding fees for parochial patients over and above the parishes' subscriptions and refusing patients who had received parish relief during three previous months. If this last stipulation was still in place eight years later, inmates in Hereford's new workhouse (established 1783) would have been effectively excluded.[48] The infirmary's governors clarified their intention to treat those "not indigent enough to be taken on the parish."[49] Evidence suggests that a regional perspective of the kind advocated by Steven King is needed to tease out the relationships between workhouses and voluntary charities throughout England.[50] In London, workhouse committees like St. Margaret's clearly faced limited and costly options when seeking hospital care for paupers. It is likely that these difficulties (and costs) quickened the medicalization of workhouses, as parishes found it often more efficient to treat sick paupers themselves.

Workhouses hoping to transfer patients to hospitals faced still further problems, and here the themes of contagion and exclusion converge. Workhouses had dubious reputations as overcrowded, filthy pits of disease. So powerful was the connection between workhouses and contagion that they had their own disease. The disease that would come to be known as typhus, and that was commonly called "jail fever," was frequently referred to by other monikers, including ship fever, hospital fever, camp fever, or indeed "workhouse fever."[51] These names were used interchangeably to refer to the infectious distemper thought to arise from the overcrowding and filth in confined spaces that caused inmates of jails and workhouses to breathe the same air over and over. With each breath they added more "effluvia" to the atmosphere, eventually rendering the air into a noxious poison. Addressing child mortality in workhouses, William Buchan declared, "Few things are more destructive to children than confined or unwholesome air. This is one reason why so few of those infants, who are put into hospitals, or parish workhouses, live. These places are generally crowded with old sickly and infirm people; by means of which the air is rendered so extremely pernicious that it becomes a poison."[52] John Barker warned of the dangers of "the corrupt even cadaverous stench . . . in workhouses and other confined places," while John Coakley Lettsom reported of a man who "having occasion to visit a miserable crowded workhouse in Spitalfields was instantly seized" with disease. Treating him, Lettsom "conclude[d] the case to be a true jail fever, or what is the same, a true workhouse fever."[53]

This worry was not unique to London, as evidenced by the claim that parochial officers in Sheffield avoided entering the workhouse at all costs: "few Officers are found hardy enough to make even an annual visit to these wretched Cabins, dreading the contagion with which they are so polluted."[54] There was no dearth of class terror about diseases bred in places like workhouses spreading far beyond their walls. The physician who in 1793 proclaimed that "prisons and charity workhouses have often become the source of the most obstinate epidemics" merely related a widely held fear.[55] Of course, hospitals could be crowded and unhealthy, but authorities like Robert Jackson pointed to workhouses and prisons as much more likely sources of contagion. "[Fever] is common in jails where men are crouded [*sic*] together, deprived of the benefit of pure air. . . . It is on the same account frequent in workhouses or poor houses. It sometimes originates, but is oftener *transplanted* to hospitals, where it spreads with rapid growth."[56]

These last words conveyed the worry vexing hospital authorities facing patients sent from workhouses. Hospital surgeon Edward Alanson advised that to protect against "importing infection," patients admitted from workhouses should be stripped, their heads shaved and their clothes baked in a special oven.[57] Hospitals made the threat of infection one of their most important admissions criteria, and on this score workhouse patients were disadvantaged. This meant, as we have seen, that workhouses often had to admit patients with infectious disorders because they had nowhere else to go, and in a classic vicious cycle this reality contributed to the wider assumptions about workhouses as contagious spaces.

It was no trifling issue. The Medical Society of London ran a competition for the best essay on diseases in workhouses and prisons. John Mason Good's winning essay emphasized fevers, syphilis, and the itch, which we have seen were indeed prevalent in workhouses like St. Margaret's. However, when explaining why these conditions predominated in workhouses he stressed neither patients' exclusion from hospitals nor the legal obligations forcing workhouses to accept them. Instead, he cited morality: "In both Prisons and Poor-Houses, which are too often the receptacles of the idle, the uncleanly, and the abandoned, nothing is more common ... than the admission of patients with the ITCH and the VENEREAL DISEASE."[58] The kind of people likely to enter workhouses were morally predisposed to odious diseases, which could then be expected to run rampant in the crowded institutions, rendering all workhouse inmates possible sources of contagion to wider society. Little surprise, then, that workhouses faced difficulties placing their inmates in hospitals and ended up treating so many of them locally. Of course, it is well established that nineteenth-century fever hospitals had close ties to, and in some cases grew out of, poor law infirmaries.[59] What is important to note is how, at least in London, workhouses served in this capacity a full century before the New Poor Law, suggesting that continuities between the Old and New Poor Law systems may deserve more attention than they have received in a field that often presents 1834 as a dramatic break. Caring for the infectious was a vital medical service but one that it is hard to imagine vestrymen provided enthusiastically.

The constant presence of contagious patients affected both the administration and even the structure of workhouses and their infirmaries. St. Margaret's had to control the movement of workhouse inmates to keep contagious patients within defined wards. Authorities even had to monitor external space for infirmary patients who, it was believed, needed fresh air but who might easily mingle with inmates from the general population. Hence in 1730 the committee ordered the steward to "take particular care that none of the Itchy Persons be suffered to go out of the Yard belonging to the Infirmary."[60]

It was bad enough that infirmary patients might infect other inmates. As the example of Sheffield's frightened vestrymen suggested, parochial officials had a deeper, more personal fear, namely that they might catch a deadly infection themselves. Discussions of "jail fever" reveal acute anxieties about spaces where elite and poor bodies came into contact. When Newgate prisoners allegedly brought the disease into the Old Bailey courthouse in 1750, fatally communicating it to magistrates, jurymen, and even the lord mayor, many people's worst fears were realized. This and other well-publicized instances of institutionally generated fever ignited a scramble to find methods to police spaces where rich and poor bodies converged. Thus we find schemes to ventilate courtrooms; to cloth paupers on trial in garments that clung tight at the neck, wrists, and ankles to trap contagion within; to clog the nostrils of court officials with vinegar-soaked lint; and to erect seating and screening to separate magistrates from potentially infected felons.[61]

Workhouses presented similar opportunities for dangerous class mixing because officials commonly used space in the workhouse for meetings of the relief committee. Respectable men thus had to enter a most frightening building, bringing themselves face-to-face with welfare applicants. Thomas Rowlandson's depiction of a relief committee shows well the proximity of rich and poor bodies witnessed in parishes across the country every week (see fig. 1.1). Poor law processes marked some of the most common cross-class encounters of the day. When viewed with the pathophobic sensibilities associating poor bodies with infection, Rowlandson's scene helps make sense of some workhouses' structural innovations. Surviving plans for St. Sepulchre's workhouse demonstrate how its design made manifest contemporary fears of interclass contagion. The architect addressed prevailing concerns about institutional contagion, dutifully placing windows in almost every room in the house. But attention to health was not met just by ventilation or by the sizable planned infirmary.[62] The fear that the poor might harbor disease informed the structure of the workhouse more broadly.

Upon admission, all inmates—not just those destined for the infirmary—were sequestered in the "Quarantine Room . . . until they are certified to be free from any disorder." Apprehension about contagion also informed the space used to process relief requests. Adjacent to the committee room was a room where pauper applicants waited until, one at a time, they moved into a third "examination and inspection" room that communicated with the committee room through a window. Thus, vestrymen and paupers never inhabited the same space, the architecture protecting committeemen from the dangerous proximity that welfare encounters commonly demanded. The rationale for the structure was expressly "intended as a Separation to prevent the liability of infection being communicated to the Committee."[63]

Similar apprehension affected St. Margaret's architecture, but differently. St. Margaret's effected a complete physical separation of its workhouse and its infirmary almost from the start. A report dated 1731 described its infirmary as a free-standing structure separate from the workhouse, potentially

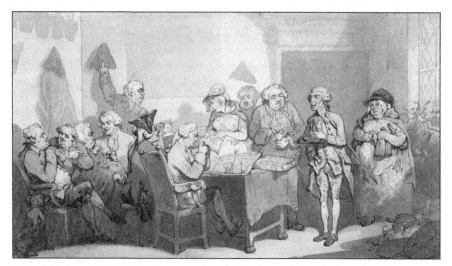

Figure 1.1. Thomas Rowlandson, *The Parish Vestry*, 1784. © Victoria and Albert Museum, London. Reproduced with permission.

in the stable mentioned earlier; the sick were "well nursed and provided for in an Infirmary taken at a little distance from the workhouse."[64] Surviving invoices for insurance policies demonstrate that right through to the late 1790s the parish insured two structures: a workhouse and an infirmary.[65]

That some infirmaries stood alone may explain the phenomenon of some workhouse infirmaries being identified without any mention of the workhouse at all. Discussions in coroner's inquests, for example, contain references to the "St. Georges' Infirmary," the location of which reveals was not the voluntary St. George's Hospital but rather the workhouse infirmary in St. George's Hanover Square.[66] A 1788 newspaper reference to "St. Ann's Infirmary" does likewise for the workhouse infirmary in St. Ann's Soho.[67] The title page of William Rowley's treatise on fevers identifying him as surgeon to the "St. Mary-le-bone Infirmary" gives the false impression that it was a voluntary hospital when it was actually St. Mary-le-bone's workhouse infirmary.[68] Notably, like St. Margaret's, it also stood detached from the workhouse (see fig. 1.2). The most common example of this phenomenon involved the workhouse in St. James Westminster, which, if coroner's inquests and newspapers are any guide, was repeatedly referred to simply as the "St. James Infirmary" with no mention of it being a workhouse at all.[69] Cartographers similarly confused terms. The same structure on Poland Street identified elsewhere as the St. James workhouse was on Richard Horwood's *Plan of the Cities of London and Westminster* merely labeled the "St. James Infirmary."[70] Thus as the century progressed some parish infirmaries acquired their own identities detached conceptually, and sometimes

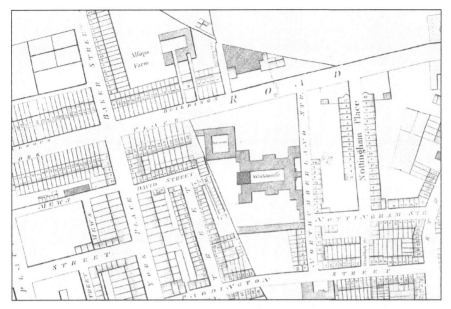

Figure 1.2. St. Marylebone's workhouse and infirmary. Detail from Horwood, *Plan of the Cities of London and Westminster*. Image by Motco Enterprises Limited, www.motco.com.

physically, from the workhouses out of which they grew. The pathophobic drive to isolate potentially contagious paupers from the general workhouse population could only have enhanced this development.

One final factor augmented the contagion anxieties surrounding workhouses. It was not uncommon to find workhouses near burial grounds. A 1732 survey shows that the workhouses in St. Andrew's Holborn, St. Dunstan in the West, St. Giles in the Fields, St. Martin in the Fields, and St. Sepulchre's were all either adjacent or in proximity to cemeteries.[71] Contagion fears may help explain the phenomenon, as the putrefaction of corpses presented a similar threat of dangerous miasma. Cemeteries were long considered possible sources of epidemics, so it is not surprising to find workhouses situated in what were assumed already to be contagious zones.[72] After all, it was not uncommon to sequester workhouses in morally dodgy or otherwise undesirable locations. Allhallows's workhouse was "formerly a tavern"; Mile End's, "formerly a Musick house of no good Repute"; and St. Sepulchre's, Middlesex, was "in a very dirty part of the Parish."[73] Situating workhouses near burial grounds likely enhanced the anxieties about contagion that surrounded them. However, the link between workhouses and cemeteries ran even deeper, stemming from yet another component of workhouses' medical services: forensics.

Workhouses dealt with death almost daily. Invoices for coffins and shrouds reveal the startling rate at which St. Margaret's workhouse bore the responsibility of burying corpses. During 1778 the workhouse bought 109 coffins over just seventy-nine days. Not a bulk purchase, an itemized bill gives the name of each deceased for whom a coffin was procured.[74] In other words, workhouse authorities buried bodies at a rate of 1.37 corpses per day. Importantly, some of these bodies underwent forensic investigation by the workhouse medical staff, something about which workhouse records are quiet but which coroner's inquests display vividly.

When corpses were discovered, in the street, in a park, or in the Thames, they were often taken to workhouses. Parishes situated on or near cemeteries made use of what was called the "bonehouse" to store bodies for inspection and forensic investigation. Thus we see parish officials in St. George's Hanover Square, St. James Westminster, and St. Martin in the Fields ordering bodies directly into the bonehouse.[75] Notably, in these cases churchwardens ordered workhouse masters to remove the bodies to the bonehouse, signaling that handling corpses was indeed the workhouse's obligation. Thus in 1768 the finder of a drowned woman in St. Martin in the Fields reported alerting "Mr. Tresslove one of the Church wardens there with, who gave [him] an Order directing the Governor of the Workhouse to fetch her to the Bone house." Bodies festered, inspiring fears that they emitted pathogenic effluvia; the convenience of a nearby bonehouse helped authorities to keep potentially contagious corpses out of the workhouse.[76]

However, other workhouses, like St. Margaret's, were not so fortunate. Such parishes seem to have taken dead bodies right into the workhouse, where medical staff could perform forensic investigations. Relating the remarkable tale of a woman who arose after appearing dead, William Watson described how her body was brought into the Clerkenwell workhouse and placed "under an open arch going into the infirmary, the usual repository for the dead before internment."[77] It was thus in the workhouse infirmary that Archdall Harris—St. Margaret's workhouse surgeon who testified in at least thirteen inquests—performed forensic examinations, including postmortem dissections.[78] Forensic duties seem to have been beyond those covered by Harris's salary, as evidenced by supplemental payments like the guinea he received on September 17, 1790, "To Attend the Jury & Opening the Body of a Male Child Math[ew] Miller at St. Marg. W[ork] H[ou]se."[79] Postmortem examinations, of course, became ever more common in the late eighteenth century and were central to the development of pathological anatomy. With so many forensic postmortems occurring in workhouses thanks to parochial responsibilities, medical historians need to recognize how workhouses made important early contributions to the development of this seismic epistemic shift usually associated only with larger hospitals.[80] Needless to say, workhouses' forensic duties could have only enhanced the contagion anxieties that this chapter has charted.

Not only did workhouses provide the space for autopsies, but coroner's juries frequently deliberated in workhouses' committee rooms. But a pattern is difficult to establish. In some cases inquests on bodies lying in workhouses were held elsewhere. But often enough, if a corpse was taken to a workhouse, the inquest "on the body" was held there. It is impossible to tell from Westminster inquests alone how commonly jurymen inspected the actual corpses, though the law required it. Coming into the workhouse at all, let alone confronting a corpse, would have again raised powerful contagion anxieties. It was no accident that parishes had traditionally given the job of examining corpses to poor, elderly women, termed "searchers of the dead."[81]

While patterns are difficult to discern, evidence suggests that coroner's juries may have arranged to sit outside of the workhouse when the possibility of contagion was acute. The body of a man named Michel Tims lay in St. James's workhouse on June 24, 1789. His putrid fever was so worrying that an apothecary ordered him "put . . . to Bed in a detached place as the Fever was of an Infectious nature." The following day, his last, Tims was taken to the workhouse either dead or dying. Even though his corpse and the medical staff who would testify were in the workhouse, and even though inquests were commonly held in St. James's workhouse committee room, the jury met instead "at the Dwelling House of Mrs. Flint . . . in Great Marlborough Street."[82]

Similar cases involve bodies of the drowned found weeks after the fact and described as exceedingly fetid. While George Jackson's "very Putri'd" corpse lay in St. Martin in the Fields workhouse, the jury commiserating on his death met safely in a private home several blocks away, as did a jury a month later investigating a drowned child not discovered until the body was similarly "putrid." Unsurprisingly, St. Margaret's witnessed the same phenomenon. In 1780 an infant was discovered weeks after being abandoned in an alley. An overseer ordered the workhouse master to send a woman, probably a parish searcher, to retrieve the body to the workhouse. Archdall Harris examined the corpse and described the body as "in a State of Putrefaction." It is probably not coincidental that the jury met not in the workhouse like many other juries, but rather "at the House of Mr. Ansley . . . in Tothill Street."[83]

One final case can perhaps bring together several of the themes this chapter has highlighted. In July 1793 an ill man named William Stephens called on his friend, John Tomkins, to help him. Tomkins and Stephens's mother loaded William into a coach and drove to the Westminster Infirmary. He was refused admission, not because he was not a proper object of charity, but because "they could not Possibly admit [him] into the Hospital by Reason of the great Danger that might possibly result from it." Tomkins and Mrs. Stephens loaded William back into the coach. Now, however, hearing of his contagions condition, they did not enter the coach themselves, choosing to walk alongside of it for their own safety. William's health was failing fast. Where were they to go? Tomkins described, "By the time the Coach had moved nearly opposite to the Warehouses in Petty France, [Stephen's] Mother . . . called to this Deponent[,] he stopped the Coach & got into it immediately & found [Stephens] to all Appearances much worse[.] They drove to the Workhouse in Dean Street."

St. Margaret's workhouse infirmary, like many across London, specialized in treating people like William Stephens. Men and women excluded from care elsewhere, whether because of economics, connections, morality, or in William's case, diagnosis, had one other option that was less likely to turn them away. It was a medical safety net, though an unpleasant one, to be sure. As they turned the coach toward the workhouse, William, his mother, and his friend likely had a confused mix of emotions: relief that there was at least some medical institution liable to admit him; worry that William might catch something even worse once inside or that his settlement details would be contested; sadness that he would have to go on the parish, accept incarceration, and don a parish uniform; but also hope that the workhouse infirmary would save him. True to form, St. Margaret's workhouse infirmary admitted him when no one else would. Sadly, the fever that so frightened the Westminster Infirmary's surgeon killed Stephens soon after admission. His infection was terrifying for workhouse authorities as well. The parish apothecary told the coroner that "he Should have this Man buried, as Soon as possible, to prevent any infection spreading thro' the house, & likewise there is no Necessity for [the] Jury to sitt on him," further advising that his body should "be directly put into a Coffin & While unburied kept in the dead hole." Tellingly, while William's dangerous corpse lay in St. Margaret's workhouse infirmary, the jury investigating his death commiserated in the safety of a nearby coffeehouse.[84]

Stephens's tale of contagion and exclusion points poignantly to some of the important ways that workhouse infirmaries differed from other kinds of hospitals. In spite of his death, and of the jury's obvious desire to get as far away from his body as possible, his story contains the kernel of a hopeful picture in which workhouse infirmaries came to the rescue of the destitute sick excluded from help elsewhere. But workhouses were reluctant saviors at best. The tales of the sick poor whose settlement claims failed and who died while being passed to other parishes, or while languishing in Bridewell waiting to be moved, or on the street after being threatened with prison if they returned seeking alms, or on overseers' doorsteps, or the stories of those who killed themselves rather than enter the workhouse at all—these tales are decidedly less sanguine.[85]

Notes

1. A notable exception for the eighteenth century is John V. Pickstone's chapter on workhouses in, *Medicine and Industrial Society: A History of Hospital Development*

in Manchester and Its Region, 1752–1946 (Manchester: Manchester University Press, 1985), 23–41.

2. Westminster City Archive Centre (hereafter WCA), St. Margaret's Westminster (hereafter Margaret's), Vestry Minutes, 1724–38, E2419, 36–37.

3. Tim Hitchcock, "Paupers and Preachers: The SPCK and the Parochial Workhouse Movement," in *Stilling the Grumbling Hive: The Response to Social and Economic Problems in England, 1689–1750*, ed. Lee Davison et al. (New York: St. Martin's Press, 1992), 145–66.

4. WCA, Margaret's, Vestry Minutes, 1724–38, E2419, 40–44.

5. Hitchcock, "Paupers and Preachers," 146.

6. WCA, Margaret's, Workhouse Committee Minutes (hereafter WCM), 1726–27, n.p., E2632, August 23, 1726.

7. WCA, Margaret's, WCM, 1727–30, E2633, October 26, 1727; November 16, 1727; August 22, 1728; October 3, 1728.

8. WCA, St. George's Hanover Square, WCM, C869, 65; Guildhall Library (hereafter GL), St. Sepulchre, London Division, WCM, MS 3137/1, 29–30, 93, 96, 101.

9. WCA, Margaret's, WCM, 1726–27, E2632, November 3, 14, 16, 1726.

10. Compiled for the year 1735 from WCA, Margaret's, WCM, 1730–36, E2634.

11. Compiled for the year 1735 from GL, St. Sepulchre, London Division, WCM, MS 3137/4, and London Metropolitan Archives, St. Luke's Chelsea Workhouse Admissions and Discharges, 1743–69, 1782–99, microfilm, x/15/37.

12. WCA, Margaret's, WCM, 1730–36, E2634, 242–43, 306.

13. The debate is extensive but well summarized in Steven King, *Poverty and Welfare in England, 1700–1850: A Regional Perspective* (Manchester: Manchester University Press, 2000), 48–76.

14. Kevin Siena, "Hospitals for the Excluded or Convalescent Homes? Workhouses, Medicalization and the Poor Law in Long Eighteenth-Century London and Pre-confederation Toronto," *Canadian Bulletin of Medical History* 27, no. 1 (2010): 5–21.

15. Tim Hitchcock, "The English Workhouse: A Study in Institutional Poor Relief in Selected Counties, 1696–1750" (DPhil diss., University of Oxford, 1985), 194–95.

16. According to the surgeon's report for 1733, the workhouse infirmary's population was 76 percent female. WCA, Margaret's, WCM, 1730–36, E2634, 242–43.

17. Kevin Siena, *Venereal Disease, Hospitals and the Urban Poor: London's 'Foul Wards' 1600–1800* (Rochester: University of Rochester Press, 2004), 75–77, 102–5.

18. Donna Andrew's *Philanthropy and Police: London Charity in the Eighteenth Century* (Princeton: Princeton University Press, 1989) remains the standard study.

19. Roy Porter, "The Gift Relation: Philanthropy and Provincial Hospitals in Eighteenth-Century England," in *The Hospital in History*, ed. Lindsay Granshaw and Roy Porter (London: Routledge, 1989), 165–66; Gunter Risse, *Mending Bodies, Saving Souls: A History of Hospitals* (Oxford: Oxford University Press, 1999), 231–34.

20. For the nineteenth century, see Jonathan Reinarz, "Investigating the 'Deserving' Poor: Charity and the Voluntary Hospitals in Nineteenth-Century Birmingham," in *Medicine, Charity and Mutual Aid: The Consumption of Health and Welfare in Britain, c. 1550–1950*, ed. Anne Borsay and Peter Shapely (Aldershot, UK: Ashgate, 2007), 111–33.

21. William Blair, *Essays on the Venereal Disease* (London, 1798), 217.

22. Siena, *Venereal Disease*, 3, 185, 223.

23. For example, the gender breakdown at both St. Thomas's and the Lock Hospital was roughly sixty to forty, male to female. Ibid., 111, 235.

24. Westminster Abbey Library and Muniments Room (hereafter WA), Westminster Coroner's Inquests, 1760–99 (hereafter Inquests), Richard Haywood, January 9, 1789.

25. WA, Inquests, Joseph Pauley, April 5, 1773.

26. On this condition, see Kevin Siena, "The Moral Biology of the Itch in Eighteenth-Century Britain," in *A Medical History of Skin: Scratching the Surface*, ed. Jonathan Reinarz and Kevin Siena (London: Pickering and Chatto, forthcoming).

27. *The Laws of the London Infirmary* (London: Henry Woodfall, 1743), 8.

28. *An Account of the Rise, Progress and State of the London-Hospital* (London: n.p., 1748), 1. See also *An Account of the Proceedings of the Governours of the Hospital near Hyde-Park-Corner* (London: n.p., 1735), 4; and *An Abstract of the Orders of St. Thomas's Hospital* (London: n.p., 1707), 1.

29. WCL, Margaret's, WCM 1730–36, E2634, 383–86.

30. WCL, Margaret's, WCM, 1726–27, E2632, February 9, 1726.

31. The phrase comes from Lynn Hollen Lees, *The Solidarities of Strangers: The English Poor Laws and the People, 1700–1948* (Cambridge: Cambridge University Press, 1998), 36.

32. WCL, Margaret's, WCM, 1726–27, E2632, September 7, 14, 1727.

33. GL, Sepulchre, WCM, 1729–30, MS 3137/2, 105, 108, 112, 115, 121, 125.

34. Royal College of Surgeons Archives, London, Lock Hospital Board Minute Book, 3:158–60.

35. For example, on Manchester, see Pickstone, *Medicine and Industrial Society*, 35.

36. *An Account of the Proceedings of the Charitable Society for Relieving the Sick and Needy at the Infirmary in Petty-France, Westminster* (London, 1723), 1.

37. That the hospital treated unsettled patients is demonstrated by lists of patients that note their parishes of origin; in 1722 well over a quarter were "stranger[s]." Ibid. 6–10.

38. London Metropolitan Archives, Westminster Infirmary, "Fair Minutes for Incurables," 1734–73, H02/WH/A29/1, May 7, 1735.

39. "Form of the Preamble to the First Subscription-Paper (According to the Manner of the Infirmary at Westminster)," reprinted in Alured Clarke, *A Sermon Preached in the Cathedral Church of Winchester, before the Governors of the County-Hospital for Sick and Lame* (London: J. and J. Pemberton, 1737), 22–23.

40. *A List of the Governors and Contributors to the Hospital, near Hyde-Park-Corner* (London: n.p., 1734), 4.

41. John Nicols, *A Sermon Preached . . . before the President, Vice-Presidents, Treasurer, and Governors of the City of London Lying-In Hospital for Married Women* (London: C. Say, 1767), 23.

42. *A Short Statement of the Nature, Objects and Proceedings of the Scottish Hospital in London* (London: n.p., 1809), 1 (emphasis in the original).

43. *Laws and Regulations of the Ossulston Dispensary* (London: J. Smeeton, 1791), 4.

44. *Account of the Kent Dispensary in the Broad-Way* (London: W. Hales, 1785), 26.

45. Siena, *Venereal Disease*, 230.

46. George Onesiphorus Paul, *Observations on the State of the Glocester Infirmary* (Glocester: n.p., 1796), 30–32, 2–4; *An Account of the Benefactions and Subscriptions to*

the Leicester General Infirmary, in John Green, *A Sermon Preached before the Governors of the Leicester General Infirmary* (Leicester: J. Gregory, 1772), 15–22; *The State of the County-Hospital at Lincoln*, in James Yorke, *A Sermon Preached in the Cathedral Church of Lincoln, on Opening the New County-Infirmary* (Lincoln: W. Wood, 1777), 24–25; *The Report of the Present State of the Publick Infirmary and Lunatic Hospital in Manchester* (Manchester: J. Harrop, 1771), 3–4.

47. Thomas Ashton, *A Sermon Preached at the Parish-Church of St. Anne, Westminster . . . before the Governors of the Middlesex-Hospital* (London: n.p., 1756), 20–24; *An Account of the Proceedings of the Governors of St. George's Hospital near Hyde-Park-Corner* (London: n.p., 1736), 2–4; Matthew Audley, *A Sermon Preached before His Grace William Duke of Devonshire, President, and the Governors of the London Hospital* (London: H. Woodfall, 1757), 29–36; *Account of the Proceedings of the Governors of the Lock Hospital* (London: n.p, 1751), 3.

48. *Rules and Orders for the Government of the General Infirmary at Hereford* (Hereford: C. Pugh, 1775), 16.

49. Thomas Talbot, *Three Addresses to the Inhabitants of the County of Hereford, in Favour of the Establishment of a Publick Infirmary* (Hereford: C. Pugh, 1774), 2.

50. S. King, *Poverty and Welfare*, 48–76.

51. Physician Lewis Mansey used ten names for this disease. *The Practical Physician* (London: J Stratford, 1800), 75.

52. William Buchan, *Domestic Medicine* (London: W. Strahan, 1772), 37.

53. John Barker, *Epidemicks* (Birmingham: E. Piercy, 1795), 63; John Coakley Lettsom, *Medical Memoirs of the General Dispensary in London* (London: Edward and Charles Dilly, 1774), 23.

54. *Observations on the Present State of the Poor of Sheffield, with Proposals for Their Future Employment and Support* (Sheffield: William Ward, 1774), 11–12.

55. Andrew Duncan, *Medical Commentaries for the Year M.DCC.XCII*, vol. 7 (Edinburgh: Peter Hill, 1793), 342.

56. Robert Jackson, *Outline of the History and Cure of Fever* (Edinburgh: Mundell and Son, 1798), 109 (emphasis added).

57. Edward Alanson, *Practical Observations on Amputation* (London: Joseph Johnson, 1782), 94.

58. John Mason Good, *Dissertation on the Diseases of Prisons and Poor Houses* (London: C. Dilly, 1795), 26–27, 33.

59. Pickstone, *Medicine and Industrial Society*, 156–83.

60. WCA, Margaret's, WCM, 1729–30, MS 3137/2, September 17, 1730.

61. James Lind, *An Essay on the Most Effectual Means of Preserving the Health of Seamen: Together with an Essay on the Jail Distemper* (London: D. Wilson and G. Nicol, 1774), 344–45; Daniel Peter Layard, *Directions to Prevent the Contagion of the Jail Distemper, Commonly Called the Jail Fever* (London: James Robson, 1772), 27–46.

62. GL, St. Sepulchre, Minutes of the Committee for Rebuilding the Workhouse, MS 3226, nos. 1–3, pp. 9, 7.

63. Ibid., 5, 3.

64. *An Account of the Work-Houses in Great Britain, in the Year M,DCC,XXXII: Shewing Their Original, Number, and the Particular Management of Them at the Above Period; With Many Other Curious and Useful Remarks upon the State of the Poor*, 3rd ed. (London: W. Brown, 1786), 65.

65. Identical policy numbers appear in invoices from 1760, 1774, and 1795 for two structures. The last identifies the second building, noting that it "pays no tax being the infirmary." See WCA, Margaret's, Workhouse Bills Bundle, E Unlisted <> 1040 (1770–74) and E Unlisted <> 1046 (1745–97).

66. WA, Inquests, Female Infant Child, February 18, 1799.

67. *Morning Post and Daily Advertiser*, February 27, 1788, refers to "the St. Ann's Infirmary, in Rose Street"; Carington Bowles, *Bowles's New London Guide* (London: Carington Bowles, 1786) confirms Rose Street as the location of the workhouse in St. Ann's Soho.

68. William Rowley, *The Causes of the Great Number of Deaths in Putrid Sore Throats, Scarlet Fevers, and Yellow Fever of the West-Indies and America* (London: E. Newberry, 1793). Rowley dedicated his treatise to his employers, "The Right Honorable and Honorable [*sic*] the Noblemen and Gentlemen, Directors and Guardians of the Poor of the Parish of St. Mary-le-bone."

69. WA, Inquests, Margaret Ball, May 31, 1790; Ann Morts, September 26, 1792; Male Infant Child, April 25, 1799. Deponents in this last case used the terms "infirmary" and "workhouse" interchangeably. Newspaper references to the "St. James Infirmary" or "St. James Parish Infirmary" on Poland Street (not to be confused with the Westminster Infirmary on James Street) include *London Daily Advertiser*, July 27, 1752; *Middlesex Journal or Chronicle of Liberty*, August 26, 1769; *Morning Chronicle and London Advertiser*, April 19, 1774; *Gazetteer and New Daily Advertiser*, May 24, 1774; *Morning Herald*, no, 1666, February 27, 1786; *General Evening Post*, September 11, 1788.

70. Richard Horwood, *Plan of the Cities of London and Westminster, the Borough of Southwark, and Parts Adjoining Shewing Every House* (London: n.p., 1792–99). For a map identifying the structure as St. James's workhouse, see Christopher Greenwood and John Greenwood, *Map of London Made from an Actual Survey in the Years 1824, 1825 and 1826* (London: n.p., 1827).

71. *Account of the Work-Houses*, 6, 25, 32, 69, 76.

72. Mark Jenner, "Death, Decomposition and Dechristianization? Public Health and Church Burial in Eighteenth-Century England," *English Historical Review* 120, no. 487 (2005): 615–32.

73. *Account of the Work-Houses*, 73, 77, 78.

74. Contained in WCA, Margaret's, Workhouse Bills Bundle, E Unlisted <> 1038 (1754–83).

75. WA, Inquests, Newborn Male Child, April 3, 1766; Man, unknown, February 16, 1770; New Born Female Child, December 4, 1780; John Coker, December 10, 1781; William Terrant, May 17, 1788; John Bradley, May 27, 1789.

76. WA, Inquests, Woman, unknown, March 18, 1768.

77. William Watson, *An Account of a Series of Experiments* (London: J. Nourse, 1768), 46–47.

78. WA, Inquests, New Born Female Child, June 19, 1769; New Born Male Child, March 4, 1771; New Born Male Child and Female Child, October 20, 1779; New Born Female Child, December 30, 1780; John Fling, February 5, 1780; Woman, unknown, October 30, 1783; Mrs. Manning, October 15, 1783; Robert Dunn, June 28, 1785; John Boulton, November 14, 1785; New Born Female Child, January 5, 1788; Thomas Perkins, January 5, 1789; New Born Female Child, February 3, 1789; New Born Female Child, March 21, 1789.

79. Contained in WCA, Margaret's, Workhouse Bills Bundle, E Unlisted <> 1045 (1790).

80. Michel Foucault, *Birth of the Clinic*, trans. Alan Sheridan (London: Tavistock 1973); William F. Bynum, *Science and the Practice of Medicine in the Nineteenth Century* (Cambridge: Cambridge University Press, 1994), 25–54.

81. Richelle Munkhoff, "Searchers of the Dead: Authority, Marginality, and the Interpretation of Plague in England, 1574–1665," *Gender and History* 11, no. 1 (1999): 1–29; Kevin Siena, "Searchers of the Dead in Long Eighteenth-Century London," in *Worth and Repute: Valuing Gender in Late Medieval and Early Modern Europe*, ed. Kim Kippen and Lori Woods (Toronto: Centre for Reformation and Renaissance Studies, 2011), 123–52.

82. WA, Inquests, Michael Tims, June 24, 1789.

83. WA, Inquests, George Jackson, February 27, 1797; Boy, unknown, March 27, 1797; New Born Female Child, December 30, 1780.

84. WA, Inquests, William Stephens, July 11, 1793.

85. WA, Inquests, William Jenkins, March 31, 1784; Sarah Huggins, August 26, 1783; Ann Slugg, January 23, 1771; Mrs. Manning, October 15, 1783; Sarah Fenwick, July 31, 1777.

Chapter Two

The Elderly in the Eighteenth-Century Workhouse

SUSANNAH OTTAWAY

In the late nineteenth century, a photograph was taken at two of London's largest workhouses. Each shows the inmates gathered to eat a meal; one is of women, the other of men. Row after row of grim-faced, uniformed elders sit despondent before identical plates of food. The images are hauntingly stark and filled with despair, and they compel the question of how British society came to adopt institutionalization of the elderly poor. But in their power to unsettle the viewer, the images also reveal the tendency of contemporaries and historians to privilege emotional responses and the historical memory of the workhouse and thus remind us of the need to examine the actual historical uses and experiences of these institutions.

Workhouses never housed more than a small proportion of the elderly of Great Britain, and conditions inside them were more often filled with tedium than abuse. Nonetheless, they were ubiquitous from the eighteenth century, and the potential of ending up in a workhouse was a very real possibility for the parish poor. Such an end not only violated personal desires for autonomy but also went against the grain of fundamental ideals of community and familial support for the aged that were deeply embedded in culture and society. Moreover, the eighteenth century was a time of increased concern for individual rights, the start of the rise of modern notions of the self, and an era that abounded with cries for human freedom. The apparent paradox of increased institutionalization for the elderly thus requires explanation. An essential component in unpacking this paradox is to situate it in the medical history of both old age and the workhouse. For the rise in institutional care for the elderly came about in part through the medicalization of both old age and the workhouse: over the eighteenth century, both this life stage and this welfare technique were increasingly associated with medicine, health, and concerns about hygiene.

This chapter traces the frequency of the use of the workhouse for the elderly, examines discussions and debates about these institutions as asylums for the aged, and seeks to understand the ways in which the incarceration of the elderly in workhouses came to make sense to the eighteenth-century parish, intellectual, and national governing elite. Throughout, we see the ways in which images of the workhouse as hospice and hospital merged with views of life extension and the medical needs of the aged to facilitate the growth of the workhouse movement. At the same time, we acknowledge the power of the opposite view: of the ubiquitous and compelling depiction of the workhouse as malodorous and unsanitary prison and of the elderly as fully deserving of comfortable retirement in their homes. These two views were utterly incompatible; the first explains the practice of institutionalizing the aged, while the second reveals the origins of the powerfully negative historical memory associated with such a phenomenon.

The Workhouse and the Elderly

Although there were large hospitals and many almshouses for the sick and aged poor throughout early modern England, and there were hospices and workhouses in frequent use on the Continent in the seventeenth century, the workhouse as old-age asylum in England was really an eighteenth-century development. The period from about 1680 to 1730 was a particularly important moment in this regard, when institutional methods (as opposed to "outdoor relief") came by many to be seen as a panacea for the problem of poverty.[1] This attitude culminated in the passage of the 1723 workhouse "test" act, often known as "Knatchbull's Act," in which parishes were allowed to mandate entry into a workhouse for any parishioner needing poor relief.

Even before this act passed Parliament, corporations of the poor had been established in fifteen cities between 1696 and 1715.[2] These large corporations, which often set up "Houses of Industry," made special provisions for including the aged poor. John Cary's account of the highly influential Bristol workhouse relates that after they had taken in the poor children, "We next took in our ancient People; and here we had principally a regard to such as were impotent, and had no Friends to help them, and to such as we could not keep from the lazy Trade of Begging: these we clothed as we saw they needed, and put on such Employment as were fit for their Ages and Strengths."[3] Here, we have an interesting juxtaposition of the elderly as both helpless and recalcitrant, suggesting that while the motivation for using the workhouse was one of pity and obligation to the physical infirmity of old age, the practical experience of housing the aged was one that pitted the disciplinary goals of the house of industry against lifelong habits of independence. For, as studies have repeatedly shown, most older people in England continued to live in their own households throughout later life.[4]

Cary's association of old age and impotence was by no means uncommon; nor should the independent-mindedness of elderly individuals have been unexpected in the early eighteenth century. While as much as 10 percent of England's population was aged sixty or more at this time, only a small fraction of those elderly men and women received formal poor relief.[5] A century of low birth rates meant that the elderly reached a proportion of the population in this period not matched until the twentieth century. While life expectancy *at birth* varied between thirty-five and forty-five over the eighteenth century, life expectancy at age thirty was about thirty to thirty-two further years for men and women, so middle-aged people could reasonably expect to survive into their old age.[6] Overall, women lived longer than men, then as well as now, and women were often more subject to poverty, a fact that was reflected in the far higher proportion of elderly women than men in most workhouses throughout the period.[7]

This is not to say that older women were unemployable, for as Schwarz and others have shown, elderly women's part-time employment was very widespread, especially in London.[8] Frequent sightings of old women employed in physically challenging tasks must have further reassured workhouse advocates that even institutions that focused on the exploitation of the labor of inmates were appropriate places for aged women. While our modern sensibilities balk at the conflation of female infirmity and manual labor, John Cary and his contemporaries were not likely to have been so nice in their thinking.

The demographic features of the period meant that the needs of the aged poor were particularly visible just as the concept of institutionalized poor relief was gaining popularity, and the need of the disabled, elderly poor for housing and assistance was a feature of both printed discussions of workhouses and account books that reveal the age structure of inmates.[9] As workhouses were increasingly used after the 1720s (some seven hundred had been erected by midcentury, with perhaps two thousand by 1800), the possibility of an old person living and dying in such institutions expanded, even as the elderly accounted for a shrinking proportion of the population in the last half of the century (down to 6–7 percent of the population by the end of the period).[10] Indeed, throughout the century, workhouses were used disproportionately to house the young and the old, and while the young entered the workhouse primarily because of their family situations, the old tended to enter because of their physical decline.[11]

Local studies have reconstructed the level of dependence on the workhouse of aged populations (here defined as those aged sixty or older). In Terling, Essex, the elderly poor were increasingly housed in the workhouse in the last decades of the century, so that by the 1790s over 70 percent of inmates were aged sixty or more. In the township of Ovenden, in Halifax parish, West Yorkshire, the figures fluctuated, with workhouse inmates who were over sixty years varying between 10 and 38 percent of inmates.[12] The massive workhouse used by the London parish of St. Martin in the Fields consistently had one-fourth to one-third of its residents aged sixty plus, and, similarly, 31.6 percent of inmates in St. James Westminster's workhouse in 1797 were elderly, and 37 to 41 percent of the inmates of London's Liberty of the Rolls workhouse were sixty or more.[13] While regional and local variations in poor relief were significant and sustained, as recent work has shown, the predominance of the elderly in workhouse populations was ubiquitous across usual regional divides.[14]

The proportion of the elderly population of these parishes in the workhouse is very difficult to determine (as it involves a detailed reconstruction of the parish populations), but as near as we can calculate, the proportion of those over sixty who spent time in the workhouse was around 6 to 9 percent in late eighteenth-century Ovenden, ranged from 2 to 14 percent in Terling, and accounted for some 11 to 37 percent of the total elderly population in St. Martin in the Fields from 1740–1800 (rising markedly from 1770 to 1800).[15] In eighteenth-century Kent, as well, many parishes used their workhouses for significant portions of their aged poor, despite the fact that some places "made the deliberate decision to leave some of the aged to continue as out-pensioners."[16] Overall, then, although it is very clear that the workhouse never housed anything close to a majority of the elderly of England, it is also evident that the presence of the workhouse would have figured significantly in the lives and imaginations of the aged poor.

Workhouses as Homes for the Elderly

To understand the paradoxical nature of the elderly's increasing institutionalization, we need to explore the basis for poor relief more generally. The rights and entitlements of the poor were centered on the barest right to subsistence and physical safety, but the vast majority of writers on the poor laws recognized special needs or privileges of the elderly.[17] Foundational texts on natural rights and the duties of society expressed unequivocally the right of all individuals to subsistence and the obligation of society to supply the means of living.[18] Frequently referenced manuals for overseers of the poor, for example, reveal an explicit statement about the need for all parishioners to ensure that no party actually died from want of food or shelter, regardless of the moral and economic value or status of the individual.[19] Even the reprobate, examples of vice and prodigality, must be "supported from Starving"; even the "lazy, thriftless" poor were to be relieved by their parish or town "in cases of manifest extremity."[20] Sermons, too, reinforced this principle; so, even though we cannot often reproduce vestry arguments, we can be certain that vestrymen did hear about their obligation to ensure the right to subsistence.[21] But while subsistence allowances were unproblematic, interpreting the subtler points of these entitlements—the "conveniences of life" to which all Englishmen had a just claim, according to John Locke—was much more difficult.[22]

For the elderly, most commentators agreed that their right to subsistence came with a presumption of entitlement to additional comforts and liberties, especially the assumption that they should be assisted *within* their communities, by both family and collectivity. Many writings on the poor articulate that the elderly possessed something above the bare rights of subsistence and preservation.[23] This presumption left promoters of workhouses with an additional need to justify imposing the workhouse test on the aged. It left opponents of the workhouse with a particularly compelling set of attacks on workhouse accommodation for the elderly—and these individuals could combine arguments about health and human rights in opposing indoor relief for old people.

Thus, even many of those who supported the workhouse in theory were evidently opposed to, or at least troubled by, its use as a home for the aged. A pamphlet published in response to a public dispute over the erection of a workhouse in Bury, Suffolk, opposed another author who "allows a house of industry [to be] a restraint upon the natural rights and liberties of the poor; That's enough." But even the author of the original pamphlet had exempted the elderly from incarceration: "I will allow that in every Parish there are some Persons, reduced by old Age, or unavoidable Calamities to a State of great Poverty. . . . Such people as these are certainly worthy of every Encouragement which Compassion can afford them: Nor would any Parish, I think, whose Poor were all like these, wish to have them removed from among them."[24] Another publication with a generally punitive attitude toward the poor in St. Giles in the Fields still asserted that a new regime would see "Those who by Age or Infirmities, are wholly incapable of Work or Labour, will be provided for and maintain'd in a regular and comfortable Manner."[25]

We cannot be surprised at the disdain of radicals like John Vancouver, who viewed workhouses as "impolitic and ruinous," forcing inmates to "a complete surrender of all property in their labour, whether of corporeal strength, or mental faculty."[26] Nor was Vancouver original; his words echo many earlier complaints not only by reformers but also by the poor. At Harborough, Leicestershire, the poor refused to enter the workhouse "because of the Confinement to which they must then be subject." Similarly, in Rumford, Essex, the poor refused to go into the house out of pride and a dislike of confinement; according to one observer, some of the poor "deem the Work-house to be a mere State of Slavery."[27] Indeed, animosity toward workhouses could reach a point of outright rebellion.[28]

Not only the poor, but also other critics of the workhouse were using the same language of the violation of rights by the end of the eighteenth century. A pamphlet writer in Kent opposed a workhouse scheme that would have used the labor of the poor during harvest with the claim: "And if the

Poor were to be let out to work as is proposed for them to be and they to take no Pay for their Labour, they would soon want Negroe-Drivers in *Kent* as well as in *America.*"[29]

Even the early voices of "political economy" displayed ambivalence about housing the aged in workhouses. Malthus argued that "it seems peculiarly hard upon old people who have perhaps been useful and respectable members of society, and in their day 'have done some service,' that as soon as they are past their work, they should be obliged to quit the village where they had always lived."[30] Jeremy Bentham's opposition to home-provision systems was clear and consistent, but even he hoped that the virtuous elderly poor could be provided with minimal pensions starting at about sixty-five years of age at the public charge, and all others could be expected to have bought into a pension scheme or benefit club.[31]

In short, if we look at the relationship of workhouses to the rhetoric of natural rights, along with assumptions about the entitlements of the elderly, the idea of confining the aged to the workhouse appears to run counter to the existing ideology of the eighteenth century. Discussions and critiques of this nature combined with concerns that centered around health and cleanliness. As Sir Frederick Morton Eden noted, "The objections which have been repeatedly urged against parochial workhouses and houses of industry; [are] that . . . under the lash of a task-master, the freedom of the British spirit is broken; and that reared in crowds, the rising generation lose the spring of health in contagion and restraint."[32]

A growing attention to health and hygiene in the workhouse occurred at the same time as the medical history of old age showed increasing optimism about the possibility of addressing health concerns in old age. Reformers' position in regard to the suitability of the workhouse for the elderly came increasingly to include an assessment of the potential of the workhouse to provide a place for health care and hospice resources for the aged. This was possible because, from the beginning of the first workhouse movement, there was a tendency to conflate all the disparate types of institutions for the poor into an ambiguous conception of houses of industry and the like.

Workhouse, Hospital, or House of Correction?

There was a tremendous amount of ambiguity not only about the term "workhouse" but about the nature of all and any institutions for the poor. Typical of the linguistic slippage at the "top" of society was the Parliamentary Act, setting up "a work-house for maintaining the poor" in Norwich in 1713. This act allowed the city to "Erect one or more Hospital or Hospitals, Workhouse or Work-houses, House or Houses of Correction within the City and to provide other convenient necessaries for setting to work and employing the Poor of what Age or Sex soever and to compel Idle or Leasy [*sic*] Poor People Begging without some lawful Imployment, or other Poor that receive Collection to Dwell or Work in such Work-Houses or elsewhere." Similar ambivalence is evident in a 1704 bill, in which any person or body politic could have full power and lawful authority to "erect, found and establish one or more Hospitals, Maisons de Dieu, Abiding Places, or Houses of Correction." Other publications called such institutions by still other names; in 1719 Laurence Braddon proposed enormous, self-sufficient corporations of the poor, which he referred to as "Collegiate Cities."[33]

This lumping tendency contrasts with the sixteenth-century founding of the Royal Hospitals, carefully differentiated in their service and methods.[34] From the mid-seventeenth century, however, as reformers increasingly sought institutional remedies for the problem of poverty, the many functions of institutions were increasingly confused and folded together. From the Bristol foundation forward, the emphasis was placed not on the different ways in which the poor needed attention in hospitals, schools, and bridewells, but on the ways in which institutionalization as a unified concept could solve the problems of the poor more generally. This allowed reformers to fold the concept of workhouse as deterrent into the concept of workhouse as hospital or asylum when encouraging the formation of such institutions.

Writers who sought to untangle the disparate functions of these institutions struggled unsuccessfully for clarity.[35] Joseph Shaw's handbook on the poor laws, on the one hand, specified, "By Workhouses I do not mean the Bridewells, or Houses of Correction established in each County . . . because the treating of them will come more properly under the Title Constables and Vagrants." But on the other hand, at one point, he slips and refers to houses of correction as workhouses.[36] This confusion was still present in the bills that went through Parliament, spearheaded by William Hay, in 1735.[37] Thomas Cooke preached a sermon that claimed, "I would have no Work-house that should not also be an Hospital; and as it contains a Bridewell to compel the Lazy, so should it have proper receptacles to succour the distressed: Aged and Impotent Persons there will be among us as long as the World endureth, and God forbid but they should be taken care of."[38] By conceptualizing workhouses as multipurpose institutions, early promoters allowed for an emphasis on the medical needs of the aged, but they also reinforced the indelible link between workhouses and punitive institutions, like houses of correction.

Health and Hygiene in the
Housing of Elderly Poor in Workhouses

It is precisely the confusion over the multipurpose nature of workhouses that Parliament sought to correct by passing Gilbert's Act in 1782. Here,

"Poor Houses" were explicitly designed to house the impotent, not the idle poor, and here, too, we see a significantly enhanced attention to the topics of health and cleanliness. Indeed, the appendix detailing the rules to be followed in these new union poor houses includes first, a stipulation that all labor must be tailored to the strength of the inmates; second, that house and inmates be kept clean; and third, that the care to be given to the elderly and sick poor should include "separate Apartments . . . provided for the Reception of the sick and distempered Poor, and an Apothecary or Surgeon to be sent for to attend them when there shall appear Necessity for it."[39] Clearly, an important part of the justification for these workhouses was precisely as a hospital or hospice for the aged.

The theme of care for the aged is ubiquitous in publications during the first workhouse movement (ca. 1690–1730), but these rarely focused on health, instead justifying the suitability of the workhouse for the aged because it allowed them to retreat from the workaday world.[40] One sermon claimed, "The Old and Infirm . . . being no longer disturb'd with worldly Cares, have Leisure and Opportunity in these happy Retirements to reflect upon their Lives past, and prepare themselves for a happy Eternity."[41] Only four of the dozens of accounts of workhouses published by the Society for the Promotion of Christian Knowledge (SPCK) in the 1720s dwelt on the issue of health for older people, and even here, the primary concern seems to have been for the health of the able-bodied. In two other cases in this account, there is specific mention of nursing for older people, but in both cases the health concerns of the elderly were actually handled in ways that pulled them out of the workhouse itself. In Barking, Essex, "There is a small Infirmary built on the Backside of the House, but the People are generally in so good Health, that there has been hitherto little Occasion to use it." In the house in Malden, Essex: "There is a large Part assign'd for an Infirmary, into which the old and infirm Persons are put; where there is a Nurse to attend them, with Firing allow'd; but the Poor there are at stated Allowances, and provide for themselves, by the same Work, or any other which they choose."[42]

The problem of the health of their inmates was addressed in vestry discussions and decisions regarding workhouses in many cases, but these do not reveal any sustained focus specifically on the nursing requirements of the elderly. As was fairly common throughout the century, the Edmonton workhouse committee in 1732 appointed a physician apothecary to a contract for the parish poor for twelve pounds per year, "for which he was required to attend free of charge to workhouse inmates and those who, though in their own homes, were chargeable to the poor rate."[43] Similarly, there was a pronounced attempt to avoid infection in larger workhouses by setting aside accommodations for the unhealthy.[44] At St. George's Hanover-Square, which housed 187 persons in 1729, "The Sicke are taken Care of by an able Physician, an Apothecary, and Surgeon, who attend daily." An SPCK correspondent from Beverley, Yorkshire, noted in 1728 that after a new workhouse was built in 1727, they delayed opening it so "that we might not hazard the Health of the Poor, by placing them in a damp House."[45] What we see in such cases is that workhouse promotion and planning exhibited a common concern about the health of the poor generally, without focusing on the specific needs of the aged.

Early sources on workhouses were more forthcoming when it came to discussions of hygiene. Indeed, a common aspect of workhouse admission for paupers would have been a ritual cleansing and reclothing. The workhouse in St. Andrew's Holborn required that new inmates' clothes be cleaned (so they could be "made useful" to the house) and that the children be "washed and cleaned" every morning. Even the provisions should be "cleanly and well dressed." Similar concerns about cleanliness (often regarding children particularly) were expressed in the early decades of the century in many workhouses including St. Giles in the Fields, where wards were to be washed weekly and inmates, according to the rules of 1731, were "examined by the Surgeon, Apothecary, or Nurse and . . . washed as soon as they are taken in, if it may be without prejudice to their Health." In St. Sepulchres without Middlesex, an SPCK correspondent in 1731 noted that "a Parcel of old Houses, in a very dirty Part of the Parish, are pulled down, and a clean, commodious Brick-House erected in the place." In this house, "the Reverend Vicar of the Parish frequently visits . . . to see that they do not neglect their Duty to God, while under the Infirmities of old Age, Poverty and Sickness, they enjoy so happy a Retirement." The Quaker workhouse at St. James, Clerkenwell, received special notice for providing "a Cold Bath for washing all that want it, for their Health or Cleanliness."[46] In all these cases, we can see that workhouses shared in the growing eighteenth-century concern for cleansing the body as a means of preserving health and combating infection.[47]

Attention to both health and hygiene increased as significant reference points in debates over the utility of the workhouse and the need to reform or abolish them in the latter half of the century. By the middle of the eighteenth century, we see a more concentrated concern for keeping the elderly away from the rabble, with more attention to their comfort and disabilities.[48] The Hundred Houses that were set up in Suffolk and Norfolk differed from earlier parish workhouses in their attention to the physical separation of the elderly poor. In Shipmeadow, for example, the plans for the new workhouse in 1766 included "an infirmary with two wards for the elderly."[49] The Isle of Wight Corporation at Newport, erected in 1791, had twenty separate rooms for couples, and two common sitting rooms adjoining them so that the aged and infirm did not have to descend stairs for their meals.[50] Indeed, an architectural historian has noted that later eighteenth- and early nineteenth-century urban workhouses "were designed to permit a high degree of classification . . . often separating the aged from the able-bodied."[51]

Earlier workhouses and houses of industry appear not to have made such efforts at segregation and separate care for the aged. The house in Half-Moon Alley set up by the London Corporation for the Poor in 1698, for example, separated the children from the "Keeper's Side," which housed vagabonds and rogues but did not specify where the elderly belonged. We also have early designs for the workhouse of St. George's Hanover Square and at Chatham, Kent, Strood, and Beverley, but here too, there is no special accommodation for the aged.[52] Indeed, for the smaller parish workhouses, it would have been impossible to set aside rooms for the aged, as there were insufficient divisions within the house rooms to make anything more than a male and female dormitory possible.[53]

Those who sought to reform the system of workhouses in the later decades of the century appear at times to have been obsessed with the health of their inmates.[54] As other historians have noted, "images of contagion were often used to describe the workhouses" of the later eighteenth and early nineteenth centuries.[55] Edmund Gillingwater's detailed reform plan for workhouses was particularly concerned with hygiene and related health issues:

> Another source of misery which too commonly disgraces our English work-houses, is the want of cleanliness. . . . The necessity and usefulness of cleanliness amongst such large bodies of people as are generally contained within such narrow limits as a parish work-house, or a house of industry, is so evident, that the directors of some of our larger repositories of the poor, in England, have wisely adopted the plan held out to them by foreigners, and have followed their excellent examples by strictly enjoining cleanliness in their respective habitations for the poor.[56]

Similarly, a critique of the Sheffield Workhouse, while praising the generosity of the town and the good intentions of the workhouse, lamented its inadequacy in terms that dwelt at particular length on problems of health and old age. "There are many accommodations essential to the comfort, the health, and even to the lives of the Poor, which to the great regret of every humane Person, the present Workhouse is utterly unable to afford them." The pamphlet particularly condemned the tiny bedrooms, which placed four to six people per bed in "the midst of unwholesome vapours" and the lack of separate accommodation for the "aged or unfortunate."[57] Conflict over the Sheffield Workhouse revolved around the issues of health and human rights a few years later as well.[58] Visitors criticized the workhouse at Oxford, where "The house is exceedingly dirty. . . . No regular quarters appropriated to the sick, aged or infirm."[59]

Evidently, those who attacked workhouses as pernicious institutions often did so through the common language of health and humanity. One bitter opponent of indoor relief wrote that we judge "institutions which are of human policy, that they approach the nearer to perfection, in proportion as they preserve to mankind their natural rights and liberties." The author specifically attacked workhouse supporters who believed that the institutions had a high "regard which is shown to the health of their inhabitants; and the excellent oeconomy and discipline of the interior of the house. As to the first, Doctor Burn seems to hold it as incompatible with such an institution, and his opinion is supported by some undeniable facts." The tract went on to describe the workhouse in Hexingham where the air was hot, and the inmates were forced to sleep nearly three a bed, and the author asserted that similar circumstances existed in "almost every one of these houses that are now established."[60] Eden's collection of information about workhouses contains numerous references to the health of inmates and the healthful situation (or lack thereof) of workhouses.[61]

After the midcentury, too, new workhouse rules often emphasized the necessity of hygiene for the inmates. The Local Act of 1756 for twenty-eight Suffolk parishes set up the first of the Hundred Houses that came to be so common in England's southeast. When this house was set up on Nacton Heath "to administer proper comfort and assistance to the sick, infirm and aged" (among other concerns), the rules mandated that before admittance into the house, the poor must be "shaved and cleansed thoroughly by washing in warm water, and then all new clothed from head to foot."[62]

Increasingly, then, whether the author of a text was interested in supporting, reforming, or abolishing the workhouse, he seems now to need to account for the health of inmates—and especially elderly inmates—in terms that assume that this issue should be a concern for those interested in poor relief more generally.[63] One reason for this was the growing focus on such institutions as asylums for the aged as a consequence of Gilbert's Act and an outgrowth of their increasing use even at the small parish level as houses for the aged. Another reason for this focus was the later eighteenth century's interest in the health of the aged.

Old Age and Medicine

Although it is difficult to pinpoint changing attitudes toward old age in English society, the long eighteenth century did exhibit signs of a more optimistic view toward preserving health in old age than was the case in the seventeenth century. In this way, the period prefigured significant changes in medical attitudes toward old age that we can find across Europe and America in the nineteenth century.[64] Medical views of the aging process in the eighteenth century still often incorporated early modern humoral theory and continued to liken old age to a disease, but there was also a growing sense of confidence regarding humanity's capacity to combat the negative effects of aging, thanks in part to new, commercialized attitudes toward marketing cures for the discomforts of old age.[65]

Medical texts cover both these elements of continuity and change, but they also often reflect the influence of Enlightenment empiricism. *A New Method of Treating Consumptions* (1727), for example, written by Nicholas Robinson (ca. 1697–1775) laid out the differences between "Decays that naturally attend Old Age" and the wasting caused by consumption. Robinson distinguished between illness and old age specifically, contrasting the rapid onset of "symptoms" of consumption, and the gradual decline and progressive muscular atrophy in the "decrepidness" of old age. Robinson explicitly calls on new scientific reasoning and method, stating that the basis of his theories on consumption "are a kind of Mathematical Reasoning, without Numbers, wherein the first Proposition is a Data consisting of self-evident Principles."[66] Robinson's observations of human bodies and use of a more modern understanding of medicine, especially new views on the nature of the circulation and regulation of fluids in the human body, led to a more diagnostic approach to aging.

Although the creation of the specific subfield of geriatrics awaited medical developments of the nineteenth century, trends in the treatment and understanding of ill health in old age indicate steps toward a more medicalized view of the last stages of life, with later eighteenth-century sources on both medicine and workhouses indicating an awareness of the specific health needs of those in old age.[67] At the same time, even in London, where disparate, specialized medical institutions were a major, growing aspect of the care of the poor and the landscape of health care, we find a keen awareness of the medical demands of the poor within workhouses by the late eighteenth and early nineteenth century. Medical personnel were hired specifically for the care of the sick poor in the workhouse, keeping health concerns in the hands of professionals rather than perpetuating older models of informal care by unskilled workhouse inmates and matrons.[68] The confluence of a more diagnostic approach to the problems of the sick, elderly poor, with the persistent awareness of the pervasive need for medical care within workhouses, set in place certain elements of the modern notions of "nursing" or "old age homes," even though the eighteenth-century workhouse was as yet far from realizing such trends.

Similarly, tracts on prolonging life in the eighteenth century continued a long tradition of faith in human ability to extend the life course, but they tended to emphasize the potential of medical intervention and physical health more than the mental, emotional, and religious focus of classical works like Cicero's *De Senectute* and its many imitations. Moreover, their brand of faith in human nature and their assertion of an individual's obligation to preserve health put a more proactive and medically involved spin on this traditional literature. Even women's particular health problems, it seems, could be "cured" by Enlightened (or patent) medicine. In the 1790s "Remarks on the Final Cessation of the Menses" offered medical nostrums to assist women in surmounting the difficulties of menopause.[69] The text is an illustration of Michael Stolberg's concept of the "irritation" model of menopause typical of the later eighteenth and early nineteenth centuries. While the "Remarks" "pathologized" this period as medically dangerous, the text also dwells on the potential of postmenopausal women's physical and intellectual vigor.[70]

Newly optimistic views on the potential of the aged to benefit by modern medicines and proper care and attention could be empowering, but they also were part of the era's new tendency to mark off this stage of life as more rigidly defined and more problematic from a social welfare standpoint. More rigid constructions of the numerical ages associated with stages of the life course and increased attention to the particular needs of the elderly characterized the later eighteenth century.[71] The meeting of these trends in the history of aging with the period's tendency to focus on institutions as potential solutions to welfare problems helps to explain the seemingly paradoxical trend of the institutionalization of the old poor that we have examined here.

Finally, the intertwining of these trends also helps to lay the groundwork for the appalling historical memory of old people in the workhouse that we touched on in the introduction to this chapter. Along with traditional views that older people had earned special treatment and community and family care, the eighteenth century introduced an element of institutional care and responsibility for the aged that destabilized these traditional norms. In this context, leaving an older person to the care of the workhouse (through the local distribution of poor relief) meant abandonment of the ideals of autonomy for that person and desertion of filial piety and norms of traditional communalism. Resolving the paradox of the institutionalization of the aged in the eighteenth-century workhouse thus does nothing to mitigate the power of the negative historical memory of these "pauper Bastilles."

Notes

1. Research for the project was funded by the American Council of Learned Societies and Carleton College. The essential study remains Tim Hitchcock, "The English Workhouse: A Study in Institutional Poor Relief in Selected Counties, 1696–1750" (DPhil diss., University of Oxford, 1985).

2. Mark Goldie, introd. to "An Essay on the Poor Law," in *Locke: Political Essays* (Cambridge: Cambridge University Press, 1997), 182–83; Tim Hitchcock, "Paupers and Preachers: The SPCK and the Parochial Workhouse Movement," in *Stilling the*

Grumbling Hive: The Response to Social and Economic Problems in England, 1689–1750, ed. Lee Davison et. al. (Stroud: Sutton, 1992), 145–66.

3. John Cary, *An Account of the Proceedings of the Corporation of Bristol, in Execution of the Acts of Parliament for the Better Employing and Maintaining the Poor of That City* (Dublin: F. Collins, 1700), 16–20. See also Sir Frederick Morton Eden, *The State of the Poor*, 3 vols. (London: Davis, 1797), 1:280–83.

4. It was not unheard of for adult children to reincorporate into parental homes, but while about half of elderly men and women in early modern English population listings lived with their children, less than a quarter of old women and no more than 7 percent of aged men lived as dependents within their children's households. Instead, those who continued to cohabit with children did so by keeping an adult child, usually a daughter, at home. The households of the elderly are discussed extensively in Susannah Ottaway, *The Decline of Life: Old Age in Eighteenth-Century England* (Cambridge: Cambridge University Press, 2004), chap. 4.

5. For the age structure of the English population, see E. Anthony Wrigley and Roger S. Schofield, *The Population History of England, 1541–1871: A Reconstruction* (Cambridge: Cambridge University Press, 1989), 216. Proportions of elderly relieved are in Lynn Botelho, *Old Age and the English Poor Law* (Rochester: Boydell and Brewer, 2004); Ottaway, *Decline of Life*.

6. The low point for life expectancy in the period was 1731, when it stood at 27.9 years, but from 1781 to 1826 life expectancy went from about 35 to about 40 years. Wrigley and Schofield, *Population History*, 236. Newer figures, based on a more limited source, are from E. Anthony Wrigley, Ros Davies, James Oeppen, and Roger S. Schofield, *English Population History from Family Reconstitution, 1580–1837* (Cambridge: Cambridge University Press, 1997), 295. The figures for average life expectancy at age thirty come from Wrigley and Schofield, *Population History*, 250, and are derived from a very rough estimate. In traditional English society, 60 percent of those who reached age fifteen survived to fifty-five; about a third of those who reached fifty-five would reach seventy-five, according to James E. Smith, "Widowhood and Ageing in Traditional English Society," *Ageing and Society* 4, no. 4 (1984): 430. Woods and Williams have pointed out that life expectancy at age twenty could have been as high as forty years even before 1650, and it increased to forty years generally between 1650 and 1850. Robert Woods and Naomi Williams, "Must the Gap Widen before It Can Be Narrowed? Long-Term Trends in Social Class Mortality Differentials," *Continuity and Change* 10, no. 1 (1995): 111.

7. See discussion in Pat Thane, *Old Age in English History: Past Experiences, Present Issues* (Oxford: Oxford University Press, 2000), 21–24. The ratio of women to men was particularly high among the oldest age groups in the London parish of St. Martin's (Leonard Schwarz, personal correspondence with author, November 1, 2009).

8. Leonard Schwarz, "English Servants and Their Employers during the Eighteenth and Nineteenth Centuries," *Economic History Review* 52, no. 2 (1999): 236–56, esp. 254; Peter Earle, "The Female Labour Market in London," in *Women's Work: The English Experience, 1650–1914*, ed. Pamela Sharpe (London: Arnold, 1998), 135–38.

9. Mary Barker-Read, "The Treatment of the Aged Poor in Five Selected West Kent Parishes from Settlement to Speenhamland (1662–1797)" (PhD diss., Open University, 1988).

10. Estimates vary between 150 and 300 parish workhouses believed to have opened in the immediate aftermath of the passage of Knatchbull's Act of 1723, with another 300 by 1750. More than a hundred private acts of Parliament authorized parishes to combine to form joint workhouses between 1601 and 1834. By 1776 there were as many as 1,970, and the 1802–3 Parliamentary returns show 3,765 parishes using a workhouse, though not necessarily in their own parish. Kathryn Morrison, *The Workhouse: A Study of Poor Law Buildings in England* (Swindon: English Heritage, 1999), 14, 29; Norman Longmate, *The Workhouse* (New York: St. Martin's Press, 1974), 24.

11. Alysa Levene and Susannah Ottaway, "Dependency, the Workhouse and Family Ties in Later Eighteenth-Century England" (unpublished paper); Steven King, *Poverty and Welfare in England, 1700–1850: A Regional Perspective* (Manchester: Manchester University Press, 2000), 204–8.

12. For the choice of the age of sixty to demarcate the elderly, see Ottaway, *Decline of Life*, 1–64, 251, 260.

13. Jeremy Boulton and Leonard Schwarz, "'The Comforts of a Private Fireside'? The Workhouse, the Elderly and the Poor Law in Georgian Westminster: St. Martin-in-the-Fields, 1725–1824," in *Accommodating Poverty: The Households of the Poor in England, c. 1650–1850*, ed. Joanne McEwan and Pamela Sharpe (Basingstoke, UK: Palgrave Macmillan, 2011), 221–45. My thanks to the authors for allowing me early access to this article. Westminster City Archives, K344–346.

14. See S. King, *Poverty and Welfare*, cf. on London: David R. Green, *Pauper Capital: London and the Poor Law, 1790–1890* (Farnham, UK: Ashgate, 2010).

15. Ottaway, *Decline of Life*, 251, 261; Boulton and Schwarz, "Comforts," table 2.

16. Barker-Read, "Treatment," 231; cf. Ethel Mary Hampson, *The Treatment of Poverty in Cambridgeshire, 1597–1834* (Cambridge: Cambridge University Press, 1934), 112.

17. John Bohstedt, *The Politics of Provisions: Food Riots, Moral Economy, and Market Transition in England, c. 1550–1850* (Farnham, UK: Ashgate, 2010).

18. James Tully, *An Approach to Political Philosophy* (Cambridge: Cambridge University Press, 1993), 111–16.

19. Michael Dalton, *The Country Justice: Containing the Practice. . . .* (London: William Rawlins and Samuel Roycroft, 1705); Joseph Shaw, *Parish Law; or, A Guide to Justices of the Peace, Ministers, Church-Wardens, Overseers of the Poor, Constables, Surveyors of the Highways, Vestry Clerks, and All Others Concerned in Parish Business* (London: Cogan, 1733), 112–13.

20. Thomas Troughear, *The Best Way of Making Our Charity Truly Beneficial to the Poor; or, the Excellency of Work-Houses in Country Parishes, to Prevent the Evil Effects of Idleness: In a Sermon Preached at Northwood in the Isle of Wight, September the 7th, 1729* (London: Downing, 1730), 13; J. P. Gent, *A New Guide for Constables* (London: Richard and Edward Atkins, 1705), 101–2.

21. William Barnes, *A Sermon Preach'd at St. Martin's Palace, in Norwich, on March 6, 1723. By the Appointment of the Right Reverend Father in God, Thomas Late Lord Bishop of That Diocese: And since at St. Mary's in White-Chapel* (London, n.p., 1727); Thomas Cooke, *Work-Houses the Best Charity: A Sermon, Preacht at the Cathedral Church of Worcester, February 2d, 1702* (London: John Butler, 1702).

22. Locke, "An Essay on the Poor Law," in Goldie, *Locke*; Thomas Horne, *Property Rights and Poverty, Political Argument in Britain, 1605–1834* (Chapel Hill: University of North Carolina Press, 1990).

23. These distinctions are clear in Giles Jacob, *The Compleat Parish-Officer*, 5th ed. ([London?], n.p., 1729), 93; Gent, *New Guide for Constables*, 101.

24. *Remarks on an Anonimous Pamphlet, Intitled, Some Account of a Meeting Held at the Guild-hall at Bury, on the 4th of November, 1771* (Ipswich: Hawes, [1772?]), 5. Cf. *Some Account of a Meeting Held at the Guild-hall in Bury St. Edmunds on the 4th of November, 1771* (Bury St. Edmunds: Green, [1771?]).

25. *The Case of the Parish of St. Giles's in the Fields, as to Their Poor, and a Work-House Designed to Be Built for Employing Them* ([London, 1725?]), 3; cf. Laurence Braddon, *An Abstract of the Draft of a Bill for Relieving, Employing and Reforming the Poor* (London, n.p., 1719).

26. John Vancouver, *An Enquiry into the Causes and Production of Poverty, and the State of the Poor: Together with the Proposed Means for Their Effectual Relief* (London: Edwards, 1796), 50–51.

27. *An Account of the Work-Houses in Great Britain, in the Year M,DCC,XXXII: Shewing Their Original, Number, and the Particular Management of Them at the Above Period; With Many Other Curious and Useful Remarks upon the State of the Poor*, 3rd ed. (London: W. Brown, 1786), 104, 53–55. Accessed through Eighteenth-Century Collections Online. Gale. Carleton College.

28. Sheila Hardy, *The House on the Hill: The Samford House of Industry, 1764–1930* (Suffolk: Gipping, 2001), 16.

29. *To the Proposers of . . . the County of Kent, and to the Inhabitants Thereof in General* ([Maidstone? 1771]), 2.

30. Richard M. Smith, "Transfer Incomes, Risk and Security: The Roles of the Family and the Collectivity in Recent Theories of Fertility Change," in *The State of Population Theory: Forward from Malthus*, ed. Donald Coleman and Roger S. Schofield (Oxford: Basil Blackwell, 1986), 191.

31. Jeremy Bentham, "Home and Community Provision Compared," in *The Collected Works of Jeremy Bentham: Writings on the Poor Laws*, 2 vols., ed. Michael Quinn (Oxford: Clarendon, 2001), 1:170, 193–96.

32. Eden, *State of the Poor*, 1:420.

33. *An Abstract of Several Acts of Parliament relating to the City of Norwich. . . .* (Norwich: Thomas Goddard, 1713), 5; Houses of Parliament Records Office, 1704 Bill, 14; Braddon, *Abstract of the Draft*.

34. Paul Slack, From *Reformation to Improvement: Public Welfare in Early Modern England* (NY: Oxford University Press, 1999), 19–21.

35. The legal writer Samuel Carter wrote, "I distinguish Work-houses from Houses of Correction, for Persons will not willingly apply themselves thither; whereas if a good Course were taken, and good Usage in Stocks and Provision, with orderly Management, it would be rather a Society or College of Artificers, than a *Bridewell*, and the Work would be cheerfully carried on S. C. [Samuel Carter], *Legal Provisions for the Poor* (London: J. Walthoe and J. Walthoe Junr., 1725), 89.

36. Shaw, *Parish Law*, 235–36, 186.

37. The committee responsible for discussing the bills sometimes used the terms "work-house," "hospital," and "house of correction" interchangeably to refer to the desired institution for the poor. Eden, *State of the Poor*, 1:303.

38. Cooke, *Work-Houses the Best Charity*, 25.

39. *The Statutes at Large, from the Twentieth Year of the Reign of King George the Third to the Twenty-Fifth Year of the Reign of King George the Third* (London: Charles Eyre and the executors of William Strahan, 1786), 14: 282. Norman Longmate has found that few Gilbert Unions were set up by 1798, but that by 1834 there were 67, for 924 parishes. *Workhouse*, 30.

40. Cooke, *Work-Houses the Best Charity*, 23.

41. Troughear, *Best Way*, preface.

42. *Account of the Work-Houses*, 51, 60. At St. Alban's, Hertfordshire (September 18, 1724): "It must be consider'd, the Men and Women are generally old and helpless, and the Children perfectly raw and unexperienced. . . . And what is still of greater Consequence is, that by keeping them employ'd, you keep them in Health, and from Idleness." Ibid., 69.

43. David Avery, "Charity Begins at Home: Edmonton Workhouse Committee, 1732–37," Occasional papers, n.s., 14, Edmonton Hundred Historical Society, 1967, 5, 19. In the early years of the workhouse, there is evidence that poor parishioners were moved into the workhouse specifically to be cared for by the parish doctor (21–22).

44. William A. Cassell, "The Parish and the Poor in New Brentford, 1720–1834," *Transactions of the London and Middlesex Archaeological Society* (1972): 179.

45. *Account of the Work-Houses*, 27, 172.

46. Ibid., 17–19, 21, 22, 30, 33, 39, 54, 55, 64, 86, 94, 77, 56.

47. Kathleen Brown, *Foul Bodies: Cleanliness in Early America* (New Haven: Yale University Press, 2009).

48. Thomas Alcock's plan in 1752, utilized by some Suffolk Hundred Houses, is an example. Morrison, *Workhouse*, 18–19.

49. Edwin A. Goodwyn, *"A Prison with a Milder Name": The Shipmeadow House of Industry, 1766–1800* (Beccles: Goodwyn, 1987), 13. The Kingston-upon-Hull workhouse added an infirmary wing in 1766 to its workhouse, and there were infirmaries in most large workhouse plans from the 1760s, but I do not know if these housed the elderly. Morrison, *Workhouse*, 17, 22–23.

50. Morrison, *Workhouse*, 25. The Sussex workhouse plans of 1793–94 in Easebourne show a separate workroom for "old people to pick wool in" (26).

51. Morrison, *Workhouse*, 30.

52. Morrison, *Workhouse*, 12, 15, 16. The building plans are from the 1720s.

53. Workhouse inventories often list the rooms in the house, and these demonstrate the paucity of separate spaces in most smaller parish houses. For example, see Calderdale District Archives, Halifax Antiquarian Society, 258/67, for Ovenden's inventory and Essex Record Office, D/P 299/8/1, on Terling's workhouse.

54. The workhouse critic Edmund Gillingwater remarked that at Mildenhall in Suffolk: "if all our parishes were as careful to promote cleanliness and industry in their own work-houses, as there is observed in this, there would have been no occasion for parishes uniting in houses of industry for a whole hundred." Edmund Gillingwater, *An Essay on Parish Workhouses* (Bury Saint Edmunds: J. Rackham, 1786), 25.

55. Morrison, *Workhouse*, 32.

56. Gillingwater, *Essay on Parish Workhouses*, 19–20.

57. *Facts and Observations Relating to the State of the Workhouse and the Poor of the Township of Sheffield, in 1789* ([Sheffield?, 1789?]).

58. William Ward, *The Substance of Mr. Ward's Speech at the Town-Hall in Sheffield, on Wednesday, April 6th, 1791, at a Meeting of the Inhabitants Who Attended . . . to Give Their Assent or Dissent to, the Bill for the Proposed New Workhouse* ([Sheffield, n.p., 1791]).

59. Cited in Longmate, *Workhouse*, 31.

60. Robert Potter, *Considerations on the Poor Laws, on the Present State of the Poor, and on Houses of Industry . . . Occasioned by a Bill Now Depending in Parliament for Establishing an House of Industry, for the Hundreds of Mitford and Launditch, in the County of Norfolk* (London: Lewis, 1775), 2–3, 4–5, 24.

61. Eden, *State of the Poor*, 1:305, 330–31, 367, 412, 420.

62. Longmate, *Workhouse*, 26.

63. Similarly, writings by and for physicians often show a concern for the health of the poor and the elderly. *Observations on the Character and Conduct of a Physician: In Twenty Letters to a Friend* (London: J. Johnson, 1772), 30.

64. Chistoph Conrad, "Old Age and the Health Care System in the Nineteenth and Twentieth Centuries," in *Old Age from Antiquity to Post-Modernity*, ed. Paul Johnson and Pat Thane (London: Routledge, 1998), 132–45; Pat Thane, "Geriatrics," in *Companion Encyclopedia of the History of Medicine*, 2 vols., ed. William F. Bynum and Roy Porter (London: Routledge, 1993), 2:1092–1115; Susannah Ottaway, "Medicine and Old Age," in *The Oxford Handbook of the History of Medicine*, ed. Mark Jackson (Oxford: Oxford University Press, 2011), 338–54.

65. Daniel Schäfer, "'That Senescence Itself Is an Illness': A Transitional Medical Concept of Age and Ageing in the Eighteenth Century," *Medical History* 46 (2002): 525–48.

66. Nicholas Robinson, *A New Method of Treating Consumptions* (London: Bettesworth, 1727), xii–xiii. Reprinted in L. A. Botelho and Susannah Ottaway, eds. *History of Old Age 1600–1800*, 8 vols. (London: Pickering and Chatto, 2008), 2:111–18.

67. Pat Thane, "Old Age," in *Medicine in the Twentieth Century*, ed. Roger Cooter and John Pickstone (Amsterdam: Harwood Academic, 2000): 617–32; David Haycock, *Mortal Coil: A Short History of Living Longer* (New Haven: Yale University Press, 2008).

68. An example is the Liberty of the Rolls workhouse, where interactions among the workhouse doctor, workhouse masters and matrons, and the workhouse committee are recorded in K344–346, Westminster City Archives.

69. "Remarks on the Final Cessation of the Menses, and on a Remedy and Method of Treatment, Adapted to Prevent or Remove the Evil Consequences Attending That Period: Together with Some Strictures on Secret and Advertised Medicines in General" (London, [1775]).

70. Michael Stolberg, "A Woman's Hell? Medical Perceptions of Menopause in Preindustrial Europe," *Bulletin of the History of Medicine* 73, no. 3 (1999): 404–28; Sara Mendelsson and Patricia Crawford, *Women in Early Modern England* (Oxford: Oxford University Press, 1998), 126.

71. Ottaway, *Decline of Life*, esp. 1–62.

Chapter Three

"These ANTE-CHAMBERS OF THE GRAVE"?

Mortality, Medicine, and the Workhouse in Georgian London, 1725–1824

Jeremy Boulton, Romola Davenport, and Leonard Schwarz

The major Part of Workhouses may be considered as composed of two
principal Divisions, *one* for the *Infirm, Sick,* and *Diseased;* and *another* for
the *Necessitous,* who notwithstanding are capable of *Labor.*

—Jonas Hanway, *Serious Considerations on the Salutary Design
of the Act of Parliament for a regular, Uniform Register of the
Parish-Poor in All the Parishes within the Bills of Mortality*

The Workhouse as an "Ante Chamber of Death" in Georgian London

It is often forgotten, or overlooked, that it was in the eighteenth century, not
the nineteenth century, that most London parishes built workhouses to house
a proportion of their parish poor. Workhouses were new institutions in the
eighteenth century, and in London at least they were large and prominent
and until recently have, on the whole, been underexplored by historians.[1]
Yet virtually all suburban parishes in the metropolis operated them in the
eighteenth century.[2] Usually built in the 1720s or 1730s, they often occupied
prime locations in the parish and might well dominate those locations, acting
prima facie as purpose-built lodging houses, complete with sick wards for the
poor, those who found themselves at the bottom of the social heap. They were
often larger than London's public hospitals, sometimes twice as large; their
total capacity was certainly far greater.[3] Despite this, it has been necessary only
recently for David Green to point out that one reason that so few London

unions erected workhouses after the 1834 New Poor Law was that a network of workhouses was already in place. In terms of poor law reform, London "led rather than followed developments elsewhere in the country."[4] The role of workhouses with regard to the nineteenth-century sick and dying poor, admitted under the New Poor Law, is thus relatively well known to historians; their predecessors have been studied far less frequently.[5]

Dying in institutions tends to be thought of as something that became common in the nineteenth century, but it was only in the twentieth century that institutional deaths in Britain *nationally* reached close to one in five of those dying. The figure today for hospitals alone, when death and dying is far more heavily medicalized and death is concentrated firmly among the very old, is about two-thirds of all deaths.[6]

Dying in a public institution was, however, always more common in Victorian London than in the provinces. By 1871 Margaret Anne Crowther estimated that 11.3 percent of all Londoners died in workhouses and other poor law institutions and a further 6.9 percent met their end in the capital's many hospitals and lunatic asylums. By 1906 the percentage of Londoners dying in institutions had doubled to 38.3, mostly due to an expansion in institutional medical provision (both public hospitals and poor law infirmaries).[7] Green's figures for deaths in workhouses alone show a similar story: that under the New Poor Law the percentage of deaths that took place in London workhouses was between 8 and 9 percent until and including 1871.

Of course, the risk of dying in an institution was age-specific and far more commonly experienced among age groups most likely to be institutionalized. In London, partly as a result of separate establishments for infants and children, death in a workhouse must been much more common at older ages. The higher percentage in London, of course, also reflected the greater emphasis (which changed over time) on indoor relief in the nation's capital. The frequency with which death took place in London institutions in the Victorian period has proved a challenging methodological problem for those undertaking demographic analysis in the capital (see table 3.1).[8] Graham Mooney, talking about the post-1837 death certification process, has argued recently that "differences in diagnostic depth depended partly on socio-demographic characteristics and area of residence within the city, but the immediate spatial context of the death was overwhelmingly vital."[9]

In addition to complicating the spatial analysis of mortality rates, the growth of institutional deaths disrupted deathbed preparation and death rituals. Famously, after 1832 death in the workhouse brought the added fear of postmortem dissection under the terms of the Anatomy Act.[10] This provided some helpful evidence regarding deaths in London's workhouses. The 1828 Select Committee on Anatomy that had heard evidence relating to the anatomy schools also reported on 3,754 workhouse deaths that had taken place in 128 London parishes in 1827. Crude though the measure is, when

Table 3.1. Deaths in the workhouse, 1841–1901 (%)

	1841	1851	1861	1871	1881	1891	1901
England and Wales	n/a	n/a	4.60	5.08	5.81	5.79	6.36
London	9.41	8.92	8.82	8.29	13.07	14.86	16.63

Source: Green, "Medical Relief and the New Poor Law in London," 228, table 11.2.

compared to the number of burials reported by each parish in the London Bills of Mortality for 1827, this can be used to generate a London-wide picture of the percentage of workhouse deaths, as in table 3.2. The table exaggerates the proportion of deaths from the workhouse, because the number of burials in the Bills of Mortality is an underestimate of the number of deaths.[11] It is probable that the figures include deaths from separate workhouse infirmaries, where these existed, and may also have included burials of the poor in private lunatic asylums, but we cannot be sure if this was so in all cases. Relatively few workhouses possessed separate purpose-built infirmaries.[12] Nonetheless, table 3.2 is suggestive. In general, the parishes with workhouses were from the suburbs, outside the old City within the Walls. In 1827, under the Old Poor Law, suburban London contained a number of large parishes, where it was not uncommon for at least 20 percent of parishioners to die in the workhouse. These percentages, of course, reflect the extent to which individual parishes favored indoor as opposed to outdoor relief, the age structure of the workhouse population, and, presumably, the extent to which other institutions might have been willing and able to house the sick and dying. Conversely, there were other parts of the capital where very few parishioners ended their days in the parish workhouse or associated institutions.

Death, Mortality, and the Parish Workhouse in St. Martin in the Fields

This chapter aims to explore the nature and impact of the rise of institutional dying in Georgian London by taking the parish of St. Martin in the Fields as a case study. In 1803 the parish housed what was the third largest workhouse in London.[13] Situated by the present-day National Portrait Gallery adjoining Trafalgar Square, it was very near Parliament and even nearer Whitehall; it could easily have been visited by members of Parliament and indeed was probably passed by some on their way home. As Jonas Hanway (who did visit it) remarked, few seem to have troubled to stop in: "How comes it to pass that many Gentlemen who attend Hospitals and other public Charities, show so little Regard to their own *Parish Workhouse*, which is

Table 3.2. Deaths from parish workhouses in the London area, 1827

	Burials reported in London Bills	Burial totals (adjusted for multiple parishes)	Deaths in workhouses	Deaths in workhouses (%)
St. Andrew Holborn	570	738	79	11
St. Sepulchre Newgate	168	168	52	31
St. Giles Cripplegate	157	157	48	31
St. Dunstan Fleet Street	151	151	13	9
St. Bartholomew the Great	62	62	6	10
St. Bartholomew the Less	8	8	0	0
St. Botolph Aldersgate	126	126	15	12
St. Botolph Bishopsgate	252	252	45	18
St. Botolph Aldgate	245	245	23	9
Trinity Minories	16	16	3	19
St. Saviours Southwark	425	425	67	16
St. Olave Southwark	290	290	34	12
St. George Southwark	773	773	74	10
St. Thomas Southwark	9	9	2	22
St. John Horsleydown	253	253	24	9
Christchurch Surrey	425	425	21	5
St. Mary Lambeth	1,953	1,953	155	8
St. Mary Newington	543	543	3	1
St. Mary Bermondsey	675	675	81	12
St. Clement Danes	340	340	53	16
St. Mary le Strand	67	67	8	12
The Savoy	34	34	0	0
St. Paul Covent Garden	143	143	27	19
St. Martin in the Fields	415	550	125	23
St. Margaret Westminster	613	?	?	?
St. John Westminster	625	1,238	168	14
St. Ann Soho	708	708	26	4
St. James Piccadilly	1,124	1,124	171	15
St. George Queen Square	168	?	?	?
St. George Bloomsbury	195	?	?	?
St. Giles in the Fields	1,040	1,235	353	29
St. James Clerkenwell	630	736	104	14
St. John Clerkenwell	106	?	?	?
St. Luke Middlesex	519	519	105	20
St. Mary Islington	547	547	44	8
St. John Hackney	390	390	40	10
St. Leonard Shoreditch	2,195	2,195	139	6
St. Katherine by the Tower	390	390	18	5
St. Paul Shadwell	339	339	38	11

(continued)

Table 3.2. Deaths from parish workhouses in the London area, 1827—*(concluded)*

	Burials reported in London Bills	Burial totals (adjusted for multiple parishes)	Deaths in workhouses	Deaths in workhouses (%)
Christchurch Spitalfields	425	425	70	16
St. Matthew Bethnal Green	569	569	144	25
St. Mary Whitechapel	645	645	200	31
St. Dunstan Stepney	547	547	78	14
St. George in the East	637	637	114	18
St. Anne Limehouse	376	376	24	6
Total	20,888	21,023	2,794	13

Source: Figures are calculated from burial totals in John Marshall, *Mortality of the Metropolis* (London: J. Haddon for Treuttel, Würtz & Richter, etc., 1832), 79; and from workhouse deaths given in appendix 18 of "Returns" in *Appendix to Report from the Select Committee on Anatomy* (London: House of Commons, 1828), 140–42.

so much nearer Home, and where much Good may be done? Among other Reasons it is very apparent that they do not chuse to attend Places which are not kept in all respects perfectly sweet and clean."[14]

In the last quarter of the eighteenth century, the workhouse often housed seven hundred inmates at any one time—many residents not staying long. After the Napoleonic Wars, admissions occasionally exceeded one thousand per year.[15] The workhouse served a parish population of between twenty-five thousand and thirty thousand and was itself situated on top of or adjacent to a large parish graveyard so overcrowded that the local vestry tried twice in the eighteenth century to ban its further use.[16] The chapter begins by explaining why workhouse mortality levels appeared to be so high and goes on to examine the impact that dying in the institution had on reporting causes of death. The chapter ends with some evidence relating to death rates in the institution.

Death in the Workhouse

Some contemporaries believed that mortality rates in parish workhouses were extremely high, due to lack of hygiene, overcrowding, and the difficulties of keeping those infected segregated from the healthy. Ruth Richardson and Brian Hurwitz note that "a recurring problem of workhouse medicine was the impossibility of segregating patients with terminal, acute, chronic, and infectious diseases. Having no casualty provision, no trained nursing staff, few drugs, and no surgical facilities, workhouses could not adequately cope with acute cases."[17] As an editorial in the Lancet commented in 1841, "The diseases which prove so fatal, therefore, assail the poor after their entrance into these ANTE-CHAMBERS OF THE GRAVE."[18]

Not surprisingly, reports of epidemics in workhouses were not uncommon and the high death rates experienced by workhouse infants were notorious in the eighteenth century. Hanway was especially colorful regarding the dangers of overcrowding:

> The custom of receiving an indefinite number, subverts the best oeconomy: it hazards the breeding an epidemical disease. I have often wondered, that the plague has not issued forth from the gates of a workhouse, to mow down the inhabitants of these vast cities. How often it really occasions disorders of the most morbific nature, particularly among the common people, is not difficult to comprehend. Take any given number of people in a workhouse, of the same age and state of health as those out of it, and see what the comparative mortality will be. Nothing can be more obvious, than that the present mode of receiving without limitation, and crouding a house with numbers, is not less dangerous to the community at large, than it is cruel to the individuals. . . . The difference of keeping a workhouse cleanly and dirty, I know in one instance, was one person in five, in the mortality of adults. I do not say but that the mortality in both cases, was very large, owing to its being crouded.[19]

More specifically, the Gilbert returns of 1772–74 on the state of the poor included a question about the number of poor who died in the workhouse, which reflects contemporary concern at the potential danger such institutions posed to their poor inmates.[20] Since the same returns also provided figures for workhouse occupancy, they provide data with which to calculate crude mortality rates in the institutions. Table 3.3 provides some metropolitan examples, estimated from a printed analysis of the Gilbert returns published in 1787. The mortality of London workhouse residents calculated from these returns appears catastrophic: overall something like one-third of all residents would seem to have died per year, and some institutions lost more than this. St. Martin's buried 226 poor people from an institution that housed on average 604 people between 1772 and 1774, an estimated crude mortality rate of 374 per 1000. The smaller workhouse of St. Giles in the Fields and St. George, Bloomsbury, seemingly experienced a staggering death rate of 558 per 1000. But such figures are highly misleading. They partly reflect the high proportion of infirm, sick, aged, newborn, and very young inmates, but still more seriously they take no account of the high turnover and relatively short stays of many workhouse residents, which makes estimating the size of the population at risk problematic. More accurate measurements of mortality in the St. Martin's workhouse are presented in table 3.3. The very high crude mortality rates seen in the table also reflect, of course, the fact that many workhouse inmates were sick, sometimes actually dying, and occasionally already dead when they entered the workhouse.

Table 3.3. Workhouse mortality rates estimated from Gilbert Returns, 1772–74

Parish	Able	Infirm	Infants	Total average number of residents in workhouses	Able	Infirm	Infants	Total average deaths per year	Total estimated death rate per 1,000 inmates
St. Andrew Holborn, &c (and St. George the Martyr)	0	273	68	341	0	113	14	127	372
Bethnal Green	104	107	20	231	0	39	10	49	212
Christchurch (Spitalfields)	0	0	0	305	0	0	0	95	311
St. Clement Danes	144	39	110	293	37	15	13	65	222
St. George Hanover Square	179	291	137	607	44	138	38	220	362
St. Giles in the Fields and St. George, Bloomsbury	163	244	32	439	0	203	42	245	558
St. James Westminster	233	452	328	1,013	0	185	105	290	286
St. John Hackney	0	0	0	140	0	0	0	23	164
St. Luke Middlesex	0	0	0	412	0	0	0	129	313
St. Margaret and St. John Westminster	195	236	8	439	34	83	26	143	326
St. Martin in the Fields	0	591	13	604	0	190	36	226	374
St. Marylebone Middlesex	69	91	76	236	21	31	33	85	360
St. Mary Whitechapel	242	60	101	403	65	54	9	128	318
St. Nicholas Deptford	30	30	33	93	7	5	7	19	204
St. Paul Shadwell	108	45	53	206	30	15	4	49	238
St. Saviour Southwark	144	49	124	317	35	52	27	114	360
St. Sepulchre Middlesex	71	22	0	93	7	11	0	18	194
Total	1,682	2,530	1,103	6,172	280	1,134	364	2,025	328

Source: *A Collection of Pamphlets concerning the Poor: With Abstracts of the Poor's Rates; Expences of Different Houses of Industry, &c. and Observations by the Editor* (London: Printed for C. Elliot, T. Kay, and Co;; and Charles Elliot, 1787), 137, 142. The number of deceased infants in St. George, Hanover Square, 38, is given as 3 in the original. The average number in St. Luke, Middlesex, 412, might be a mistake for 442, the average suggested by the original returns. Total death rate calculated by the authors.

Death Comes to the Workhouse

Given the presence of the workhouse surgeon and apothecary and the fact that sickness was a common cause of destitution, it quickly became common practice for sick and dying paupers—or those whom it was suspected would soon become paupers—to be carried straight to the workhouse.[21] Before 1725, when the workhouse was constructed, such individuals were sent to a network of parish nurses.[22] Staffed in the eighteenth century by unpaid ward nurses, a salaried surgeon, and an apothecary, the workhouse provided a significant level of health care for inmates. Moreover, the medical functions of St. Martin's workhouse seem to have increased after a major 1772 rebuilding, with significantly less use made thereafter of public hospitals to care for seriously ill paupers (and lunatics), who were instead cared for in-house. The workhouse had a number of designated sick wards throughout the period, but, like many other workhouses, no separate infirmary. Unfortunately, it is rather difficult to know what proportion of the inmates were sick at any one time, since the admission registers do not give such information.[23] An indirect estimate for 1817–18, when the workhouse was under considerable pressure and admissions unusually high, suggests that the sick might have formed just 20 percent of those admitted, but together with the infirm, nursing mothers and infant children the proportion of dependents would have been about 40 percent. It is possible that the proportion of sick entering the workhouse would have been higher in the eighteenth century, since the admission figures in 1817–18 may have been swelled by an influx of casual poor.[24]

For the early period of our project we can also link workhouse records of admission and discharge to itemized payments made by the overseers of the poor. This enables us to make limited "patient narratives" to reconstruct the "pathways" by which individuals came into contact with the local poor law. What follows is the result of limited linkage with an early set of overseers' accounts for 1726–27 and the workhouse admission and discharge registers. Here, the fifty or so paupers who were stated to have been explicitly transported at parish cost to the workhouse have been examined in some detail. Clearly, this exercise tells us only about those paupers unable to make it to the workhouse under their own steam, but it does have the advantage that, in many cases, we have a modest history of poor law payments made to the same individual prior to their admission and sometimes after their discharge. What does this tell us?

To begin with, of course, those of the sick poor who were taken to the workhouse did not necessarily die there. They might be simply discharged after a period of residence or sent on to another institution. Some might even have been "cured," that is, some or all of their symptoms disappeared or were alleviated.[25] For example, the parish spent a shilling for "Coach hire for Mr Barnard to the Workhouse he having broke his Legg" on May 25, 1726. William Bernard, aged sixty-five, was admitted on May 26. He left the house on August 20, 1726, his leg presumably having mended. A number of those carried to the workhouse were women in labor rather than the sick. It is also the case, of course, that many sick paupers were never admitted to the workhouse, for a range of reasons that would have included their age, ability to sustain an independent existence, and the presence of family members able to care for them. Others might be sent directly to a hospital, bypassing the workhouse, particularly if specialist care was required or the pauper suffered from a dangerous infectious disease. After 1746, for example, smallpox sufferers could be sent directly to the new London Smallpox Hospital. Thus, one Anne Benge recalled in 1765 that she

> was a yearly hired servant to Mrs Burnett a Victualler at the sign of the Black Boy and Apple Tree the corner of the Hop Garden in St Martin's Lane in the said Parish of St Martin in the Fields for the space of one whole year at the yearly wages of 4 pounds diet and lodging, and then was taken ill with the smallpox and was by the officers of the Parish of St Martin in the Fields sent to the Smallpox Hospital, and when she was recovered returned to her said place again and continued for the space of 12 months longer.

Benge was admitted to the workhouse for a week after her examination and then dismissed.[26]

What sort of illnesses did the workhouse treat? Our workhouse admissions registers are largely silent on this, but there are significant exceptions. A number of sick paupers were in their last illness. Dorothy Grigson received two shillings and sixpence from the parish and was described as "aged" on April 28, 1726. The parish then paid sixpence "for carrying her to the Workhouse she being sick" on May 3, 1726. Admitted a few days later, the registers show that the then seventy-four-year-old Dorothy stayed until August, dying in the institution on August 11, 1726. Again, the parish was charged twelvepence for "carrying Ursula Evans sick to the Workhouse" on June 2, 1726. Aged only twenty-seven, she died six days later in the workhouse. So sick were some paupers that they died en route to the workhouse. Thus, in 1741, the fifty-five-year-old Gabriel Delmanzie "Dead Dyed in ye. Chair a Coming in" and the fifty-year-old Thomas Barry, "Dyed the same Day as He was coming in the Chair." This case was not unique. Not all sick paupers carried to the workhouse at the expense of the parish overseers were adults—although most were. The parish paid just threepence to "a Woman for carrying Henry Jones ill to the Workhouse" on June 16, 1726. Henry, a one-week-old boy, was admitted on June 17, 1726, and died there on July 9, 1726. Again, Anne (Amy) Granger, a fourteen-year-old girl, was taken by chair "sick" to the workhouse on July 15, 1726, stayed a month and then left the house never to return.[27] In most cases, however, small children would not have required parish-funded transport.

In other cases, the admission of a sick pauper to the workhouse was only part of far more complex patient narratives. For example, the forty-eight-year-old Frances Eldridge was sent by coach to the workhouse at parish expense when she was ill on May 26, 1726. She was admitted to St. Bartholomew's Hospital from the workhouse on September 28, 1726. She was sent back from this hospital on October 28, 1726, and spent an additional five months in the workhouse until she was dismissed on March 23, 1727. Francis was readmitted within a week and died in the workhouse on August 11, 1727. In fact, her initial admission to the workhouse might have been prompted by the final illness of her husband, William Eldridge, who, like Frances from the Long Acre division of the parish, had received two payments of a shilling each in May 1726, "his wife ill of a Fever." William, a sixty-four-year-old, was himself admitted to the workhouse (without any need for financial assistance from the parish to do so) on June 1, 1726, and died there four days later.[28]

Another striking case that illustrates the complex relationships between pauper illness and the workhouse was that of thirty-eight-year-old Mary Nightingale, carried by coach "ill to the workhouse" in 1726. Although this illness prompted her first entry into the workhouse, Mary had relatively protracted contact with the institution, as well as with at least two of London's public hospitals. Admitted to the workhouse on account of her undisclosed sickness on October 20, 1726, she was sent to St. Thomas's Hospital in November. On New Year's Day, 1727, the overseers gave her five shillings "to put her into Business," but she clearly did not prosper, since she was readmitted to the workhouse on January 19 and admitted to St. Bartholomew's Hospital from the workhouse a month later on February 16. This was not the end of Mary's contact with the workhouse, since she was readmitted no less than five times between September 1727 and January 1729, finally dying there over three months later on April 26, 1729, at the age of about forty. Mary's stays in London's public hospitals (which also seem to have included a short stay at Guy's Hospital) are also documented elsewhere in the overseers' accounts, although throughout there is no clue as to what must have been a chronic, and perhaps ultimately fatal, condition.[29]

We know more about Mary's circumstances, which helps us to further contextualize her contact with the parish. She was examined under the settlement laws shortly after her first entrance into the workhouse, having been passed from St. Botolph without Aldersgate:

Mary Nightingall aged about 30 [*sic*] Years at the Workhouse, Saith she is the Wife of Thomas Nightingall who is in the Country as she hath heard, That she was Married to him at the Parish Church of Alhallows on London Wall Eleven Years last February, Saith he is by Trade a Printer. That he Served his Apprenticeship with one Mr Iliff in Aldersgate Street in the Parish of St.

> Botolph Aldersgate from whence she was passed, Saith since the Expiracon of
> his Apprenticeship they kept house in Drury Lane between Russell Court and
> Vinegar Yard upwards of a Year, paid £20 Pr Ann Rent and to the poor as she
> believeth left the same about five years ago and never kept house since as she
> knoweth or ever heard, or Rented £10 Pr Ann or paid any Parochial Taxes to
> any Parish since, hath two Children Mary aged eight Years and Thomas aged 6
> Years the 31st of this Instant October with her Friends.[30]

Although there is no sign of her daughter, her "friends" must have let
Mary down, since in all probability it was her son, Thomas Nightingale, aged
seven, who was admitted into the workhouse May 4, 1727, and died there on
January 8, 1728: a good example of how poorly developed social networks
might lead to incarceration and death in a parish workhouse.[31]

Other paupers developed symptoms of chronic disease that required specialist hospital treatment after admittance. For example, it was ordered by
the churchwardens and governors of the workhouse in September 1755 that
William Gregory "a poor person in this House having the falling sickness be
forthwith sent to the Hospital." Gregory had been admitted in August 1755
and was sent to Guy's Hospital shortly thereafter. He returned to the workhouse on January 15, 1756, dying there nine months later.[32]

Cases from the Westminster Coroner's Inquisitions put further flesh on
these usually laconic bones.[33] Thus the twenty-year-old Elizabeth Poole,
recorded as entering the workhouse in March 1767 and dying the following
day, was found by a coroner's jury to have "died suddenly in Convulsions, at
the Workhouse."[34] William Norton "of the Strand in the parish of St. Martin
in the Fields Surgeon" examined her body and confirmed that this was a
natural death and that she "appears to this Deponent to have died in convulsions."[35] How did Elizabeth end up in the workhouse? Her admission was
described at the coroner's inquest:

> Joseph Steele one of the Beadles of St. Martins . . . on his Oath deposed that A
> woman come to the [Workhouse] of said Parish on Saturday last [at a quarter
> to noon] & desired this Deponent to come to a woman that was in a Fit in
> Crown Court Russell Street in said Parish, says that he went there and found
> the Deceased on the Floor one pair of Stairs in a house there, being in a
> Fit . . . and foaming at the Mouth, Says that he got an Order from the Overseer
> and had her carried in a Chair to the workhouse of St. Martin's.[36]

Take the case of Thomas Iton, a forty-one-year-old man buried in St.
Martin's on June 11, 1776. Formally admitted to Workhouse Ward 14 on
June 4, Thomas threw himself out of a workhouse window while in the grip
of a fever-induced delirium. A long-time inmate of the workhouse, William
Glasscock, deposed that on "Monday last June 3d. in the Afternoon Thomas
Iton the Deceased was brought to said Workhouse by two Men, having a

Fever as Deponent understood . . . that the Deceased was in the same Ward (being the Sick Ward) with Deponent."[37] The Workhouse Surgeon dealt with the aftermath of Thomas's suicidal leap:

> He found the Deceased in the Sick Ward in Bed raving and Swearing, being quite Delirious Sayd that he bled the Deceased, and found a Light Wound upon the top of Deceased's Head which bled a Little and Deponent Bathed the Wound Says that the Deceased was restless & Delirious, which [caused?] Deponent to order a strait Waistcoat for him which was put on and Deceased died in about two hours, Says that he Examined the Deceased's Head today, and found the Skull much Depressed but not Fractured, Says that he believes "there was a Concussion of the Brain, which caused the Deceased's Death.[38]

So, within months of its opening, the parish workhouse acted simultaneously as a hospital and a hospice for the sick poor; it was also a "diagnostic conduit" through which many of the poor sent to hospitals first passed, and it soon came to act as a morgue for the parish.

Since the sick and dying were taken routinely to the parish workhouse, it is unsurprising that some paupers were dead on arrival, as we have seen. However, the workhouse site complex also included the parish bonehouse, a structure used to house those found dead in the parish or dragged from the Thames or from ponds, ditches, and privies in the parish. This seems to have been located somewhere in the "New Ground" adjacent to the workhouse. Before 1764 there are few references to this structure, although it is clear that a bonehouse was in operation well before this date.[39] From 1764, however, the workhouse registers begin recording paupers deposited or transferred to the bonehouse, treating it in effect as a separate workhouse ward. Between 1764 and 1824 a total of 312 individuals, almost all of them adults, were "brought in dead" to the workhouse, and nearly all (86 percent) of these were recorded as being deposited in the "Bone House." The workhouse surgeon would often be called on to examine corpses.[40] Sixty corpses put there were anonymous. Those without an identity would be exposed to public view so that the bodies could be claimed. Not all corpses found in the parish, one should add, were accepted by the workhouse authorities.[41]

Quantifying Workhouse Mortality

Data derived from parish burial books shows that in most years at least 15 percent of *all* burials in the parish were coming from the institution (see fig. 3.1). The proportion of the population living in the workhouse at any one time, in stark contrast, was between 2 and 3 percent. Its disproportionate share of local mortality was precisely because the workhouse drew in the streams of sick and dying paupers described earlier. The relatively modest

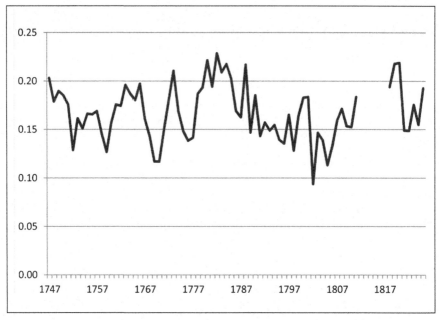

Figure 3.1. Workhouse burials as a proportion of all burials in the parish (including burials of nonresidents and residents buried elsewhere), St. Martin in the Fields, 1747–1824. St. Martin in the Fields sextons' burial books, COWAC, 419/123, 233–44; Accession, 419/265–69, F2465, F2467, F2469.

percentage fluctuations in figure 3.1 suggest, at least on the face of it, that there were few occasions when the workhouse experienced dramatic leaps in mortality that were not part of local mortality surges.

To understand the exceptional mortality patterns of the workhouse, it is necessary to view the high death rates observed in the context of patterns of admissions and residence in the workhouse. Figure 3.2 illustrates the age pattern of burials in the workhouse as a proportion of those buried in the parish as a whole. The workhouse accounted for around 10 percent of infant burials in the parish, and for fully 40 percent of burials of older adults. Burial patterns were similar by sex in childhood but diverged by sex from the age of around fifteen, reflecting both workhouse admission policies in favor of women and the composition of the population of the parish as a whole. Adult women were overrepresented in the population of St. Martin's, as a consequence of the preponderance of women in domestic service. However, this excess of women in the living population was reflected in the dead only among paupers. Fee-paying burials were sex-balanced. Thus the excess female population of St. Martin's was confined almost entirely to the pauper population (and therefore, in death, among the workhouse burials).

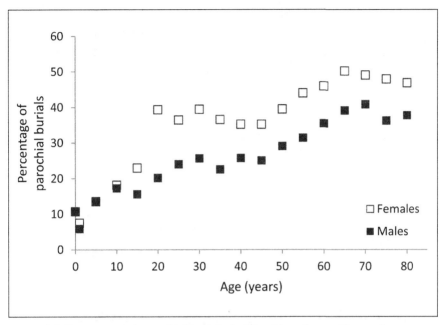

Figure 3.2. Percentage of parochial burials deriving from the workhouse, by age and sex of decedent, St. Martin in the Fields, 1752–1824. Burial totals are derived from the sextons' burial books and include only burials of residents in the parish (burials of corpses imported from other parishes and exported to other parishes are excluded). St. Martin in the Fields sextons' burial books, COWAC, 419/123, 233–44; Accession, 419/265–69, F2465, F2467, F2469.

Figure 3.3 indicates the extent to which those paupers who died in the workhouse did so shortly after entry. Over half of all deaths in infancy and young adulthood occurred within a month of admission. The differences in the workhouse burial patterns by age reflect to some extent the different uses of the workhouse by age. The proportion of those admitted to the workhouse for reasons of acute illness, as opposed to financial or other reasons, varied by age and sex, as did the propensity to remain in the workhouse. Infants and young adults did not tend to stay long in the workhouse if they survived, and therefore most deaths in these age groups perforce occurred shortly after admission. Turnover of young adult males was especially high, with very high death rates in the first weeks after admission, but also very high rates of discharge. In contrast, many children remained in the workhouse until apprenticed, if they survived, and deaths in these age groups were accordingly distributed over a number of years. Similarly, although elderly adults were more likely to die in the workhouse than inmates at other ages, a relatively small proportion died soon after entry, because most

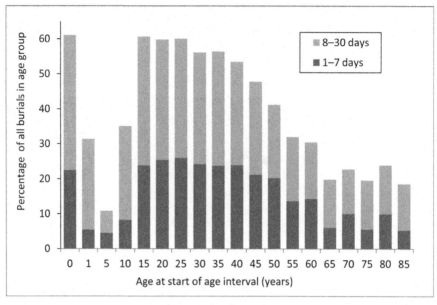

Figure 3.3. Percentage of all deaths in the workhouse in each age group that occurred in the first week and first month after admission, sexes combined, St. Martin in the Fields, 1725–1824. St. Martin in the Fields workhouse admission and discharge registers, COWAC, F4002–5, F4007–9, F4022, F4073–81.

entering at aged sixty or older entered for reasons of poverty rather than acute illness and most remained until they died.

Thus the patterns in figure 3.3 are in part an obvious consequence of the average length of stay in the workhouse. However, figure 3.4 reveals that the concentration of burials in the first weeks after admission was in fact primarily a product of the extraordinarily high mortality experienced in this period. The death rates calculated in figure 3.4 take into account the numbers of inmates still resident in the workhouse at each duration after admission and the time spent in the workhouse by inmates in each interval (the time "at risk"), so these rates are not affected by differences in residence patterns by age and sex. They indicate that mortality was extremely severe in the first weeks after admission, especially in the case of males. The pattern is shown here for young adults, but similar patterns held at all ages. Among males aged twenty to forty-nine, mortality rates exceeded four deaths per person-year, in the first week after admission. This apparently nonsensical value, which would yield a crude rate of 400 percent mortality, reflects the short length of time contributed by each individual to the rate (a maximum of one person-week) and the exceptionally high risk of death in this period. Mortality also declined more than exponentially with length of stay in the

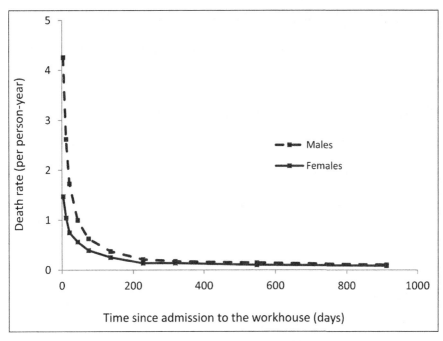

Figure 3.4. Mortality rates by duration of stay in the workhouse, adults aged twenty to forty-nine, St. Martin in the Fields, 1725–1824. St. Martin in the Fields workhouse admission and discharge registers, COWAC, F4002–5, F4007–9, F4022, F4073–81. Data were analyzed using st commands in STATA 9.2 software.

workhouse. That is, the chances of survival improved with increasing length of stay in the workhouse. Therefore, the longer one stayed in the workhouse, the lower the risk of death.

While this progressive improvement in survival chances could be viewed as a Darwinian process of survival of only those most inured to conditions in the workhouse, it should be borne in mind that there was a constant (voluntary or involuntary) outflow of the more able-bodied in search of employment, so long-term residents of the workhouse hardly constituted a selected group of robust survivors. Rather the pattern is likely to indicate that, as Timothy Guinnane and Cormac Ó Gráda found to be the case in Dublin workhouses during the Irish famine, a significant proportion of inmates resorted to the workhouse in a state of acute illness, and many died shortly after entry.[42] The extraordinary mortality rates in the first weeks after admission, with rates exceeding one death per person-year at risk, are the major cause of the breathtaking crude mortality rates calculated using admissions and deaths in the workhouse. While overcrowding and lack of hygiene may have elevated workhouse mortality, as claimed by contemporary observers cited earlier, these were not the main reasons for the workhouse's excessive share of parochial burials.

It is reasonably clear therefore that the high death rates one finds in this, and probably many other workhouses, were partly caused by the admission of people that were very young, very old, sick, dying, or even dead. This does not exclude the possibility, however, that some diseases might have spread within the workhouse. One might anticipate, like Hanway and others, that workhouses would have acted as centers of infection and had in other ways a measurable demographic impact on their localities.[43] Mary Dobson has noted that the "medical accounts of institutions—gaols, ships, workhouses, poorhouses, houses of correction—and in military stations at home and overseas give a vivid, if depressing, insight into the toll of death and disease amongst the criminal, the poor and the diseased."[44] What part, if any, did the eighteenth-century London workhouse play in the transmission and hosting of disease? Did these institutions act as a "gateway to death" for previously healthy inmates? Were workhouse inmates vulnerable to diseases such as the lethal outbreaks of "gaol fever," which are known to have been rife in London's prisons at this time?[45] Since many sick people were admitted, one would have expected this to cause regular epidemics in the workhouse, as incoming sick paupers infected healthy inmates. Was the workhouse itself a site or focus of infectious disease?

Although there is anecdotal evidence for the lethal nature of institutions, recent research has painted a far more optimistic picture of institutional mortality. In the mid-nineteenth century both hospitals and workhouses appear to have been relatively efficient when it came to excluding those suffering from infectious disease (thus improving their death rates while allowing infectious diseases to spread in the general population). The idea that hospitals (and come to that workhouses) "raised local mortality rates by bringing infected patients together with non-infected ones" is not supported by some studies, despite claims made by contemporaries at the time and some historians since.[46] Despite what contemporaries and some later historians might suppose, many eighteenth-century London workhouses took precautions to limit levels of dirt, sickness, and disease. It is impossible to know whether such measures were carried out consistently or even at all, but it should not be thought that those who ran these institutions invariably ignored questions of hygiene, ventilation, cleanliness, and the dangers of the infected.

Awareness of such problems might, in fact, have been especially high in large metropolitan institutions, where the threats to health were plain to see and the amount of local expertise available was exceptionally high.[47] At the very least, one suspects that the conditions in overcrowded tenements might often have been markedly inferior in terms of overall cleanliness and hygiene. The governors of the workhouse of the two parishes of St. Giles in the Fields (which shared a boundary with St. Martin's) and St. George Bloomsbury, for example, ordered in 1726 that

> all Persons, as soon as there is an Opportunity, after their Admission, be viewed and examined by the Surgeon, Apothecary or Nurse, whether they have any infectious Distemper, and be washed, as soon as they are taken in, if it may be without prejudice to their Health. And that such as are found to be lousy or to have the Itch, be put into the particular Wards assigned for them, and not be removed, till perfectly clean. . . . That separate Wards be also assigned for the Foul-Disease, Small-Pox, Malignant Fevers, and all other infectious Distempers, and that Care be taken to convey and remove all who are so afflicted in due Time thither, for preserving others from Infection.

Later orders called for the regular fumigation of wards, rooms, infirmaries, and bedsheets with wormwood. Workhouse nurses were to

> take care to search all the Beds for Fleas, Buggs and other Vermin, once a Week, or oftener if occasion, and to have all their Beds made, and to sweep and clean their respective Wards, every Morning between the Hours of Eight and Ten; that every Ward be washed once a Week, or oftener as Need shall require; and the Windows be kept open in all, except the Sick Wards, every Day during Dinner, to air the Rooms, except in very rainy Weather.[48]

We know that a churchwarden of St. Martin's visited St. Giles's workhouse in 1725 and since both workhouses were, in fact, initially operated by the same entrepreneur it is very possible that similar regulations were followed at St. Martin's. Although no comparable set of rules survives for St. Martin's in that period there is plenty of evidence of concern to preserve the health of inmates, including the provision of separate wards for the sick. Orders for the first workhouse, among other features, included that "a sink for washing of hands, be made in the Dining Room."[49] Regulations relating to health and cleanliness are found in St. Martin's in 1775. By 1805 the workhouse seems to have had its own baths, and in that year the parish authorities enacted specific measures to ensure that the wards were kept clean, well ventilated, and regularly white-washed and "that Two Wards be appropriated for the reception of Paupers upon their Admission previous to their being Warded which shall in no case be, until first examined by the Surgeon & properly cleaned, then to be cloathed with the Parish Garments." In 1814 an official was thanked by the workhouse governors "for superintending and enforcing the good Government of the Workhouse, particularly in the essential point of its cleanliness, and in doing which a considerable saving of Expence has been effected by his employing Persons in the House to white wash and clean the Wards under his own direction and personal inspection."[50]

Did Georgian London's large parish workhouses then have any measurable effect on the health of inmates? John Landers suggested, after all, that it was the crowding of the poor of the metropolis into substandard accommodation that produced peculiar susceptibility to the "price shock" of the early 1740s. Where they were built, lodging houses and night shelters helped to increase the "effective density of population" "with all that that implies for levels of potential exposure to infection."[51] On the face of it, parish workhouses would surely have acted in precisely the way that Hanway and others thought. To examine this crucial question we need to look in more detail at the role of the workhouse as a transmitter and harborer of disease.

The role the workhouse played in local mortality experience can be examined in further detail because of the survival of the parish burial books, or "Sexton's notebooks," that are extant (with only two short breaks) between 1747 and 1824. These books supply the names, ages, addresses, burial fees, and causes of death for almost all of those dying or buried in the parish. These notebooks have been further amplified by the addition of a burial register for a burying ground at Camden Town, which opened in 1805. This latter register does not, unfortunately, give cause of death. For this reason, analysis of causes of death excludes the period after 1805. From 1747 to 1805 there are just over sixty thousand burials.[52]

Space precludes a full discussion of the different patterns of causes of death in the workhouse compared with the rest of the parochial population. Causes of death vary by age and sex, and therefore any analysis of cause-specific mortality must take into account the differences in the composition of the workhouse compared with that of the parish population as a whole. It must suffice here to note that of the causes of death recorded in the parish, two stood out as overrepresented in the workhouse: "Fever," and "Foul Disease."

"Fever" was a very common descriptor, accounting for around 12 percent of all burials in the parish. Typhus, the classic disease of overcrowded institutions and the poor, would have been included among fevers, in the absence of a more specific descriptor in the St. Martin's records. Figure 3.5 plots the percentage of fever deaths in the parish buried from the workhouse and suggests that fevers may have been particularly mortal in the workhouse in the 1780s, when its population peaked. To test whether the high levels of fever mortality in the workhouse in this period were a function of conditions within the institution, we analyzed the distribution of fever deaths by time after admission, compared with nonfever deaths in the workhouse, for the period 1775–94, when fevers accounted for 22 percent of all deaths in the workhouse.

Figure 3.6 shows cause-specific death rates by length of stay in the workhouse, for adults aged twenty to forty-nine. It was necessary to select a restricted age range to be confident that any patterns specific to fever were not simply a function of the age-specific patterns of fevers compared with other causes of death. In this period 65 percent of all workhouse fever

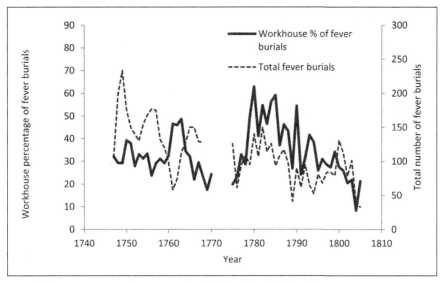

Figure 3.5. Counts of total fever burials and fever burials from the workhouse as a percentage of all fever burials in parish, St. Martin in the Fields, 1752–1805. Figure 3.5 may exclude some of the more specialized subdivisions of "fever" subsequently introduced but is most unlikely to do so on a large scale. St. Martin in the Fields sextons' burial books, COWAC, 419/123, 233–44; Accession, 419/265–69, F2465, F2467, F2469.

deaths occurred at ages twenty to forty-nine, and fevers accounted for 41 percent of the deaths at these ages (only 2.4 percent of linked deaths were not ascribed a cause). Figure 3.6 indicates that death rates from fever showed the same more-than-exponential decline with length of residency in this period as mortality from other causes and a similar degree of male bias (data not shown). Thus most fever deaths in this period occurred within the first month of admission to the workhouse and were therefore probably largely the result of infections contracted outside the institution (and which may have prompted admission). The higher death rates of men in the workhouse compared with women accord with overall sex differences in mortality in the workhouse and therefore probably reflect the higher ratio of ill to simply destitute paupers among male admissions. By contrast, infections of workhouse origin might be expected to have produced a less sex-selective mortality pattern. Therefore, the high contribution of workhouse fever deaths to parochial totals in this period is probably a reflection of the expansion of the hospital function of the workhouse after the rebuilding in the early 1770s rather than a period of institutional epidemics. Importantly, the total number of fever burials in the parish was not unusually high in the 1780s. Therefore, whatever the role of the workhouse in fever mortality in this period, it does not appear to have had a major impact on mortality in the parish as a whole.

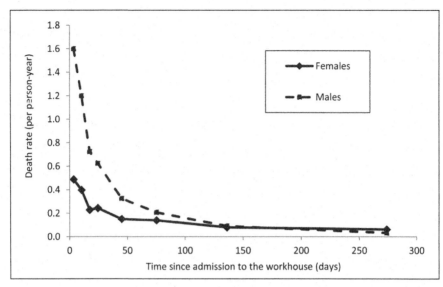

Figure 3.6. Mortality rates from fever by duration of stay in the workhouse, adults aged twenty to forty-nine, St. Martin in the Fields, 1775–94. Data are derived from the workhouse registers and from workhouse inmates linked to burial records by cause in the sextons' burial books of the parish. They were analyzed using st commands in STATA 9.2 software. St. Martin in the Fields sextons' burial books, COWAC, 419/123, 233–44; Accession, 419/265–69, F2465, F2467, F2469; St. Martin in the Fields workhouse admission and discharge registers, COWAC, F4002–5, F4007–9, F4022, F4073–81.

"Foul Disease," a term describing various causes of presumed venereal origin, was apparently confined almost completely to the workhouse, which contributed 84 percent of all foul disease burials recorded in the parish. In this case, the preponderance of foul disease burials in the workhouse probably reflects the different "diagnostic space" that the workhouse occupied. It can be assumed that the friends and relatives of most of those dying elsewhere took care to have their death classified under a different heading, as John Graunt described a century previously.[53] Mirroring the acute male bias of foul disease cases in London hospitals, 88 percent of adult foul disease burials from the workhouse were female and 37 percent were children (29 percent under the age of one).

Conclusions and Speculations

We have sought to tease out the impact of just one of the large workhouses erected in England's capital city during the eighteenth century. By the middle of that century, almost every suburban parish had erected an institution that served as a hospital, hospice, and mortuary. Workhouses were more common in the capital than hospitals. St. Martin's workhouse was an unusually large institution and it played what might have been an exceptionally large role in the parish's welfare system. In other parishes the balance between indoor and outdoor relief must have tilted far more strongly toward the latter, as the 1803 returns suggest and the 1827 figures confirm. Yet one of the larger institutions in London and—what is more—an institution that, in purpose and location, might have been specifically designed to *raise* the local death rate, did not obviously do so.

Of course, St. Martin in the Fields may have been exceptional. Each parish and workhouse must have had its own history, with cycles of growth, reconfiguration, neglect, and decline. Their impact on local mortality patterns is measurable in a number of different ways. Because so many individuals sought admission or were taken to the workhouse due to serious illness, the proportion buried from the local workhouse was always much higher than the small proportion of the population living there at any one point in time. Moreover, the potential age-specific impact could have been high. In St. Martin's it was older adults who were most likely to die in the workhouse. Across London the local impact of each of these institutions must have varied according to the nature of the workhouse regime, the funds and expertise available, the extent to which workhouses were medicalized, and so on.

Although death rates in this workhouse appeared catastrophically high, a more complex picture emerges when mortality is analyzed by methods that take into account the time spent by inmates in the workhouse. Mortality rates within the first days of entry were extreme, reflecting the influx of seriously ill paupers to the workhouse. However, the risk of death fell continuously with increasing length of stay in the workhouse. The mortality of those who survived their first six months was, notwithstanding, still much higher than found in the wider population. Whether this was because the workhouse was relatively unhealthy or because (perhaps more likely) inmates were unusually likely to be chronically ill and otherwise in a poor condition is a matter that requires further investigation.

The very high crude death rates in workhouses therefore seem to have been caused by the admission of the elderly, the fragile, and those already seriously ill. More sophisticated and detailed work on those admitted and their residential and life histories can shed light on the extent to which workhouses exacerbated mortality rates by killing previously healthy inmates. However, this preliminary analysis suggests that St. Martin's workhouse was a passive rather than an active demographic agent, at any rate over the long term. More work needs to be done on the local medical regime, the role of the workhouse as a lying-in hospital for poor women, the treatment of infants and young children in the workhouse, and the extent to which vulnerable age groups were evacuated to nurses in the country.[54] What seems striking, at least at this preliminary stage, is the relative *absence* of epidemics focused on the workhouse. Whether this was so for the other metropolitan workhouses also remains to be seen. If workhouses did not significantly boost the mortality rates of healthy residents, this does raise the intriguing possibility that they actually had a *positive* effect on local mortality by removing infectious individuals from their families.

This study suggests other future lines of inquiry. One is struck by the extensive medical experience that workhouses provided for their staff, notably the workhouse apothecary and surgeon. The workhouse played a significant part in sending paupers to the public hospitals, and thus it is likely that many of those who ended up in public hospitals had already been seen and assessed by workhouse medical personnel. One also wonders about the nature of the workhouse death. A significant proportion of the poor, after 1725, died in a workhouse ward, not in their own dwellings. One wonders how involved, if at all, were other family members and how death rituals and customs were affected by this new institutional context of death and dying.

Notes

The authors would like to thank Drs. Peter Jones and John Black for their data input. Further thanks are due to Joanna Innes for her suggested references and two anonymous readers. The research for this paper was funded by Welcome Trust Research Grant, No. 081508 and by the ESRC Research Grant, RES-000-23-0250. We would like to thank both bodies for their support.

1. For instance, John Landers's pioneering book makes no mention of them; see *Death and the Metropolis: Studies in the Demographic History of London, 1670–1830* (Cambridge: University of Cambridge Press, 1993). The Webbs included a substantial chapter about workhouses, which is still worth consulting; see Sidney Webb and Beatrice Webb, *English Local Government: English Poor Law History*, pt. 1, *The Old Poor Law* (London, Longmans, Green, 1927), 215–304. The most recent, as yet unpublished, full-length treatment remains Tim Hitchcock, "The English Workhouse: A Study in Institutional Poor Relief in Selected Counties, 1696–1750" (DPhil diss., University of Oxford, 1985). See also Tim Hitchcock, "Paupers and Preachers: The SPCK and the Parochial Workhouse Movement," in *Stilling the Grumbling Hive: The Response to Social and Economic Problems in England, 1689–1750*, ed. Lee Davison et al. (London: St. Martin's Press, 1992), 145–66. More recent studies of workhouses include, in particular, an important chapter in Alannah Tomkins, *The Experience of Urban Poverty, 1723–82: Parish, Charity and Credit* (Manchester: Manchester University Press, 2006), 37–72; for later eighteenth- and nineteenth-century London, see David R. Green's magisterial *Pauper Capital: London and the Poor Law, 1790–1870* (Farnham, UK: Ashgate, 2010).

2. "London" is here taken as referring to the entire metropolis, not the square mile of the city alone. For the individual workhouses, see particularly *Report from*

the Committee Appointed to Inspect and Consider the Returns Made by the Overseers of the Poor . . . reported . . . 15th May 1777, 396–404.

3. Susan C. Lawrence has surveyed the capacity of London hospitals in 1788 in *Charitable Knowledge: Hospital Pupils and Practitioners in Eighteenth Century London* (Cambridge: Cambridge University Press, 1996), 39. There is a count on the night of June 6, 1841, of London's hospitals and workhouses: the hospital total was less than 14 percent of that of the workhouses; see appendix to *Fifth Annual Report of the Registrar General of Births, Deaths, and Marriages in England* (London: HMSO, 1843), 228.

4. David R. Green, "Icons of the New System: Workhouse Construction and Relief Practices in London under the Old and New Poor Law," *London Journal* 34 (2009): 264.

5. For instance Anne Digby, *Pauper Palaces* (London: Routledge and Kegan Paul, 1978), 166–79; Margaret Anne Crowther, "Health Care and Poor Relief in Provincial England," and David Green, "Medical Relief and the New Poor Law in London," both in *Health Care and Poor Relief in 18th and 19th Century Northern Europe*, ed. Ole P. Grell, Andrew Cunningham, and Robert Jütte (Aldershot, UK: Ashgate, 2002), 203–19 and 220–45.

6. Tony Walter, *The Revival of Death* (London: Routledge, 1994), 13.

7. Margaret Anne Crowther, *The Workhouse System, 1834–1929: The History of an English Social Institution* (Cambridge: Methuen, 1983), 57–58. For deaths in the workhouse after the New Poor Law, see "Death in the Workhouse," accessed September 3, 2011, http://www.workhouses.org.uk/life/death.shtml.

8. Graham Mooney, Bill Luckin, and Andrea Tanner, "Patient Pathways: Solving the Problem of Institutional Mortality in London during the Later Nineteenth Century," *Social History of Medicine* 12 (1999): 227–69.

9. Graham Mooney, "Diagnostic Spaces: Workhouse, Hospital and Home in Mid-Victorian London," *Social Science History* 33 (2009): 379.

10. Ruth Richardson, *Death, Dissection and the Destitute* (Chicago: University of Chicago Press, 2011).

11. For the reasons that lie behind such underregistration, see Jeremy Boulton and Leonard Schwarz, "Yet Another Inquiry into the Trustworthiness of Eighteenth-Century London's Bills of Mortality," *Local Population Studies* 85 (2010): 28–45.

12. The returns report 424 burials from the workhouse of St. Marylebone. A more detailed description of these figures is contained in Mooney, Luckin, and Tanner, "Patient Pathways," 232.

13. "Abstract of the Answers and Returns Made Pursuant to an Act, Passed in the 43d Year of His Majesty King George III. . . ." *Parl. Papers*, 1803–4, 13:717–26.

14. Jonas Hanway, *Serious Considerations on the Salutary Design of the Act of Parliament for a Regular, Uniform Register of the Parish-Poor in All the Parishes within the Bills of Mortality* (London, 1762), 65, 68.

15. For a detailed treatment of the post-Napoleonic period, see Lynn MacKay's work on St. Martin's: "A Culture of Poverty? The St. Martin in the Fields Workhouse, 1817," *Journal of Interdisciplinary History* 26, no. 2 (1995): 209–31; MacKay, "Moral Paupers: The Poor Men of St. Martin's, 1815–1819," *Social History of Medicine* 34 (2001): 115–31.

16. Orders passed in 1766 proved abortive, but it was successfully closed in 1778. City of Westminster Archives Centre (hereafter COWAC), F2007/351, 35, F2008/13.

It reopened briefly in the early nineteenth century. For Hanway's comments on the proximity of the workhouse to burial grounds, see Jonas Hanway, *The Citizen's Monitor* (London: Dodsley, Sewell, and New, 1780), 174.

17. Ruth Richardson and Brian Hurwitz, "Joseph Rogers and the reform of workhouse medicine," *British Medical Journal* 299 (1989): 1508.

18. Thomas Wakley, editorial in *The Lancet* (May 1, 1841), 194.

19. Hanway, *Citizen's Monitor*, 106–7. As is well known, Hanway made it part of his life's work to reduce the mortality of London's children; see Dorothy George, *London Life in the Eighteenth Century* (London; Kegan Paul, 1925), 213–61, 401–5; James S. Taylor, *Jonas Hanway: Founder of the Marine Society* (Farnham, UK: Ashgate, 1985), 102–17.

20. We would like to thank Joanna Innes for drawing our attention to this source.

21. Medical facilities and policies in the workhouse have been described in detail elsewhere; see Jeremy Boulton and Leonard Schwarz, "The Parish Workhouse, the Parish and Parochial Medical Provision in Eighteenth-Century London," working paper at: http://research.ncl.ac.uk/pauperlives/workhousemedicalisation.pdf.

22. Jeremy Boulton "Welfare Systems and the Parish Nurse in Early Modern London, 1650–1725," *Family and Community History* 10 (2007): 127–51.

23. For some estimates of sickness levels in the very early years of the workhouse, see Boulton and Schwarz "Parish Workhouse."

24. The estimate of sickness in the workhouse was based on a report of a Workhouse Sub-Committee, which detailed each ward and its function in 1817. This was then mapped onto admissions from 1817 to 1818. For the report, see COWAC, F3914. For a comparable exercise for this period, see MacKay, "Culture of Poverty," 215–23.

25. For the ambiguities of the term "cured," see Philip K. Wilson, *Surgery, Skin and Syphilis: Daniel Turner's London (1667–1741)* (Amsterdam: Rodopi, 1999), 54, 158–61.

26. COWAC, William Bernard, F462/278, F4002/30; Anne Benge, F5054/3, F4076/6.

27. COWAC, Dorothy Grigson, F462/196, F4002/36; Ursula Evans, F462/198, F4002/34; Gabriel Delmanzie, F4073; Thomas Barry, unpaginated; Henry Jones, F462/255; Henry, F4002/39; Anne (Amy) Granger, F462/202, F4002/36.

28. COWAC, Frances Eldridge, F462/338, 278; F4002/6A, 34; William Eldridge, F462/277–78, F4002/34.

29. COWAC, Mary Nightingale, F462/267–68; F4002/16, 54, 92. For expenses incurred in her hospital stays, 1726–27, see F462/342, 343, 345, 346, 347, 348, 350, 355, 356, 358, F467/273.

30. COWAC, Mary Nightingall, F5020/66. Thomas Nightingale married Mary Swancoat at Allhallows, London Wall, February 27, 1714/15, IGI. Spelling modernized, here and subsequently.

31. COWAC, Thomas Nightingale, F4002/16.

32. COWAC, William Gregory, F4008/183–207; F2225/16, 58. Gregory, reported to be a lunatic, was included among three workhouse paupers intended for a madhouse at Bethnal Green on July 27, 1756.

33. These cases were generously made available by Professors Tim Hitchcock and Robert Shoemaker, directors of the *Plebeian Lives Project*. They are now available at "London Lives," accessed November 18, 2011, http://www.londonlives.org/index.

jsp. The originals are held at Lambeth Palace Library, London, uncataloged but arranged chronologically. It is expected that researchers who wish to follow this up will go to the relevant point on the website.

34. City of Westminster Coroners' Inquests into Suspicious Deaths (hereafter CWCISD), January 2, 1767–December 30, 1767, *London Lives* (hereafter *LL*), *1690–1800*, WACWIC652070145, accessed June 17, 2012, http://www.londonlives.org, version 1.1. Manuscripts housed in Westminster Abbey Muniments Room.

35. William Norton was the workhouse surgeon, on a salary of forty-five pounds a year at this time.

36. CWCISD, January 2, 1767– December 30, 1767, *LL*, WACWIC652070150.

37. For Glasscock's evidence at Thomas Iton's inquest, see CWCISD, January 11, 1776–December 30, 1776, *LL*, WACWIC652160229, June 5, 1776.

38. Ibid., WACWIC652160230, June 5 1776. Evidence of Jarvis, who became workhouse surgeon on Norton's retirement.

39. References to the St. Martin's Bone House occur before they were in the workhouse admission records. *London Journal*, October 18, 1729, no. 533, refers to "the corpse of a young Woman, pretty bulky, was found drowned at Salisbury Stairs in the Strand: her Body (which was almost naked) was carried to St Martin's Bone House, but not being own'd on Thursday Night, and the Coroner's Warrant coming down, the Overseers thought fit to bury it." Another similar item in the *Westminster Journal*, January 17, 1747, no. 268, refers to a man found dead in the Strand "afterwards carried to the Bone-house in St Martin's in the Fields, and exposed to public view." The "Bone-House of St. Martin's Church-yard" was also referred to in the trial of William Byrd, t17420909-37, September 9, 1742, Old Bailey Proceedings Online, http://www.oldbaileyonline.org. This trial was part of the "St Martin's Roundhouse Disaster of 1742," for which see Tim Hitchcock, "'You Bitches . . . Die and Be Damned': Gender, Authority and the Mob in St. Martin's Roundhouse Disaster of 1742," in *The Streets of London*, ed. Tim Hitchcock and Heather Shore (London: Oram, 2003), 69–91.

40. CWCISD, *LL*, WACWIC652070566, September 25, 1767; WACWIC652170251, June 13, 1777; WACWIC652230281, July 3, 1783. For an apothecary called on to determine a death, see WACWIC652290329, May 29, 1789.

41. For exposing corpses to view, see previous note. CWCISD, *LL*, WACWIC652240021, January 5, 1784, reported the finding of a dead child floating in the Thames. One Mary Barker deposed that she "took the Child to the Place where she Works in Hungerford Washed it and in the Evening carried it to Mr. Atkins the Beadle, who went with her to the Workhouse in St. Martins Lane, but the Governor refused to take in the Child [telling this] Dept. that she must carry it to the Publick House nearest to the Place she brought it from and Dept. accordingly carried the Child to the Merry Watermen in Charles Court where she left it."

42. Timothy Guinnane and Cormac Ó Gráda, "Mortality in the North Dublin Union during the Great Famine," *Economic History Review* 55, no. 3 (2002): 487–506.

43. For two venerable revisionist studies, see John Woodward, *To Do the Sick No Harm: A Study of the British Voluntary Hospital System to 1875* (London: Routledge and Kegan Paul, 1974); and Eric M. Sigsworth, "Gateways to Death? Medicine, Hospitals and Mortality, 1700–1850," in *Science and Society, 1600–1900*, ed. Peter Mathias (London: Cambridge University Press, 1972), 97–110. For an early Victorian view, see Thomas Wakley's condemnation of high workhouse mortality, in his editorial, *Lancet*,

May 1, 1841, 194. Jonas Hanway condemned bed sharing in London workhouses in the following terms: "It is well known that two or three adults are often crouded into a bed, tho' they hazard the poisoning each other. Sometimes two sick persons are put into the same bed; at others, one sick and the other in health; a proceeding which kicks at all pretensions to policy or humanity." *Citizen's Monitor*, 127. For epidemics in the Foundling Hospital, see Alysa Levene, *Childcare, Health, and Mortality at the London Foundling Hospital* (Manchester: University of Manchester Press, 2007), 155–62. It should be noted that case-fatality rates of many infectious diseases were quite low. Thus a measles epidemic at the Foundling Hospital in 1768 infected 139 of the 438 children—but only 6 died (158). Studies based on mortality alone therefore may well underplay or completely miss substantial outbreaks of infectious disease.

44. Mary J. Dobson, *Contours of Death and Disease in Early Modern England* (Cambridge: Cambridge University Press, 1997), 248; see also pages 249 and 267.

45. This was particularly true in 1753, when gaol fever infected and killed some Old Bailey judges and counsel. *Gentleman's Magazine*, February 1753. See also John Howard's remarks on gaol fever in *An Account of the Principal Lazarettos in Europe: With Various Papers Relative to the Plague: Together with Further Observations on Some Foreign Prisons and Hospitals; and Additional Remarks on the Present State of Those in Great Britain and Ireland* (Warrington, n.p., 1789), 231–32. Howard doubted that some disorders were "proper gaol fever, produced in and peculiar to such situations; or an epidemic disease, which attacked prisoners only in common with other inhabitants of the same town" (232).

46. Mooney, Luckin, and Tanner, "Patient Pathways," 242–45, and esp. note 66.

47. Boulton and Schwarz, "Parish Workhouse."

48. *Regulations Agreed Upon and Established This Twelfth Day of July 1726 by the Gentlemen of the Vestry Then Present, for the Better Government and Management of the Work-House Belonging to the Parish of St. Giles in the Fields* (London, n.p., 1726), 2–4, 14.

49. COWAC, vestry minutes, F2006/201.

50. Boulton and Schwarz, "Parish Workhouse." *Rules and Regulations for the Government of the Workhouse, of the Parish of St. Martin in the Fields, and of the Infant Poor-House at Highwood Hill* (London: n.p., 1828) included regulations to keep the house clean and the inspection of the sick; see esp., 5–6, 10–11, 13. For the visit of the churchwarden to St. Giles, see the following payment of two shillings in his accounts. "To the Servants of St Giles's Workhouse Shewing Me the House and the Severall Offices," COWAC, F83/32. It was ordered in 1725 that "Mr Marriot be Employed in ordering and furnishing provisions for the poor in the Workhouse in this parish and providing other necessarys in the same manner as he does in the Workhouse in the Parish of St. Giles in the Fields." COWAC, F2006/194. The parish agreed to pay Marriot a salary equivalent to that which he received in St. Giles. 259–60. Marriot was dismissed following complaints of mismanagement and neglect in October 1727 (289–90). For the 1775 and 1805 regulations and efforts to achieve cleanliness, see COWAC, F2072/32r.–34r; F2076/19, 309.

51. Landers, *Death and the Metropolis*, 88, 353–54.

52. The Sexton's notebooks and the Camden Town burial registers are housed in the Westminster Archives Centre: WAC 419/123, 419/233, 419/234, 419/235, 419/236, 419/236N, 419/237, 419/238, 419/239, 419/240, 419/241, 419/242, 419/243, 419/244, F2469. For St. Martin's workhouse, see Boulton and Schwarz,

"Parish Workhouse"; Jeremy Boulton and Leonard Schwarz "'The Comforts of a Private Fireside'? The Workhouse, the Elderly and the Poor Law in Georgian Westminster: St. Martin-in-the-Fields, 1725–1824," in *Accommodating Poverty: The Households of the Poor in England, c. 1650–1850*, ed. Joanne McEwan and Pamela Sharpe (Basingstoke, UK: Palgrave Macmillan, 2011), 221–45.

53. "Chap. III. of Particular Casualties," in John Graunt, *Natural and Political Observations Made Upon the Bills of Mortality* (London: n.p., 1662), accessed September 3, 2011, http://www.edstephan.org/Graunt/0.html. For the misreporting and concealment of the "secret malady," see also, Kevin Siena, *Venereal Disease, Hospitals and the Urban Poor: London's "Foul Wards," 1600–1800* (Rochester: University of Rochester Press, 2004), 30–61; Jeremy Boulton and John Black, "'Those That Die by Reason of Their Madness': Dying Insane in London, 1629–1830," *History of Psychiatry* 23, no. 1 (2012): 27–39.

54. For the nursing of foundlings outside London, see the fine recent study by Levene, *Childcare, Health, and Mortality*, 90–144.

Chapter Four

Workhouse Medical Care from Working-Class Autobiographies, 1750–1834

ALANNAH TOMKINS

Historians of the workhouse under England's Old Poor Law who wish to move beyond the generalities of returns to Parliament and examine the daily lived experience of workhouse life must generally turn to one of two sources. The policy intentions at the time a parish workhouse was opened are occasionally accessible in vestry minutes, workhouse rules, dietaries, or daily schedules. Alternatively, there are the entries in parish overseers' accounts, which show the practical result of accommodating the poor and sometimes generated itemized shopping lists of goods and services supplied to the house. At their best, the latter might include the bills submitted by surgeon-apothecaries for treatments supplied to named workhouse inmates. Fortuitous survivals of both types of material for the same place and period can yield valuable insights.[1] Pauper letters constitute an exciting source for English poor relief, and their potential has been elaborated of late, but these are not likely to augment the options substantially for research on workhouse life, since few or no letters were written by paupers while they were inmates.[2]

The working-class autobiography comprises one further, plausible genre for evidence of workhouse treatment. Autobiographies per se have secured extensive scholarly attention, at first from John Burnett, and then with David Vincent and David Mayall, who published their collective *Bibliography* in 1985.[3] While other texts have come to light since 1985, the Vincent-Mayall *Bibliography* remains indispensable for two reasons. First, the calendar of autobiographies includes details about the location of copies, which cements its ongoing value as a research tool. Second, the index is a meticulous and reliable guide to the calendared content of the individual narratives. The potential of this genre (and of the array of thematic ways into it) are now being explored. Jane Humphries has made the fullest use of this type of material to date.[4] Where pertinent autobiographical evidence survives, it should not surprise us if health, illness, and workhouse medicine formed a prominent and recurrent motif. There is some evidence (even prior to the collection of chapters for this volume) that workhouses under the Old Poor Law routinely operated as venues for the delivery of medical goods and services to paupers and might be used explicitly and consistently for housing, nursing, and treating the sick.[5] This could even prove the case where management of the workhouse was farmed out to a contractor.[6]

This chapter uses the *Bibliography* to access working-class contacts with workhouses under the Old Poor Law. There are twelve such texts, of which five have something substantive to say about medical arrangements in workhouses before 1834. Clearly, working-class autobiographies are quantitatively insignificant, yet qualitatively they add something distinctive to the familiar run of workhouse sources. They provide first-person testimony of the experience of life within workhouses, where their production was not a function of the workings of the law; in this respect they are unique. They shed light on medical relief in workhouses that delineates the variable details of that relief, which are interesting if isolated examples in themselves; more important, they evaluate the material and emotional impact of medical relief from the point of view of—to use the modern terminology—a service user.

There are contextual issues that impinge on the application of the five relevant narratives. In no case can an autobiography be connected to the independent survival of workhouse records that identify the writers as inmates. In one case only are there vestry minutes contemporaneous with an autobiographer's admission.[7] This means that there is no way to check for the occurrence, date, or duration of the alleged admission. Furthermore, the relevant texts are skewed in terms of date, gender, and geographic coverage. There are no autobiographies that relate to the period before 1770 and none written by women. This is in line with the genre of working-class autobiographies as a whole, which rarely allude to earlier decades and where female writers are vastly outnumbered by their male counterparts.[8] The featured workhouses cluster in the North Midlands (Nottingham, Salford, Bradford, and Heywood) with only one house in the south of England (Warminster in Wiltshire). London is entirely unrepresented. The limitations of this physical bias are perhaps mitigated by the realities of research to date (and the other chapters in this volume), which have tended to promote a focus on London and the southeast of England.

Furthermore, the accounts coalesce in terms of the life cycles of their authors; four spent time in workhouse as children or adolescents, but not as adults, and their memoirs were in every case written or dictated decades later. Jonathan Saville (1759–1842) spent a short time in the workhouse at Horton near Bradford up to 1766 (aged around seven) but was then readmitted to the same house (aged around fourteen) for one or two years. In later life he worked as a weaver but was also very active as a Methodist preacher, activities that had implications for the capture of his autobiography. He dictated his life story to a fellow Congregationalist, who published the narrative after Saville's death. Samuel Bamford (1788–1872) moved to the Salford workhouse in around 1794, when his father was made master of the house. He experienced direct exposure to workhouse life as the resident child of a parish employee for approximately five years (aged between approximately six and eleven); he wrote up these experiences fifty years later as the first volume of his autobiography. William Marcroft (1822–94) spent a brief period in the Heywood workhouse near Bury (aged just three) with his mother, Sally. Therefore, his account is predicated on his own earliest memories and, presumably (given the detail he employs), on his mother's account of the same period. Henry Price (b. 1824) was admitted to the workhouse in Warminster when his mother married and moved, with Price's stepfather, to Monmouthshire. Price remained in the house for around three years (aged ten to thirteen) from 1834 onward but did not put pen to paper until the twentieth century. Only one autobiographer offers a view of the workhouse from a more mature perspective, and then published his account within a short time. David Love (1750–1827) was an itinerant bookseller, among other occupations, and spent time in St. Mary's workhouse, Nottingham, in 1814 (aged sixty-four); his life history was published less than a decade later.[9]

These contextual issues gesture toward the multitude of theoretical problems with using texts as ambiguous as autobiographies in the capacity of historical sources and with using them for the specific purpose of examining workhouse life.[10] At its broadest, this is a problem of the recording of a public or semipublic transcript wherein the writer has engaged in a conscious act of self-fashioning.[11] The process of self-presentation is likely to influence the inclusion and omission of events or reflections to be drawn from the entirety of a writer's lived experience (that would be impossible to narrate in full). It is likely that such a text pursues one or more established motifs and that descriptions of lived experience are shaped to some extent to fit the genre. By the date of the earliest publication used here, that of David Love, there were a number of models that might have been adopted by a literate and aspiring literary writer. These included the spiritual autobiography initiated and exemplified by seventeenth-century nonconformists and the warning to others perhaps best represented by the confessions of condemned felons selected for publication by the Ordinary of Newgate prison.[12] The eighteenth and nineteenth centuries saw the evolution and proliferation of such narratives, including the secular hagiography and the Methodist life story.[13] This is not to claim that all autobiographers were engaged in an explicit attempt to deceive. It does, however, require the researcher to read the text in the light of narrative conventions within genres to frame the resulting text appropriately.

One trait shared by all the writers considered here is their desire to communicate. They all volunteered autobiographical information, and none were compelled to share their life history. Therefore, the act of writing (or in one case dictating) is evidence of a measure of agency; most people either could not write or did not choose to do so, whereas these men had the resources and the motivation to share their stories. This means that the events or processes they described were governed by fundamentally different drives than those behind other semi- or partially autobiographical narratives forced from people by the workings of the poor law, chiefly in the form of settlement or bastardy examinations. It also opens the possibility that authors had diverse audiences and future effects in mind (rather than narrow, instrumental ones). Agency among the parish poor has formed a discernible refrain in recent scholarship on the Old Poor Law, and so autobiographies provide another genre in which to test its extent.[14]

The life-cycle emphasis of these particular autobiographies introduces another issue. Experiences during childhood are formative and are likely to make a deep-seated and long-lasting impact on individuals and their later adult perceptions. Therefore, it is important to give due weight to the way that child development (as we currently apprehend it) impinged on people's memories of institutional life. Some children are now known to have a strong capacity for attachment to people and places, even in less-than-ideal circumstances.[15] This suggests that children who spent some time in workhouses *might* give an unduly positive account of the institution. At the same time, there is good evidence to suggest that children who experience drastic risk (engendered by deprivation, family disharmony and violence, substance abuse, or the absence of a stable adult, parent-type figure) might construe their circumstances as "normal" at the time but be predisposed to realization and negative reaction in later life.[16] Thus, the disruption to domestic and family life resulting from admission to a workhouse (as an exacerbation of experiences associated with household poverty) might realistically be supposed to have put children at risk in a way that might later give rise to anxiety or mental health problems.

Conversely, children who possessed one or more protective factors in their lives (including continuity of care from an adult acting in a parental role, affection expressed by other family members or the wider community, and other positive attributes) would have been well placed to navigate risk and avoid negative outcomes as adults.[17] Evidence of resilience engendered by protective factors can include deliberate planning for the future to ensure that adult lives avoid the kinds of risk endured as children, and this is exactly the kind of resilience advertised in working-class autobiographies.[18] Individuals who, according to their own criteria, "made good" were perhaps particularly likely to stress the difficulties they struggled with or suffered under as children to emphasize their later success in escaping risk and establishing satisfactory alternatives (in terms of family life, employment history, quality of housing, political power, or other forms of social well-being). And then there is the workhouse itself, an institution replete with negative associations. The agenda of the Poor Law Commission of 1834, with its explicit aim to render the workhouse as a punitive option for the poor, did not succeed in deterring all entrants, but it was wildly successful in terms of stigmatizing the institution.[19] This stigma extended forward into the twentieth century, such that workhouses inspired shudders among the working class long after their technical closure.[20] This is surely proof, if any were needed, that "historical epochs may delineate or structure our emotional transactions."[21] Stigma has also been projected back into the eighteenth century by historians anxious to see the workhouse from below and presumably determined not to risk injustice to the voiceless poor through a patronizing assumption of mute contentment.[22] Susannah Ottaway has reinforced this projection, having argued that the reputation of the eighteenth-century workhouse was initially damaged by the institution's association with houses of correction.[23] The question remains, though, to what *extent* the eighteenth-century and early nineteenth-century poor regarded admission to a workhouse as a stigmatizing event. If a punitive design predated 1834 (in individual parishes or across the nation), did this impinge on the perceptions of the workhouse poor?

Given the potency of the workhouse in English social history for inspiring certain types of image and response, this makes childhood memories a matter of particular concern. For example, some nineteenth- and twentieth-century writers who recalled the post-1834 workhouse clearly described their exposure in culturally identifiable terms, and specifically they evoked the *Oliver Twist* story, which swiftly entered the public consciousness after its publication in 1837. Henry Price recalled, "There were times when I felt very lonely and forsaken and had a good cry. Oliver Twist like one day a carpenter in want of an apprentice came to the House."[24] Will Crooks apparently made frequent use of the term "Bumbledom" to characterize officious groups of poor law guardians or penny-pinching policies.[25] Therefore, in light of social and class-conscious imperatives to the contrary, it seems highly unlikely that writers alluding to post-1834 houses would have been unduly falsely positive. Indeed, any positive recollection of the workhouse under the New Poor Law is of considerable interest, given the strong potential for opprobrium to be directed at the author.[26] The question remains as to whether any sort of steer might have influenced reminiscences of houses before 1834.

The workhouse motif might have been mobilized to boost the apparent sensibility or political credentials of a writer. The commentary of some authors includes clear points of self-approval if not aggrandizement; Bamford and Price, for example, both refer to their defense of weak or insane workhouse inmates and, in Bamford's case, this could legitimately be viewed as an attempt to position his younger self as affiliated to the defense of the poor. This sort of stance could certainly have been advertised or potentially fabricated as a coherent precursor to his politically radical career. Saville dwells at some length on his relative isolation from close family members and on recurrent stays in the workhouse, a device that amplifies the trajectory of his progress toward independence and self-improvement in the face of his orphan status, poverty, and disability. Even so, it is not obvious why a *beneficent* workhouse would be integral to this story. The critical reader is left with two broad conclusions: either Saville's memoirs are rendered with the intention of veracity (with all deference to modern understanding of the variability of memory) or he was constructing a consciously varied account wherein the qualities of the workhouse, its staff, and inmates were determined by contextual events, namely the need to avoid an unreservedly grim depiction of his entire childhood.

The remainder of this chapter offers a view of indoor, medical welfare under the Old Poor Law. In the process, it argues that accounts of pre-1834 houses were routinely neutral or upbeat and that this attitude can reasonably be ascribed to readily identifiable aspects of the authors' experience or to the contexts of narrative production. In each case, however, it is not obvious that they yield a falsely positive illustration of workhouse life or that they comprise a grotesque distortion of the experiences of their nonliterate fellow residents. Collectively, they permit the speculation that perceptions of workhouse life before 1834 were not so laden with stigma and that the institution was not viewed with such resentment and fear before the successful injection of these attributes through the designs of the Poor Law Commission.

The physical manifestations of medical welfare dispensed in workhouses and reported by autobiographers are limited in range and unsurprising in content. Smaller houses provided domestic care and a tailored diet augmented by occasional visits from medical practitioners, while larger houses had the scope to specialize and offer continuity of medical attention by salaried practitioners and dedicated wards or a workhouse infirmary for the sick poor.[27] The former is well represented by the Heywood workhouse, which initially tried to accommodate William Marcroft's "disordered" mother in the same room as a young man apparently deranged through disappointment in love. This closeting of disturbed persons in one room may have seemed appropriate and rational in anticipation of Sally Marcroft's admission, but the presence of her young son (and the violence of her intended roommate) rendered the arrangement immediately impracticable. The workhouse staff responded promptly and found the Marcrofts space in an alternative room.

In contrast, the large, differentiated house is best exemplified by the St. Mary's workhouse in Nottingham. St. Mary's was an extensive parish, and poor relief constituted welfare activity with an enormous turnover, of between fifteen and twenty-five thousand pounds per annum in the decade 1815–25. In light of this responsibility, the parish had elected to reorganize medical relief in 1813, switching from a contract system of payment per item (of attendance or treatment) to a salaried, full-time surgeon under the superintendence of an honorary physician. The new system initially attracted much criticism on the grounds of the likely increase in cost, but fears of raised expenses proved, in the short term at least, unfounded. Furthermore, "under the old plan the Poor complained very much of being badly attended, under the present establishment we believe they have seldom had any just reason to complain."[28] The surgeon was given quarters in the workhouse and, according to temporary inmate David Love, ample resources for dosing the paupers.

The emotional *responses* of writers to medical welfare in workhouses, though, are surprising for their endorsements, which range in tone from cautious approval to evident affection and enthusiasm. Clearly this is a problematic claim, given the temporal contingency of expressions of feeling and the tentative place of emotions in history more generally. Even so, we can theorize about why this should be so and find reinforcement for the idea that a positive response to the workhouse could be deemed rational if each author's emotion derives from perception, appraisal, and judgment about personal well-being.[29]

It is plain that one reason for this stance was the challenge and risk presented by life outside the workhouse. Domestic life for the working poor and their children was at best materially deprived and, at worst, characterized by sustained cruelty.[30] Perhaps the most potent example of suffering on this score is that of Jonathan Saville. He was apprenticed at a young age but, owing to the alleged cruelty of his master's family, his placement entailed his suffering a broken thigh, which went untreated for four years. The injury was the cause of a lifelong disability. Saville characterized his return to the workhouse in early 1770s as a return home, a move away from violence and neglect and toward kindness.

> At length, my master wishing to get rid of me, applied to the Thornton overseers, who told him to send me to Horton workhouse. The Horton and Thornton overseers came to see what condition I was in. They said they thought I should not live a month; but if I did, I was to come to the workhouse. I survived the month; and never did prince long for his crown so much as I did to get there. . . . When we got to the Workhouse, they set me down on the floor; and no sooner was it told about the house that little Jonathan was come back, than all the old women left their spinning and came to see me. I believe if my master had not got out of the way, they would have done him an injury.[31]

The contrast between Saville's life as an apprentice and as an adolescent inmate of the workhouse was drastic and encouraged him to reflect

on acts of kindness that subsequently cemented his perception of the
workhouse residents as a substitute family. The workhouse master apparently engaged in voluntary acts of personal care when he carried Saville
to a local spring in the hopes that bathing might prove recuperative. The
task involved dressing and undressing the young Saville, an intimacy that
the author later recalled with affection and, as importantly, with no hint
of fear or intimation of abuse. A fellow inmate fashioned him a pair of
crutches to improve his mobility. If Saville proffered a personal history
that even approximated to his lived experience—and he certainly did not
feign his permanent disability—then his positive response to the workhouse is entirely coherent. It was, arguably, the workhouse inmates and
staff who supplied or augmented his resilience factors, enabling him to
fulfill an active and apparently confident adulthood. This is not to say that
he did not write in a recognizable strain. His is an explicitly Methodist life
story, but this mode would not have inhibited him from characterizing the
workhouse a cheerless and deprived environment if this was his perception. Instead, Saville went out of his way to credit the workhouse both with
his recovery and the fostering of his intellectual abilities, claiming, "If you
want to know where I got my education, where my college was, it was in the
workhouse yonder."[32]

Positive reflections might also arise where people were able to consider
not just their individual response to a single institution but the place of
the workhouse in the poor law more broadly. David Love's enthusiasm
was spurred by his time in St. Mary's workhouse in Nottingham, and he
made explicit comparisons between welfare in England with what the
poor might expect elsewhere in Europe. Love entered the workhouse
in 1814, shortly after the institution of the new medical system, and so
perhaps saw it at its best. He remained there for several months and, on
his departure, he wrote a panegyric in verse to its virtues. In addition to
other apartments in the workhouse, he described the medical infrastructure as munificent:

> The Doctor's room is nigh at hand,
> Where drugs are given at his command;
> There powders, pills and laudanum keep,
> To cause the sick and weak to sleep,
> With boluses of every kind,
> And finest drops to break the wind;
> And many drugs together mix,
> From four-score to the age of six.[33]

Arguably, Love was describing the kind of care package delineated in the
introduction to this volume. But his praise was for the general system, as well
as for specifics that pertained in St. Mary's. He went on:

> Now highly-favoured England see
> Such good and wholesome laws for thee:
> Thy poor and helpless comfort find,
> The sick, the weak, the lame, the blind:
> Not Scotland, Ireland, France nor Spain,
> Nor other places o'er the main,
> Make such provision for their poor,
> As England does for its procure;
> In other Kingdoms, wretchedness,
> Misery, want and deep distress,
> For refuge have nowhere to fly,
> Perhaps in grief and anguish die.
> I cannot write without applause,
> On such a good and worthy cause;
> We see and feel the bless'd effect
> Better the poor could not expect[34]

Love is remembered in the *Oxford Dictionary of National Biography* as the author of rather lame verse, but when viewed as an historical artifact rather than the object of literary criticism, his poem may well be unique.[35] Other authors paid literary tribute to charitable giving, and there is even a poem that purports to reflect on the institutional excellence of the Royal Devon and Exeter Hospital, but no one else attempted to ascribe such beneficence to the workhouse in rhyme.[36] Love's comparison is given a modicum of force by virtue of his own status; he was a Scotsman by birth and an inveterate wanderer, so he could speak from direct comparison of Scotland with England and possibly other locations.

Twenty-first-century readers of Love's poem might reasonably wonder how far his verse was merely a paean to the benefits of a paternalist culture and, therefore, whether it could have been a fair reflection of life within the workhouse in Nottingham. He had clearly internalized the gratitude that commentators on parish relief and charity hoped would be the response of the poor to benefits of all kinds (but that was more notable by its absence, namely in the affront expressed when paupers asserted their rights to relief).[37] Nonetheless, was his effusion the overheated construction of a pliant and compliant elderly man or a moderate exaggeration of institutional adequacy?

The workhouse under the Old Poor Law might also be compared favorably, in retrospect, with the more restricted regime in operation after 1834. Henry Price's residence in Warminster workhouse spanned the last year of the Old Poor Law and the first years of the New. When he arrived in Wiltshire—he had been sent from London to his place of legal settlement—he apparently found an acceptable or even welcome retreat. He was covered with smallpox sores, following his recent recovery from the still-common disease, and, as a result of his gruesome appearance, the other workhouse children initially ran away from him. Even so, he had nothing but benign and nostalgic generalities for the Warminster house prior to 1834: "I must say that the Poor House at that time for the infirm and the Fatherless and Motherless children was a real refuge from the stormy blast and a thoroughly good Home." His favorable memories of medical care are summarized by the recollection that inmates were "well fed, nurs'd and doctor'd";[38] in contrast, he found a great deal to say against the workhouse after unionization, when the house regime became markedly punitive. Price's testimony emanates from a nonpublic transcript that was not apparently written for publication and still survives only in manuscript, so he was patently unafraid of official reprisals for his frankness.[39] It was, however, written at least six decades after the events of 1834. This means that Price had witnessed over half a century of negative responses to the workhouse under the New Poor Law from his social peers and had potentially internalized and incorporated these into his own life story.

Autobiographers went beyond praise of the workhouse in contrast with turbulent life experiences to express direct, positive reasons for their favorable descriptions of workhouse medicine and care. The most striking aspect here, repeated in three of the texts, is the importance of personnel or the personalities of staff in rendering the experience of workhouse life advantageous or better than it might have been. Warm depictions of institutional employees are all the more notable for their contrast with literary counterparts, who were rarely rendered in upbeat terms.[40] Saville reflected favorably on the three workhouse masters incumbent at Horton during the span of his stay and obtained his start in weaving owing to a variety of social capital accruing to his antecedents; his father's devout reputation was a deciding factor. Similarly, Marcroft's family benefited from a combination of a responsive workhouse mistress and her knowledge of other generations of his family. Sally Marcroft was admitted to the Heywood poorhouse some time before 1825, following postpartum dizziness and strange behavior. She was recognized by the workhouse governess as the daughter of William Marcroft Sr., and, in consideration of this connection, the official attitude toward her softened. The governess reputedly said, "we will make you as comfortable as things will let us," a pledge that, in the short term, included provision of peppermint tea and permission to sleep with her child while keeping a candle at bedtime, favors presumably denied to other pauper inhabitants.[41] Sally Marcroft was given work in the house as a servant and, later, as a seamstress, and her proficiency at both plain sewing and embroidery were allegedly the means for her full rehabilitation in the minds of workhouse staff; in other words, she ceased to be treated as an insane person for the duration of that admission. Unfortunately for Sally, she was seemingly subject to repeated bouts of mental disturbance, and she experienced a number of later admissions and died in the Heywood poorhouse in 1841.

The house, therefore, comprised an ongoing source of residential care and a facility for a troubled family under the auspices of both the Old and New Poor Laws. Marcroft himself was not subject to readmission, and he did not speculate on the conditions of the post-1834 regime. Even so, it seems reasonable to assume that, like Henry Price, Marcroft's account was influenced by the fifty years that intervened between his workhouse admission and the composition of his memoirs. His is the most neutral depiction of the five texts in relation to the tone of his discussion about the qualities of workhouse welfare. Marcroft was clearly proud of his mother and her being deemed worthy of special treatment in the workhouse, through the recognition given to her first for her lineage and then for the quality of her needlework, but, also, he was publishing at a time when an ultranegative image of workhouse had been in place for fifty years. Here, then, the sketch of the Heywood workhouse may benefit from his desire to defend his mother's memory.

One narrative depicts the extreme and even fatal challenge presented by the workhouse to the autobiographer's health and family. Yet the text reflects favorably on the community of care potentially on offer to workhouse residents, be they paupers or parish employees. Samuel Bamford removed to Salford workhouse in the mid-1790s with both of his parents, his uncle Thomas, and four siblings.[42] His father had been appointed as the workhouse master, while his uncle was placed in charge of house manufactures. Two of the youngest Bamfords died of smallpox soon after their arrival in the house. Given what is now understood about the respiratory transmission of smallpox, it seems likely that domestic conditions in the Salford workhouse facilitated their contracting the disease, although perhaps they were not necessarily responsible for the fatal outcome in these two specific cases. Soon thereafter, both Samuel and his uncle contracted typhus, of which the uncle then died. Nursing duties performed by both of Samuel's parents meant that they too fell ill of the same infection, and Samuel's mother died. In this way, the Bamford family was halved in size by diseases contracted at the workhouse within around twelve months. Bamford would have been forgiven for recalling this as a period of unalleviated misery.

Yet Bamford's autobiography does not dwell exclusively on loss and bereavement. It tacitly describes an atmosphere in the workhouse of dutiful care of the sick by employees and, in the aftermath of typhus, the support of the inmates for the beleaguered master's family. Bamford described the workhouse as "a theatre for the active habits and kindly feelings of my dear parents and my uncle"; he is quite lyrical on the subject of the beneficial influence of his parents on the lives of workhouse inmates. Given his mother's early death, he may perhaps be expected to have been nostalgic and poignant on this subject. The woman judged to have carried typhus to the workhouse was not neglected; rather, "everything was done for her which good nursing and the medical skill of those days could effect." Tellingly though, his account is not limited to benign generalities but is permeated with convincing detail. After his mother had died in the same room where he slept, Bamford recalled being immediately comforted by the women employed as nurses or layers-out in the house, "kind-hearted creatures. . . . I felt that all friends were not yet lost to me."[43] The first nurse employed to attend the young Samuel and his father at night during their convalescence was notable for her callous, unfeeling attitude; her drunkenness; and, on one occasion, her murderous rage. When she turned violent, however, Samuel and his father were rescued from her, presumably by interim staff but potentially by the inmates, and, thereafter, replacement nurses were described as very good.

The Salford house was one of the larger workhouses at this time, and while not one of the vast urban houses of industry, the township could afford salaries for additional workhouse staff.[44] The "little cheerful old man" who filled the unusual post of house apothecary was described as a beneficial character for the inmates: "his walk was almost a kind of dance, it was so lightsome, and he went tripping round to his patients, as he called them, every morning, with a smart saying or a cheerful word for every one." Salford also employed a stout assistant with some responsibility for the management of lunatics, so "there was no lack of power for coercion when it was necessary, but that was seldom the case except with the unfortunate insane."[45]

During his convalescence, Samuel found "sympathisers" among the inmates. As he writes,

> And though they were of the humblest station of their race, their friendship was probably not the least sincere, nor, consequently, ought it to be the least regarded. When I got strong enough to falter into the yard, I was surrounded by the pleased countenances of children who accompanied me with every demonstration of joy. . . . The mature and elderly paupers also, would stop, look at me, and walk away invoking blessings on "the poor motherless boy."[46]

He recalled his playmates among the pauper children by name and imagined himself as having fulfilled the role of a younger brother to those who had none. He considered himself to have friends throughout the house, including in the lunatic ward.

Bamford's testimony may be regarded as suspiciously favorable. Is it possible that the workhouse, an institution that came to be hated quite viscerally in the 1830s and beyond, could have been so inclusive and welcoming in earlier decades? In later life, and certainly by the time he wrote his autobiography, Samuel Bamford became alienated from the more strenuous aspects of the radical agenda, but it is still reasonable to suppose that he continued to have a vested interest in the favorable representation of workhouse life.[47] Nostalgia for his early life, memories of his mother, and ongoing filial respect quite possibly contributed to his valorization of his parents' incumbency in Salford. One of his explicit intentions in writing this section of his reminiscences was to emphasize that an association with the workhouse poor did nothing to corrupt him. This was important because nineteenth-century sentiments toward the workhouse poor were typically skeptical and judgmental. These attitudes had their origins in the eighteenth century but replaced an older view of the poor that was more generous.[48] For Bamford, writing about the 1790s in the context of 1849, this meant he arguably acted as an apologist for older, gentler assessments of the workhouse poor. He emphasized that his exposure to workhouse inmates gave rise to no inducement to vice; instead, the inmates of the Salford workhouse are represented as poor but compassionate and amiable rather than deserving of condemnation. It is highly likely that he had his mid-nineteenth-century readership in mind, and their suspicions of the workhouse poor, when he framed this account.

The historiography, which spans the intersection of medicine and poor relief, tends to supply case studies pointing to either generosity of treatment or meanness, deriving from a parochial desire to distribute or save taxpayers' money. The quality of pauper experience is, therefore, attributable to timing, location, and personality. Did the poor present themselves to parish authorities during years of plenty or austerity? What was their parish's policy in relation to their type of poverty? Were they able to articulate a convincing account of deserving poverty to a responsive individual or collective, or did they struggle to escape the category of undeserving in the face of a stony and judgmental vestry? Evidence drawn from working-class autobiographies tends to reinforce these generalizations, but with the emphasis firmly placed on the positive likelihood of good fortune and decent outcomes. This is in many ways an uncomfortable conclusion, and one that is at odds with long-standing assumptions about workhouses per se, whether emanating from the Old or New Poor Laws. It cannot be dismissed, however, as an erroneous impression derived from sources so problematic that they are drained of all authority.

At first sight, these narratives draw their authenticity from their composition by key actors, the poor participating in relief systems, expressing viewpoints that are not yielded by other genres. As such, they bring something unique to the array of sources for the study of the poor. They are akin to pauper letters in that they are strategic writings, where the nature of the strategy in play is sometimes much less obvious than is the case with correspondence. Yet a systematic methodology or methodologies can amplify our appreciation of autobiographical narratives and shore up their value as historical testimony. A close consideration of the autobiography alongside what is known of the author's life from the historical record can deepen our understanding of their perspective. Authorial motivations can also be interpreted in the light of modern notions of child psychology, contextual chronology, social convention, and literary tradition. These approaches do not diminish the authenticity of the texts but provide qualified reinforcement for trusting the author, while benefiting from the numerous advantages of hindsight. In this way, it is possible to read working-class autobiographies as providing an overriding (if not overwhelming) endorsement of medical relief in the workhouse before 1834, delivered in a manner that was deemed both materially and emotionally satisfactory and reported in an age when cultural perceptions of the workhouse were indivisible from the story of Oliver Twist. Disconcerting as this may seem, it is perhaps one of the more surprising consequences (and proofs) of pauper agency.

Notes

1. Alannah Tomkins, *The Experience of Urban Poverty, 1723–82: Parish, Charity and Credit* (Manchester: Manchester University Press, 2006), 50–56, in relation to workhouse diets.

2. Thomas Sokoll, ed., *Essex Pauper Letters, 1731–1837* (Oxford: Oxford University Press, 2001), for example, 97, 178, 469. Paupers allude to the workhouse as their possible future destination or as a place that they have worked hard to avoid. No letters are written by paupers resident in the workhouse at the time of writing or reflecting on their experiences in workhouses. The same is true in Steven King, Thomas Nutt, and Alannah Tomkins, eds., *Narratives of the Poor in Eighteenth-Century Britain*, vol. 1, *Voices of the Poor: Poor Law Depositions and Letters* (London: Pickering and Chatto, 2006).

3. John Burnett, David Mayall, and David Vincent, eds., *The Autobiography of the Working Class: An Annotated Critical Bibliography*, 3 vols. (Brighton: Harvester, 1985–87). See also the Burnett Archive of Working-Class Autobiographies held at Brunel University Library, with online index, http://www.brunel.ac.uk/services/library/research/special-collections/burnett-archive-of-working-class-autobiographies.

4. Jane Humphries, *Childhood and Child Labour in the British Industrial Revolution* (Cambridge: Cambridge University Press, 2010).

5. See Elizabeth Melling, ed., *Kentish Sources*, vol. 4, *The Poor* (Maidstone: Kent County Council, 1964), 102, 105, for a pauper being given a cold bath in the Dartford workhouse in 1732, and wine being issued for a smallpox victim in the same house in 1736. Lynn MacKay, "A Culture of Poverty? The St. Martin in the Fields Workhouse, 1817," *Journal of Interdisciplinary History* 26, no. 2 (1995): 221–6; Philip Anderson, "The Leeds Workhouse under the Old Poor Law: 1726–1834," *Publications of the Thoresby Society* 56, no. 2 (1980): 88.

6. Tomkins, *Experience of Urban Poverty*, 69–71, 148.

7. Nottinghamshire Record Office, PR Addit 9739, Nottingham, St. Mary vestry minutes, 1807–33.

8. David Vincent, *Bread, Knowledge and Freedom: A Study of Nineteenth-Century Working-Class Autobiography* (London: Methuen, 1982), 8.

9. Francis Athow West, ed., *Memoirs of Jonathan Saville of Halifax* (London: Hamilton, Adams, and Co., 1848); Samuel Bamford, *The Autobiography of Samuel*

Bamford, vol. 1, *Early Days* (London: Frank Cass, 1967); William Marcroft, *The Marcroft Family* (Manchester: J. Heywood and Co., 1886); Price, "My Diary"; David Love, *The Life and Adventures of David Love* (Nottingham: Sutton & Son, 1823).

10. Regina Gagnier, "Social Atoms: Working-Class Autobiography, Subjectivity, and Gender," *Victorian Studies* 30, no. 3 (1987): 335–63.

11. James Scott, *Domination and the Arts of Resistance* (New Haven: Yale University Press, 1990), 86–87.

12. Paul Delany, *British Autobiography in the Seventeenth Century* (London: Routledge and Kegan Paul, 1969), esp. chap. 5; Michael Mascuch, *Origins of the Individualist Self: Autobiography and Self-Identity in England, 1591–1791* (Stanford: Stanford University Press, 1997), esp. chap. 7.

13. Isabel Rivers, "'Strangers and Pilgrims': Sources and Patterns of Methodist Narrative," in *Augustan Worlds: Essays in Honour of A. R. Humphreys*, ed. J. C. Hilson, M. Monica B. Jones, and John R. Watson (Leicester: Leicester University Press, 1978). Among many possible examples, see William MacMichael, *The Gold-Headed Cane* (London: Royal College of Physicians, 1968); Hannah Ball, *Memoirs of Miss Hannah Ball of High Wycombe in Buckinghamshire: Extracted from Her Diary* (York: Wilson, Spence, and Mawman, 1796). I am indebted to Susannah Ottaway for the latter reference.

14. For paupers' capacity to negotiate the terms of their parochial relief, see, among others, Steven King, "'Stop This Overwhelming Torment of Destiny': Negotiating Financial Aid at Times of Sickness under the English Old Poor Law, 1800–1840," *Bulletin of the History of Medicine*, 79, no. 2 (2005): 228–60.

15. John Bowlby, "The Nature of the Child's Tie to His Mother," *International Journal of Psychoanalysis* 39, no. 5 (1958): 350–79; William Damon, *Social Personality and Development: Infancy through adolescence* (New York: Norton, 1983), 44.

16. Patricia Mrazek and David Mrazek, "Resilience in Child Maltreatment Victims: A Conceptual Exploration," *Child Abuse and Neglect* 11, no. 3 (1987): 357–66, with reference to the author J. G. Ballard.

17. Edith Grotberg, *A Guide to Promoting Resilience in Children*, International Resilience Project, 1995, http://resilnet.uiuc.edu/library/grotb95b.html#chapter1.

18. European Network for Children Affected by Risky Environments within the Family (ENCARE), "Risk, Protective and Resilience Factors for Children," December 14, 2009, http://www.encare.info/riskyenvironments/resilience/factors; I am grateful to Dr. Lisetta Lovett, consultant psychiatrist, for direction on this point.

19. Margaret Anne Crowther, *The Workhouse System, 1834–1929: The History of an English Social Institution* (London: Routledge, 1983), 30–33, and chap. 9.

20. Simon Fowler, *The Workhouse: The People, the Places, the Life behind Doors* (Kew: National Archives, 2007), 7.

21. Jefferson Singer, "Putting Emotion in Context," *Journal of Narrative and Life History* 5, no. 3 (1995): 262.

22. This is usually implied rather than argued, but see, for example, the uniformly pejorative context of references to the workhouse in Edward P. Thompson, *The Making of the English Working Class* (London: Penguin, 1980).

23. Susannah Ottaway, "Hygiene and Humanitarianism in the Eighteenth-Century Workhouse" (paper delivered at the Medicine and the Workhouse Conference, Birmingham Medical Institute, October 31, 2008); chapter 2 in this volume.

24. Price, "My Diary," 16.

25. George Haw, *From Workhouse to Westminster: The Life Story of Will Crooks, MP* (London: Cassell, 1907).

26. I shall be considering the role of the post-1834 workhouse in autobiographies in Alannah Tomkins, "'Hell with the Lid Off': Re-evaluating the English Workhouse from Working-Class Autobiographies," *Social History of Medicine* (forthcoming).

27. The largest London workhouses offered a range of options for the sick poor within and beyond the workhouse walls; see Jeremy Boulton and Leonard Schwarz, "The Parish Workhouse, the Parish and Parochial Medical Provision in Eighteenth-Century London," in *Narratives of Sickness and Poverty in Europe*, ed. Steven King and A. Gestrich (Amsterdam: Rodopi, forthcoming).

28. Nottinghamshire Record Office, PR Addit, 9739, Nottingham, St. Mary vestry minutes, 1807–33, Copy of the [fifth] medical report addressed to the overseers and parishioners, March 25, 1818.

29. Barbara Rosenwein, "Worrying about Emotions in History," *American Historical Review* 107 (2002): 836.

30. Humphries, *Childhood and Child Labor*, 134–35; Katrina Honeyman, *Child Workers in England, 1780–1820: Parish Apprentices and the Making of the Early Industrial Labour Force* (Aldershot, UK: Ashgate, 2007), 201–7.

31. West, *Memoirs of Jonathan Saville*, 6, 8–9.

32. Ibid., 28.

33. Love, *Life and Adventures*, 143.

34. Ibid., 144–45.

35. James Sambrook, "Love, David (1750–1827)," *Oxford Dictionary of National Biography* (London: Oxford University Press, 2004), accessed November 16, 2011, http://www.oxforddnb.com/view/article/17039.

36. Joseph Wilde, *The Hospital, a Poem in Three Books, Written in the Devon and Exeter Hospital, 1809* (Norwich: Stevenson, Matchett, and Stevenson, 1809), quoted in Roy Porter, "The Gift Relation: Philanthropy and Provincial Hospitals in Eighteenth-Century England," in *The Hospital in History*, ed. Lindsay Granshaw and Roy Porter (London: Routledge, 1989), 169–72.

37. Scott, *Domination*, 86–87; S. King, Nutt, and Tomkins, eds., *Narratives* Vol. 1, 7. For an eighteenth-century directive to exact gratitude, see James Stonhouse, *Friendly Advice to a Patient* (London: printed for John Rivington and James Rivington, 1748).

38. Islington Public Library, Henry Price, "My Diary" c. 1904.

39. Price, "My Diary."

40. Even Wilde's poem on the Royal Devon and Exeter Hospital condemned the nurses as unfeeling; see *Hospital*, 58.

41. Marcroft, *Marcroft Family*, 22–23.

42. Bamford, *Autobiography of Samuel Bamford*, 1:54.

43. Ibid., 57, 58, 62.

44. *Abstract of Answers and Returns under Act for Procuring Returns Relative to Expense and Maintenance of Poor in England*, Parliamentary Papers, 1803–4 (175), 247, gives the occupancy of the Salford workhouse as fifty-four persons.

45. Bamford, *Autobiography of Samuel Bamford*, 1:67–68.

46. Ibid., 64–65.

47. Peter Spence, "Bamford, Samuel (1788–1872)," *Oxford Dictionary of National Biography* (London: Oxford University Press, 2004), October 2009, http://www. oxforddnb.com/view/article/1256.

48. See, among others, Lynn Hollen Lees, *The Solidarities of Strangers: The English Poor Laws and the People, 1700–1948* (Cambridge: Cambridge University Press, 1998), chap. 3.

Chapter Five

"A Sad Spectacle of Hopeless Mental Degradation"

The Management of the Insane in West Midlands Workhouses, 1815–60

LEONARD SMITH

The significance of the workhouse in the tapestry of care for mentally disordered people in England has tended to be underestimated by historians.[1] The nineteenth century has been regarded principally as the era of the rise and triumph of the universal, monolithic public lunatic asylum system.[2] County authorities were first empowered to establish a pauper lunatic asylum as early as 1808. Several had taken the opportunity before the key legislation of 1845 mandated counties and boroughs to provide an asylum.[3] Within a decade almost every county had built an asylum, on its own or in conjunction with others, or was in the process of doing so. These great "museums of madness," as Andrew Scull has evocatively styled them, laid the basis of institutional provision for generations to come.[4] Between 1850 and 1900 the numbers and size of the county asylums continued to expand steadily, as did the numbers of people confined within them.[5]

The purpose-designed county lunatic asylum was, however, never the sole institutional receptacle. During the eighteenth century and the first half of the nineteenth, there had been a considerable growth of provision in the private and voluntary sectors. Private madhouses had originally catered to the insane members of the wealthier classes, but some were increasingly providing for pauper lunatics funded by their parishes.[6] Lunatic hospitals, financed by voluntary subscription, had been established in several major cities, and these also accepted some paupers among their clientele.[7] In fact, by 1834 there was an extensive range of specialist provision in England, which has been characterized as a "mixed economy of care" for the insane.[8] From the outset, the workhouse also constituted an important constituent of this mixed economy.

In 1847 there were nearly nine thousand mentally disordered people in workhouses. Down to 1890, the proportions of people deemed insane residing in them remained at a consistent 25 percent of the overall number.[9] Nevertheless, there has been a tendency only to acknowledge rather dismissively that the workhouse had some place in the overall pattern of provision. Certain perceived truisms, highlighted by Peter Bartlett, have tended to be applied to workhouse management of mentally disordered people. The first of these was that the main motivation for keeping people in the workhouse was to avoid the expense of placement in an asylum. The second was that those retained there were chronic, hopeless cases, usually either elderly or people considered to be "idiots" or "imbeciles." The third was that a lack of capacity in asylums, due largely to overcrowding, was a key factor leading to people remaining in workhouses.[10] Bartlett acknowledged that these contentions were somewhat simplistic. Nevertheless, evidence from the West Midlands confirms that there is more than an element of justification for each of them.

This chapter explores features of the care and management of mentally disordered people in workhouses in late Georgian and early Victorian England, utilizing the West Midlands as a case study. The region was notable for containing large urban concentrations, small manufacturing towns, and old market towns, as well as extensive rural areas, composing a variegated patchwork of industrial, commercial, and agricultural districts. Given its complex social and economic geography, the West Midlands provided examples of the various patterns of development in institutional provision for the insane. The part played by boards of guardians and workhouses varied markedly between places and over time, similar to what Bill Forsythe and others have described for Devon.[11] In examining this more closely, consideration will be given to three main aspects. The first of these is the nature of the people designated insane who were admitted and confined, and the changing rationales for them being kept in the workhouse or removed to some form of lunatic asylum. The second aspect is the nature of care provided for them and the early development within workhouses of specific facilities for the insane. The third part of the chapter deals with the effect on the workhouse system of the rise of the national network of county lunatic asylums after 1845, particularly the incipient development of quasi-asylums within larger urban workhouses.

The Workhouse Insane

The Poor Law Amendment Act of 1834 marked a significant watershed in the nature of workhouse provision for mentally disordered people. The inquiry commissioners who had surveyed existing arrangements throughout the country had been perturbed by evidence that some very disturbed individuals were present in various workhouses. They were often forcibly restrained and confined in squalid conditions, their consequently deteriorating mental health causing disruption to other inmates.[12] Such situations had been long prevalent, to judge from evidence given to the Select Committee on Madhouses in 1815. The private madhouse proprietor, William Ricketts of Droitwich, referring to workhouses in Worcestershire, spoke graphically about the circumstances:

> When a pauper becomes insane, the parish officers are unwilling to believe that it is a mental disease, and seldom or ever take notice of it until it becomes dangerous; in most cases he is then consigned to the workhouse, where he is chained down, and nothing done for him until he becomes a raving maniac; and it very often happens that he is not removed from the workhouse until they are incapable of keeping him from his being in a state of violence.

Ricketts had little doubt that parish authorities' practice of keeping disturbed and dangerous lunatics in the workhouse was primarily intended to save the expense of paying for places in asylums, such as his own.[13]

Circumstances differed significantly among counties following the passage of the County Asylums Act (often referred to as Wynn's Act) of 1808. This laid down that, in counties where an asylum had been established, overseers were required to ensure conveyance to the asylum of "any lunatic, insane person, or dangerous idiot" at the expense of the parish to whom he was chargeable. Neglect to do so could incur a fine of between forty shillings and ten pounds.[14] Staffordshire was one of the first counties to adopt the legislation, opening its own lunatic asylum in 1818. The county justices were relatively efficient in ensuring that the parochial authorities complied with the act, which largely ensured that only harmless "idiots" remained in the workhouses.[15] The parishes of those other West Midlands counties that lacked their own asylum were not subject to the same requirements and were therefore far less constrained in retaining a range of mentally disordered people within their workhouses.

Those confined in workhouses generally comprised both lunatics and idiots. Overall figures extant for Worcestershire in 1829 show 135 lunatics and 133 idiots belonging to the county. Of these, 176 were in institutions—30 in a county asylum (probably Stafford, with which the Worcestershire magistrates had made an agreement), 1 in a lunatic hospital, 27 in private madhouses, and the majority, amounting to 118, in workhouses.[16] In Warwick a survey of the inmates of St. Mary's workhouse in 1819 had indicated that, out of 79 inmates, there were 3 designated as lunatics, 4 as idiots, and 1 as "childish." One of the female idiots, Ann Allen, had been in the house for forty-five years, and two others, Elizabeth

Toney and Ann Crook, for forty years—they were all still there six years later in 1825. Of the lunatics Sarah Hitchcox had been there for eighteen years in 1819, and she was also still there in 1825; another had been in the house for seven years in 1819 and remained in 1825. In that latter year, there were 6 women in the house designated as insane and a further 4 as idiots, in addition to 1 male lunatic and 1 idiot.[17]

Some returns for Shropshire from 1829 show an interesting mixture. In the Market Drayton workhouse there were 5 lunatics and 6 idiots, while in the Ludlow workhouse there were 5 idiots, and in the Newport workhouse 2 idiots. In addition, 8 people were recorded as being at a county asylum (probably Stafford). Care in the community also remained significant, with as many as 43 people from various parishes recorded as being on out-relief, 7 of whom were boarded out with people other than family members.[18] Elsewhere within the county, in the more populous towns of Oswestry and Shrewsbury, specific provision had been made in 1821 within their work-houses. In 1825 there were 5 insane patients in the Oswestry House of Industry, and by 1838 this had risen to 18.[19] At the Shrewsbury House of Industry there were 11 lunatics and idiots confined in 1826. By 1839 the numbers there had risen to 50, and to more than 80 by the mid-1840s.[20]

Well before the Poor Law Amendment Act of 1834, there had been a fairly wide consensus that an asylum was the proper institution for lunatics. However, attitudes were much more equivocal as to whether idiots needed to be in an asylum or whether they could be appropriately looked after in the workhouse. The stipulation of the 1808 County Asylums Act that luna-tics and "dangerous" idiots should be committed to an asylum was taken as affirmation that those not viewed as dangerous might appropriately remain in the workhouse.[21] Section 45 of the 1834 act sought to rationalize the situ-ation, laying down that lunatics or idiots who were dangerous were not to be kept in a workhouse for longer than fourteen days before being sent to a lunatic asylum.[22] This contained sufficient ambiguity to give scope for poor law unions to adopt varying solutions. First, it was generally taken to mean that it was legitimate to keep quiet, withdrawn, or depressed lunatics, as well as idiots, in the workhouse, however unwell. Second, it was now appar-ently acceptable for dangerous mentally ill people to remain for a limited period—this potentially enabled the workhouse to be used for a trial period to see if the acutely insane person might calm down within a few days. It effectively sanctioned the use of the workhouse as a holding center between community and asylum, pending further assessment. There was at least now, though, a reasonably clear criterion that would determine whether a person could remain in the workhouse or be transferred to an asylum, and that was dangerousness. But this concept was open to widely differing interpretation.

In practice, the determination of dangerousness was much influenced by a paramount consideration of local poor law authorities—the pursuit of economy. Placement in a lunatic asylum was relatively expensive in the 1830s and 1840s, when compared to basic maintenance costs in the workhouse. In areas with a county lunatic asylum, such as Staffordshire, the costs tended to be lower than in counties like Warwickshire and Worcestershire, where poor law authorities mainly had to have recourse to private asylums. The provisions of the 1834 act had, indeed, actually provided a stimulus to the private sector. Some existing private asylums, like those at Droitwich, Hereford, and Lichfield, were joined by new ones geared to cater to the growing demand for accommodation of disorderly pauper lunatics.[23] One of these was Duddeston Hall, in the Birmingham suburbs, opened in 1835. Its proprietor, the surgeon Thomas Lewis, contracted with the guardians of Birmingham and Aston to receive dangerous lunatics from their workhouses and to return them once they were calmer and more settled.[24] He built up a thriving and lucrative trade by this means. As well as Birmingham and Aston, several other midland unions, such as Warwick, Solihull, Rugby, and Nuneaton in Warwickshire, and Kidderminster and Bromsgrove in Worcestershire, were sending their unmanageable lunatics to Duddeston.[25]

The temptation for poor law unions to find ways to avoid this expense was considerable.[26] They might persevere with disruptive, disorderly, and "refractory" behavior in the workhouse for some time before concluding that the stage had been reached to transfer the culprit to an asylum, as case examples clearly demonstrate. The governor of the Warwick workhouse, in May 1839, expressed great concern about an inmate named Williams, whom he considered a dangerous lunatic and who had tried several times to injure those attending him. However, rather than arrange admission to an asylum, the board of guardians advised the governor "to restrain the pauper by use of the Straitwaistcoat" and "to adopt necessary measures of coercion." They rationalized their response with a suggestion that Williams's violent behavior may have been under the influence of "passion" rather than insanity.[27] A similar reluctance to take other action was apparent in two cases in the Wolverhampton workhouse in 1842. It was reported at the beginning of October that an idiot named William Walton was subject to "fits of violence," which had recently increased very much in ferocity. He had without warning kicked another inmate and seriously injured him. This was apparently allowed to pass, and it took a savage attack on another inmate, whom Walton both kicked and bit, before the workhouse master sought his removal to the county asylum for fear of fatal consequences. Three months later there was similar dilatoriness in regard to Henry Swift, a lunatic, who was "at times so violent that it has required several men to hold him," causing people to be terrified of him. Eventually, he was sent to Stafford Asylum.[28] These instances indicated, at best, a lack of adherence to the law.

Faced with such infractions, the Poor Law commissioners periodically exhorted or even instructed local unions to comply with the law.

For example, in March 1840 the commissioners wrote to the Bromsgrove Board of Guardians regarding John Hall, who had previously been a patient at the private Droitwich Lunatic Asylum, to urge "careful consideration whether Hall is a fit person to remain an inmate of the Workhouse." The guardians took advice from the union surgeon and the workhouse master, before responding that "the Pauper is not that dangerous Lunatic, insane person, or Idiot contemplated by the 45th Section of the Poor Law Amendment Act." The commissioners reluctantly conceded that the decision lay with the guardians and their medical officers but warned that they "will bear in mind the responsibility they incur."[29] In September 1842, having noticed that the master of the Nuneaton workhouse had reported Elizabeth Pearson to be "an Idiot dangerous at times," the Poor Law commissioners wrote to the Nuneaton guardians requiring her removal to an asylum, who in turn ordered the relieving officer to arrange it.[30] At the beginning of 1844 Edwin Chadwick, on behalf of the commissioners, intervened with the Birmingham guardians, following a report that there were several people deemed dangerous in the workhouse. He referred particularly to two cases, Emma Bailey and Martha Gould, both of whom were being kept under mechanical restraint, and suggested that the onus was on the guardians to show that they were not dangerous. After investigation by their surgeons, the guardians stood firm on Emma Bailey, but unenthusiastically agreed to send Martha Gould to an asylum, even though they questioned the degree of her mental disorder.[31]

The practice of keeping disturbed, and often dangerous, lunatics in the workhouse continued, despite the interventions of the Poor Law commissioners. The problems were highlighted by the Metropolitan Commissioners in Lunacy, whose detailed national survey in 1842–43 comprised all types of institutions in which the insane were being managed, including county asylums, public lunatic hospitals, private asylums, and workhouses. Their findings formed the basis of a seminal report in 1844, which was the precursor to the major lunacy legislation of 1845.[32] The commissioners deplored the short-term pecuniary motivations of guardians and pointed out the likely future consequences, both financial and therapeutic:

> It has been the practice, in numerous instances, to detain the insane pauper at the workhouse . . . , until he becomes dangerous or unmanageable; and then, when his disease is beyond all medical relief, to send him to a Lunatic Asylum where he may remain during the rest of his life, a pensioner on the public. This practice, which has been carried on for the sake of saving, in the first instance, to each parish some small expense, has confirmed the malady of many poor persons, has destroyed the comfort of families, has ultimately imposed a heavy burthen upon parishes and counties and has, in a great measure, nullified the utility of Public Lunatic Asylums.[33]

The main concern of the commissioners, led by Lord Ashley (later the Earl of Shaftesbury), was to advocate for the dissemination of a comprehensive public asylum system and to ensure that people were sent to an asylum while their illness was still at a curable stage. The overall tenor of their report was highly critical of the role of workhouses, as well as private asylums, in managing and caring for pauper patients.

The attempts to economize occurred also at a later stage of the person's mental disorder. Guardians and relieving officers throughout the region remained in regular contact, both with the managers of the county asylum at Stafford and with the proprietors of private asylums, on the state of their institutionalized pauper lunatics. Periodic visits might be undertaken to monitor progress. Any sign that the patient had become settled and less dangerous was likely to lead to removal from the asylum and a return to the workhouse, even if he or she still remained mentally unwell. Records from diverse unions, such as Birmingham, Aston, Warwick, Bromsgrove, and Dudley, confirm this process.[34] For example, in April 1835 the surgeon Edward Cox, having visited Stafford Asylum, advised the Birmingham guardians that he considered John Timms, Charlotte Westwood, and Ann Green "though not properly restored may be brought back as manageable and harmless cases, and submitted to the Superintendence and humane care of Mr Allcock the Governor."[35] In December 1839 the Bromsgrove guardians were advised by their surgeon, Mr. Fletcher, that J. Hall and G. Smith "now at the Droitwich Lunatic Asylum may be removed with perfect safety"; they were duly brought back to the workhouse. In March 1842 Fletcher visited Duddeston Hall and examined all the Bromsgrove lunatics, as a result of which three were removed back to the workhouse.[36] It perhaps needs to be stressed, however, that decisions on removal from asylums were not necessarily motivated solely by monetary considerations. Reports in some instances did indicate that either the person had recovered or that their condition had become more settled.

Inside the Workhouse

The nature of provision for lunatics and idiots in workhouses differed markedly, both over time and between locations. Evidence given to the 1815 Select Committee indicated that their treatment in parish workhouses, under the Old Poor Law, ranged from benign neglect to outright ill-treatment. According to the lunacy reformer Edward Wakefield, the insane were "under the care of persons totally and entirely ignorant of the proper treatment of Lunatics in general; . . . the rooms in which they are kept are ill adapted to the confinement of such persons, and because in some cases which I have seen from those causes, those unfortunate persons have been constantly confined in strait-waistcoats, frequently kept in bed night and day." He noted also that "lunatics in workhouses are an extreme annoyance to the other inhabitants of the house" and were treated accordingly. Specific and graphic evidence regarding poor conditions for the insane in parish workhouses in the west of England was given by Henry Alexander. Other witnesses also testified to neglect and mistreatment, including the Staffordshire madhouse proprietor Thomas Bakewell, who claimed that those in parish workhouses in the area were "very improperly treated." His fellow madhouse keeper, William Ricketts of Droitwich, exclaimed that "it would be useless for me to repeat to you the cruelty daily exercised on lunatics in workhouses." He spoke of workhouses in Worcestershire where they were "miserably treated," with many "chained down to their beds for weeks together."[37]

In most workhouses in the early decades of the century, lunatics and idiots were accommodated with the general inmate population rather than in separate facilities. One exception was in Shropshire, where rather unique arrangements were developed. In 1821 and 1822 respectively, the directors of the Houses of Industry in Oswestry and Shrewsbury obtained licenses from the justices to undertake "the care, cure and maintenance" of pauper lunatics. In effect, a dedicated lunatic asylum was created within parts of each workhouse. The medical officers at the Shrewsbury house in 1826 reported reassuringly that "proper modes of treatment have been from time to time adopted for their cure."[38] By 1839 it had actually been named the Kingsland Asylum and effectively functioned as a private lunatic asylum, despite its location within the workhouse walls.[39] Conditions in the 1840s, particularly the widespread use of mechanical restraint and the chaining of patients into their beds at night, brought condemnation from the Commissioners in Lunacy, and it was finally closed in 1852.[40] At Oswestry, the main shortcoming was the extremely poor standard of staff, recruited from among destitute workhouse inmates and paid one shilling per week.[41] Indeed, the use of other paupers to look after the lunatics and idiots became common practice in most workhouses.

By the 1830s the larger urban unions were increasingly making direct provision for their insane paupers, primarily with a view to a financial saving. This normally took the form of establishing specific insane wards inside the workhouse itself. Birmingham had embarked on this process well before 1834. Two new buildings were added in 1835, and the whole facility was reorganized. There were in excess of sixty inmates, including both idiotic cases and others described as "suffering from mental aberration which are perfectly manageable," who might otherwise have had to be sent to an asylum. The authorities congratulated themselves on the "great pecuniary retrenchment resulting to the Parish," notwithstanding the expense of erecting additional rooms.[42] The guardians of neighboring Aston, doubtless influenced by what had been achieved by their neighbors, took steps to make provision within their workhouse. With seventeen paupers placed at Duddeston Hall in May 1837, they were very conscious of the cost implications. They anticipated that, following building alterations, "some of the cases now existing and others that may occur would be provided for better and at far less expense, in the House than sending them . . . to an Asylum for the reception of Lunatics."[43]

The provision of insane wards led to a growing belief by guardians that they could manage a wider range of conditions and behavioral presentations within the workhouse. An apparent preparedness to flout the law brought places like Birmingham into conflict with the Poor Law commissioners over the interpretation and implementation of section 45 of the 1834 act. The matter was also taken up by the Metropolitan Commissioners in Lunacy in their national survey of 1842–43 and in their ensuing report. They were especially critical of the Birmingham workhouse and of the type of patients there, which included epileptics "liable to fits of raving madness, during which they were excessively violent," people who were "occasionally under great excitement and furiously maniacal," and two females with "strong suicidal propensities."[44] Following publication of the 1844 report, the alarmed Poor Law commissioners instituted a special investigation of facilities for the insane in the Birmingham and Leicester workhouses, appointing Samuel Hitch, the respected medical superintendent of Gloucestershire County Asylum, as a temporary assistant Poor Law commissioner for the purpose.[45]

Hitch described the accommodation appropriated to the insane in the Birmingham workhouse as "the most secluded, and the most remote from the supervision," compared to other parts of the house. There were two distinct parts, known as the "Asylum Ward" and the "Mad Garret," the latter being exclusively for females. The lunatic wards were located in lofty buildings, facing each other across a courtyard divided by iron railings; the other two sides of the yard were enclosed by high walls. The courtyard was approached by a "long narrow and tortuous passage" from the main part of the workhouse. On the men's side there were five single rooms without windows, for refractory patients. The stone-floored dining hall was furnished only with benches round the walls, "each patient taking his rations in his hands and sitting down where he can find a convenient place"; it doubled as an exercise area on wet days. Passage ways were used both as sleeping quarters and day rooms. Restraint equipment was spread around the various parts of the buildings. There was a general absence of sanitary and washing facilities. Rooms were generally small and ill-ventilated, and overcrowding was endemic. Hitch construed the accommodation as "most defective" and was concerned particularly about the therapeutic and moral implications, there being

no place for exercise, none for occupation, neither for amusement, no means for keeping separate the clean and dirty, the noisy and quiet, the vicious and the moral, the disgusting and the approaching to convalescent—no means whatever of classification, but all are either circumscribed within high walls or shut up in a garret—When freed from the latter, the two sexes are so exposed to each other that the grossest immorality may take place unless more than a common supervision is kept over them.

Hitch at least managed to comment favorably on the cleanliness and order of the wards, and also observed that the patients appeared to be generally well treated. He assessed the condition of each individual, recommending several for transfer to an asylum. His overall conclusion, however, was that most of the inmates presented as "a sad spectacle of hopeless mental degradation," their condition hardly amenable to asylum treatment.[46]

During 1845, in the aftermath of Hitch's special report, a range of reforms and improvements were implemented in the Birmingham workhouse. The guardians effectively established a formalized lunatic asylum within its walls, with the surgeon Thomas Green acting as its dedicated medical officer.[47] In practice, this meant the continued frequent contravention of section 45, though the most dangerous and unmanageable patients were periodically dispatched to private asylums, including Hunningham Hall, near Leamington Spa, and Haydock Lodge in Lancashire.[48] Green, in effect, operated the wards as a testing ground for the projected Birmingham Borough Lunatic Asylum. When it opened in 1850, he was appointed as its medical superintendent and took many of the workhouse patients with him.[49]

Although in the early 1840s poor law unions were being regularly castigated for not sending even dangerous people to an asylum, it was not always entirely their fault. Despite the opening of more private asylums, the demand from unions to place disorderly lunatics was outstripping supply. County asylums like that at Stafford were severely overcrowded, notwithstanding programs of building expansion, rendering them often physically unable to accept any more referrals from workhouses and even leading them to seek to send back "harmless" lunatics.[50] Some private asylum proprietors, like Thomas Lewis at Duddeston Hall, were refusing admissions due to being full to capacity.[51] The complaint increasingly came both from public asylum superintendents and from local poor law authorities that the asylums were silting up with hopeless chronic cases, who could be managed in workhouses, while there was no room for the more acutely ill who required an asylum place.[52]

Toward the Workhouse Asylum

The lunacy legislation of 1845 mandated the universal establishment of public asylums for every county and county borough in England and Wales, either on their own or in combination with others.[53] The whole nature of provision for pauper lunatics was quite rapidly transformed as a consequence. A series of new county asylums were opened to cover the West Midlands region—Shropshire in 1845; Herefordshire in 1851; Warwickshire and Worcestershire, both in 1852.[54] The first borough lunatic asylum in England opened in Birmingham in 1850.[55] Each of these asylums was set up on the model of a therapeutic, "curative" institution, based on the approved practices of "moral management." Significant numbers of people were transferred into these institutions from private asylums and from workhouses, and these included both those deemed to have the potential for recovery and many whose conditions were considered chronic and "incurable."[56]

The new county and borough asylums, however, never had the capacity to provide for all mentally disordered people. The legislation had to be amended as early as 1846 to allow for some people to remain in workhouses.[57] Those left behind were primarily the idiots, imbeciles, and elderly demented people, who were not dangerous and for whom there was no prospect of "cure." As accommodation in the county asylums steadily became filled up, despite regular programs of building extensions and additions, most of them became seriously overcrowded.[58] By the late 1850s the old problems had reemerged, and growing numbers were again accumulating in workhouses. The phenomenon was evident in most of the main towns of the West Midlands, including Birmingham, Wolverhampton, West Bromwich, Stoke-on-Trent, Bromsgrove, Stourbridge, Coventry, and Worcester.[59] It was also becoming apparent that the workhouses were filling up not only with idiots and imbeciles but also with lunatics whose presentation was considered "harmless."[60]

However, not all of the insane population of the workhouses were "harmless." In some places, the workhouse was still being utilized as a receiving and assessment facility before a decision was made on committal to the asylum.[61] Thomas Green, in 1856, protested bitterly that this was standard practice in Birmingham and that it was highly detrimental to many patients. He contended that the incidence of insanity was often related to the trade cycle and cited a typical scenario: "A working man, or little tradesman, hitherto in flourishing circumstances, suddenly finds his means so far curtailed, that he is compelled to resort to his hard earned savings, which are soon exhausted. With the fear of poverty ever before him, he broods over his altered prospects—it may be that he takes to drinking, which hastens the catastrophe; finally the mind gives way, and he is a lunatic." The consequence, according to Green, was that the unfortunate man was then brought to the workhouse, "the very place, the dread of which has been the source of his malady."[62] He pointed out that the practice of detaining people in the workhouse was positively countertherapeutic, the orthodox view being that early intervention and treatment in the asylum offered the best prospects for cure.[63] He was not alone in his protestations. William Parsey, the medical superintendent of the Warwickshire Asylum, complained in 1858 that the custom was prevalent of sending pauper lunatics to the workhouse in the first place, "under short-sighted notions of economy." They would be sent on to the county asylum only when "difficulty of management" rendered further detention impracticable.[64] Similar complaints had been made by his counterpart at the Worcestershire Asylum, James Sherlock, in 1856.[65]

The national Commissioners in Lunacy, formed after the legislation of 1845, took an increasing interest in the problem and progressively included workhouse insane wards within their schedules of inspection visits. They would lodge criticisms about poor conditions or inappropriate accommodation and make representations to guardians about individuals who appeared unsuitable for the workhouse and required transfer to an asylum.[66] A public debate developed, involving asylum medical men, lunacy commissioners, and poor law commissioners, as to which people were most appropriate to be admitted into scarce and expensive asylum places and who could be catered to adequately in workhouses.[67] A growing consensus was emerging that the asylum should be for those who were acutely mentally ill, deemed curable, or disorderly and violent. The widespread reality of overcrowded county asylums must certainly have helped to concentrate minds.[68] It increasingly came to be considered not unreasonable for the workhouse to cater to people whose mental disorder was congenital or chronic, who were deemed incurable, who posed no threat to themselves or to others, and who mainly required basic care and attention. In some instances allegedly harmless pauper lunatics were being sent back to workhouses from public asylums, partly to relieve overcrowding in the latter. For example, the Birmingham Borough Asylum in 1859 was reported to be "so much crowded that it has been difficult to maintain the atmosphere of the different apartments sweet and pure enough for healthy respiration." Some relief was provided by the removal of twelve patients to the borough workhouse.[69]

The Commissioners in Lunacy were extremely reluctant to move from their premise that the public lunatic asylum was the appropriate place for the confinement of the insane. Their distaste for provision in the workhouse was made clear in their 1858 report, which condemned almost every aspect of it, including poor physical conditions, the low caliber of staff, lack of exercise facilities, meager dietary, excessive use of mechanical restraint, and so on. They were particularly unimpressed with the principle and practices of designated insane wards.[70] A visit to the lunatic wards of the Wolverhampton workhouse in May 1858 resulted in some fairly trenchant criticisms. The pauper patients were described as "dirty in their persons and dress; their clothes are in many instances ragged, and generally they present a listless and neglected appearance." The people attending them were "quite unfitted for such responsible duties"; the female ward attendant was "a rough and dirty young woman." There were no means of occupation or amusement. Several of the patients were considered to require immediate removal to an asylum.[71] The commissioners' intervention had some effect, for the Wolverhampton guardians were stung into action. Most of the defects were quickly remedied, including the replacement of the unsatisfactory pauper attendants with paid staff, improvements to the accommodation, enlargement of the airing courts, and a better dietary. Having made these changes, the guardians considered that they had done enough and were now providing satisfactory facilities, even comparable to those in a county asylum. Tellingly, their view was endorsed by Andrew Doyle, the Poor Law Board's inspector.[72]

Conclusion: Pragmatism and Economy

Throughout the period under consideration, under Old and New Poor Laws, the parish or union workhouse constituted an important element in the care of mentally disordered people, both in the West Midlands and elsewhere. Although a substantial proportion of the clientele provided for might have been "idiots" or "imbeciles," there was a continually fluctuating but often significant number of "lunatics" within many workhouses. If there was a consistent threshold for determining when a person became unsuitable for the workhouse and required a specialist lunatic asylum placement, it was dangerousness rather than diagnosis. Once an individual posed significant risks to staff and other inmates, or to themselves, creating management problems beyond the capability of workhouse staff, they were likely to be transferred. Forsythe and others have demonstrated in their important Devon study that some poor law unions were more flexible than others in determining when a person required transfer to an asylum, with therapeutic considerations prevailing in some instances.[73] There is some evidence that this sort of differential decision making also took place in parts of the West Midlands. However, despite such exceptions, considerations of economy remained the key determinant, exemplified particularly by the traffic of individuals back and forth between workhouse and asylum, according to their behavioral presentation. The creation of insane wards within some workhouses, despite the ongoing risk of conflict with legality, demonstrated the lengths to which guardians were prepared to go to minimize the use of public or private asylums.

By 1860 a number of factors had coalesced to confirm the position of the workhouse in the fabric of services for the insane. Some of these were external and related to the county lunatic asylums. It was becoming apparent that the high hopes and expectations that had surrounded the development of the public asylum system, particularly as regards the achievement of recoveries and "cures," were not being realized. Associated with this was the accumulation of chronic and hopeless patients, leading to asylums silting up and becoming overcrowded, which in turn restricted the numbers of new patients who could be received into them. These difficulties played into the hands of boards of guardians determined to resist unnecessary expenditure on expensive asylum care, especially if it now appeared that people were unlikely to benefit from it. Commissioners and inspectors found that they had to shift their emphasis from discouragement of provision in workhouses to the promotion and enforcement of basic standards within them. The insane ward, once frowned on, was to gradually become the accepted way of managing and caring for lunatics in the urban workhouse. That having been established, the basis was laid for the permeation of a system of what were, in effect, workhouse asylums. The integral role of workhouses in institutional provision for mentally disordered people, in the West Midlands and beyond, would be assured for decades to come.[74]

Notes

1. I have, in this chapter, largely used the contemporary terminology of "lunatic" for mentally ill person, and "idiot" and "imbecile" for people with what would now be called a learning disability, while "insane" tended to be used as a blanket term to cover all forms of mental disorders.

2. Andrew Scull, *The Most Solitary of Afflictions: Madness and Society in Britain, 1700–1900* (New Haven: Yale University Press, 1993); Joseph Melling and Bill Forsythe, *The Politics of Madness: The State, Insanity and Society in England, 1845–1914* (London: Routledge, 2006).

3. *An Act for the Better Care and Maintenance of Lunatics, Being Paupers or Criminals in England*, 1808, 48 Geo. 3, Cap. 96; *An Act for the Regulation of the Care and Treatment of Lunatics*, 1845, 8 and 9 Vic., Cap. 100; *An Act to Amend the Laws for the Provision and Regulation of Lunatic Asylums for Counties and Boroughs, and for the Maintenance and Care of Pauper Lunatics, in England*, 1845, 8 and 9 Vic., Cap. 126; Kathleen Jones, *A History of Mental Health Services* (London: Routledge and Kegan Paul, 1972); Leonard Smith, *"Cure, Comfort and Safe Custody": Public Lunatic Asylums in Early Nineteenth-Century England* (London: Leicester University Press, 1999).

4. Andrew Scull, *Museums of Madness: The Social Organisation of Insanity in Nineteenth-Century England* (London: Allen Lane, 1979).

5. Scull, *Most Solitary of Afflictions*, 334–74.

6. William L. Parry-Jones, *The Trade in Lunacy* (London: Routledge and Kegan Paul, 1972); Charlotte Mackenzie, *Psychiatry for the Rich: A History of Ticehurst Asylum, 1792–1917* (London: Routledge and Kegan Paul, 1992).

7. Roy Porter, *Mind Forg'd Manacles: A History of Madness in England from the Restoration to the Regency* (Cambridge: Cambridge University Press, 1987), 129–33; Anne Digby, *From York Lunatic Asylum to Bootham Park Hospital* (York: University of York, Borthwick Papers, 1986); Leonard Smith, *Lunatic Hospitals in Georgian England, 1750–1830* (London: Routledge, 2007).

8. Leonard Smith, "The County Asylum in the 'Mixed Economy of Care,'" in *Insanity, Institutions and Society, 1800–1914: A Social History of Madness in Comparative Perspective*, ed. Joseph Melling and Bill Forsythe (London: Routledge, 1999), 23–47.

9. David J. Mellett, *The Prerogative of Asylumdom: Social, Cultural and Administrative Aspects of the Institutional Treatment of the Insane in Nineteenth-Century Britain* (New York: Garland, 1982), 137; Peter Bartlett, *The Poor Law of Lunacy: The Administration of Pauper Lunatics in Mid-Nineteenth-Century England* (London: Leicester University Press, 1999).

10. Bartlett, *Poor Law of Lunacy*, 51–55.

11. Bill Forsythe, Jospeh Melling, and Robert Adair, "The New Poor Law and the County Pauper Lunatic Asylum: The Devon Experience, 1834–1884," *Social History of Medicine* 9, no. 3 (1996): 335–55.

12. British Parliamentary Papers (hereafter BPP), 1834 (27), *Report from His Majesty's Commissioners for Inquiring into the Administration and Practical Consequences of the Poor Laws*, app. A, 171 A, 266 A, 429 A, 527 A, 662 A, app. C, 168c.

13. BPP, 1816 (6), *Select Committee on Madhouses in England*, 54.

14. *An Act for the Better Care and Maintenance of Lunatics, Being Paupers or Criminals in England*, 1808, 48 Geo. 3, sec. 18.

15. *Wolverhampton Chronicle*, October 7, 28, 1818; William White, *History, Gazetteer and Directory of Staffordshire* (Sheffield: privately printed, 1834), 136.

16. Worcestershire County Record Office (hereafter CRO), QS 92j/35/6; Staffordshire CRO, D550/1, Staffordshire General Lunatic Asylum, Minute Book of Visitors, July 11, 1821.

17. Warwickshire CRO, DR 126/687, List of the Poor in St. Mary's Workhouse, 1819, 1825.

18. Shropshire CRO, QS/122, "Returns of Insane Paupers," February 1, 1829.

19. BPP, 1826 (21), *Lunatics (Returns)*, 90, 91. For further discussion of the unusual arrangements that developed in Shropshire, see Shropshire CRO, QS/122, "Draft Return to Secretary of State Relative to Oswestry Lunatic Asylum," November 6, 1841.

20. BPP, 1826 (21), *Lunatics (Returns)*, 91; Shropshire CRO, QS 183/1, Reports of Visiting Justices, April 8, 1839; *Report of the Metropolitan Commissioners in Lunacy to the Lord Chancellor* (London: Bradbury and Evans, 1844), add., 43.

21. *An Act for the Better Care and Maintenance of Lunatics, Being Paupers or Criminals in England*, 1808, 48 Geo. 3, sec. 18.

22. Jones, *Mental Health Services*, 124–25; Mellett, *Prerogative of Asylumdom*, 136–37.

23. For the development of private madhouses and asylums in the West Midlands, see Leonard Smith, "The Pauper Lunatic Problem in the West Midlands, 1818–1850," *Midland History* 21 (1996): 106–13; L. Smith, "Eighteenth-Century Madhouse Practice: The Prouds of Bilston," *History of Psychiatry* 3 (1992): 45–52; L. Smith, "To Cure Those Afflicted with the Disease of Insanity: Thomas Bakewell and Spring Vale Asylum," *History of Psychiatry* 4 (1993): 107–27; L. Smith, "Duddeston Hall and the 'Trade in Lunacy,' 1835–65," *Birmingham Historian* 8 (1992): 16–22; L. Smith, "Sandfield House Lunatic Asylum, Lichfield, 1820–1856," *Staffordshire Studies* 10 (1998): 71–75.

24. L. Smith, "Duddeston Hall," 16–17; *Metropolitan Commissioners*, 42, 230–31.

25. Birmingham Archives (hereafter BA), Birmingham Union Board of Guardians (hereafter UBG), minutes, for example, July 2, 1839, April 7, July 7, 1840; Aston

UBG, minutes, for example, May 16, August 29, 1837, January 9, 1838, April 9, 1839; Warwickshire CRO, CR 51/1581, Warwick Union: Minute Book, July 11, 1837; CR 51/218, Solihull Union: Minute Book, November 9, 1836, June 28, 1837, January 3, 1838, CR 51/219, April 3, September 25, 1839; CR 51/299, Nuneaton Board of Guardians, minutes, December 23, 1840; CR 51/549, Rugby UBG, July 2, 1842; Worcestershire CRO, Kidderminster Board of Guardians, Union Letter Book, April 16, 1840, April 16, October 10, 1843; Bromsgrove Board of Guardians, 251/400/1 (ii), May 11, November 23, 1840, December 27, 1841; March 7, 1842, 251/400/2 (ii), August 29, 1842, March 27, May 1, June 26, December 4, 1843; October 7, 1844.

26. Kathleen Jones, *Lunacy, Law and Conscience* (London: Routledge & Kegan Paul, 1955), 161–62; Ruth G. Hodgkinson, "Provision for Pauper Lunatics, 1834–1871," *Medical History* 10 (1966): 138–54; Michael Donnelly, *Managing the Mind: A Study of Medical Psychology in Early Nineteenth-Century Britain* (London: Tavistock, 1983), 13–15.

27. Warwickshire CRO, CR 51/1581, Warwick Union: Minute Book, May 18, 1839.

28. Wolverhampton City Library Archives, Wolverhampton Board of Guardians, "Report of the Workhouse Master, 1842–5," October 1, 1842; December 31, 1842.

29. Worcestershire CRO, 251/400/1(ii), December 23, 1839, March 23, April 6, 1840.

30. Warwickshire CRO, CR 51/299, Nuneaton Board of Guardians, minutes, September 8, 1842.

31. BA, Birmingham UBG, minutes, January 15, 1844, 2.

32. Jones, *Mental Health Services*, 132–49.

33. *Metropolitan Commissioners*, 6–7.

34. BA, Birmingham UBG, minutes, April 20, 1836; Aston UBG, minutes, March 29, 1842; Warwickshire CRO, CR 51/1581, June 6, 1837, June 25, 1839; Dudley Reference Library, Dudley Board of Guardians, minutes, March 2, 1846.

35. Birmingham Guardians, April 7, 1835.

36. Worcestershire CRO, 251/400/1 (ii), December 23, 1839, 251/400/2 (i), March 7, 1842.

37. BPP, 1816 (6), *Madhouses in England*, 46, 54.

38. BPP, 1826 (21), 90–91.

39. Shropshire CRO, 183/1, Reports of Visiting Justices, April 8, 1839.

40. *Metropolitan Commissioners*, 43; *Further Report of the Commissioners in Lunacy*, 1847, 107; *Fifth Annual Report of the Commissioners in Lunacy*, 1850, 7; *Seventh Annual Report of the Commissioners in Lunacy*, 1852, 7. Shropshire CRO, Kingsland Asylum: Justices Reports, July 29, 1852, October 26, 1853.

41. Shropshire CRO, Reports of Visiting Justices, April 8, 1839. One of the assistants "appears to be suffering from scrofula and has been brought up in the Workhouse which she has never left"; the other was "a young woman who was described as having been taken into the house quite destitute and having gone out was unable to obtain employment and was therefore again admitted into the Workhouse."

42. BA, Birmingham UBG, minutes, April 7, 1835.

43. BA, Aston UBG, minutes, May 16, 1837.

44. *Metropolitan Commissioners*, 1844, 10, 98–9, 136, 234–35.

45. For Hitch, see Leonard Smith, "'A Worthy Feeling Gentleman': Samuel Hitch at Gloucester Asylum, 1828–1847," in *150 Years of British Psychiatry*, vol. 2, *The Aftermath*, ed. Hugh Freeman and German Berrios (London: Athlone, 1996), 479–99.

46. National Archives, MH 12/13288/18261, Samuel Hitch, "Report of the Insane Poor Confined in the Workhouse Birmingham," October 31, 1844.

47. BA, Birmingham UBG, minutes, January 27, July 22, 1845.

48. BA, MS 344, CB1 A, Male and Female Casebooks, 1845–50.

49. Birmingham Guardians, minutes, October 30, 1849, May 22, June 5, 1850.

50. L. Smith, *Safe Custody*, 65, 71–72, 79–82, 172–74; British Library, Additional Manuscripts, 40, 429, Peel Papers, vol. 249, fos. 114–15, February 23, 1841, Garrett to Peel.

51. Birmingham Guardians, minutes, August 6, 1844.

52. National Archives, MH 50/1, Commissioners in Lunacy, Minute books, December 10, 1845, February 12, 1846.

53. *An Act for the Regulation of the Care and Treatment of Lunatics*, 1845, 8 and 9 Vic., Cap. 100; *An Act to Amend the Laws for the Provision and Regulation of Lunatic Asylums for Counties and Boroughs, and for the Maintenance and Care of Pauper Lunatics, in England*, 1845, 8 and 9 Vic., Cap. 126.

54. Shropshire CRO, QS 183/4, April 7, 1845. The Shropshire and Montgomery Lunatic Asylum was built under the legislation of 1808.

55. *Sixth Annual Report of Commissioners in Lunacy*, 1851, 23; *Seventh Annual Report of Commissioners in Lunacy*, 1852, 5, app. A39. Herefordshire did not have its own asylum but participated with Monmouthshire, Radnorshire, and Breconshire in the Joint Counties Lunatic Asylum, at Abergavenny.

56. Scull, *Most Solitary of Afflictions*, 266–93; Peter McCandless, "Insanity and Society: A Study of the English Lunacy Reform Movement, 1815–1870" (PhD diss., University of Wisconsin, 1974), 253–54, 270.

57. McCandless, "Insanity and Society," 271.

58. Scull, *Most Solitary of Afflictions*, 268–81; Peter McCandless, "'Build! Build!' The Controversy over the Care of the Chronically Insane in England, 1855–70," *Bulletin of the History of Medicine* 53 (1979): 553–74.

59. Janet Saunders, "Quarantining the Weak-Minded: Psychiatric Definitions of Degeneracy and the Late-Victorian Workhouse," in *The Anatomy of Madness: Essays in the History of Psychiatry*, vol. 3, *The Asylum and Its Psychiatry*, ed. William F. Bynum, Roy Porter, and Michael Shepherd (London: Routledge, 1988), 273–96; *Fifth Report of the Commissioners in Lunacy* (1850), app. A, 28; *Sixth Report* (1851), app. D, 46; *Ninth Report* (1855), app. C; *Tenth Report* (1856), app. C; *Eleventh Report* (1857), app. F.

60. McCandless, "Insanity and Society," 275–83.

61. Bartlett, *Poor Law of Lunacy*, 155.

62. Birmingham City Library, Local Studies Section, Birmingham Borough Lunatic Asylum, Fifth Annual Report, January 1856, 33.

63. Ibid., Sixth Annual Report, January 1857, 26.

64. Warwickshire CRO, CR 1664/30, County Lunatic Asylum, Annual Report, 1858, 5.

65. Worcestershire CRO, BA 8343, Third Annual Report of the County and City Lunatic Asylum, 1856, 29.

66. David J. Mellett, "Bureaucracy and Mental Illness: The Commissioners in Lunacy, 1845–90," *Medical History* 25 (1981): 221–50.

67. Bartlett, *Poor Law of Lunacy*, 45–6, 206–23; McCandless, "Insanity and Society," 281–308; Mellett, "Bureaucracy and Mental Illness," 236–39; Mellett, *Prerogative of Asylumdom*, 137–57.

68. Hodgkinson, "Provision for Pauper Lunatics," 150.

69. Birmingham Borough Lunatic Asylum, Ninth Annual Report, January 1860, 32.

70. *Twelfth Annual Report of the Commissioners in Lunacy*, 1858, supplement, April 15, 1859, "On the Condition, Character, and Treatment of Lunatics in Workhouses," 1–33.

71. *Twelfth Annual Report of the Commissioners in Lunacy*, app. to supplement, 1859, 61.

72. BPP, 1859 (7), *Select Committee on Care and Treatment of Lunatics*, 128–30, 137, 150–51, 128, 135, 137.

73. Forsythe, Melling, and Adair, "New Poor Law," 339–52.

74. For examples, see Edward Myers, "Lunacy in the Stoke-upon-Trent Workhouse, 1834–1900," *Psychiatric Bulletin* 18 (1994): 492–94; Edward Myers, *A History of Psychiatry in North Staffordshire* (Leek: Churnet Valley Books, 1997), chap. 3, 65–115.

Part Two

The New Poor Law

Chapter Six

Workhouse Medicine in Ireland

A Preliminary Analysis, 1850–1914

Virginia Crossman

Introducing his *Guide for Irish Medical Practitioners* (1889), Professor Richard J. Kinkead noted that care of the sick population in Ireland devolved on state-supported functionaries to a far greater extent than in England or other European countries. In England, he observed, none but the actually destitute were entitled to medical relief, and therefore the artisan class "provided for themselves in sickness by the agency of co-operative organizations such as 'clubs' or by resort to cheap practitioners. In Ireland, on the contrary, all such citizens look as a matter of course to the tax-payer for medical relief." Kinkead calculated that the Irish poor law provided medical aid to over 840,000 people each year, or nearly one fifth of the population. Such dependency on state help in times of sickness was, he suspected, far from "beneficial for any community . . . because of the want of self-reliance and domestic providence which it inculcates, but as the system is such, the medical practitioner naturally assumes an importance in Ireland in advance of that which attaches to this position in other countries." Poor law medical officers were "incomparably the most important servants of the community . . . exercising the most direct and lasting influence upon the prosperity and happiness of the Irish people."[1] Yet despite the centrality of the poor law to the development of medical provision in Ireland, the history of Irish poor law medical services remains to be written. Recent research has begun to explore the evolution and administration of the dispensary system, but the operation of and treatment provided in workhouse infirmaries have received no detailed examination.[2] This chapter offers a preliminary analysis. It gives a concise overview of medical services under the Irish poor law, highlights a number of central developments, and provides an administrative and analytic context in which these developments might be explored further.

From the mid-nineteenth century, the hospital function of English workhouses acquired increasing importance as inmate populations came to be dominated by the sick, elderly, and infirm. By the late 1860s around

90 percent of workhouse inmates in the London area were either sick or elderly or both.[3] The proportion was lower in provincial workhouses but was still significant. The period after 1860 saw the gradual professionalization of workhouse nursing and improvements in medical facilities. Medical matters became a regular item on the agenda of boards of guardians, who found it increasingly difficult to ignore the advice of their medical officers.[4] From the later part of the nineteenth century, stricter classification and improved standards of care helped to lessen the stigma associated with treatment in workhouse hospitals; paupers became patients.[5] Progress was not uniform, however. As Alysa Levene has noted, "medical services for the poor were *ad hoc* and variable in coverage and quality . . . local services relied on the initiative of individual officers and long-held expectations on entitlements as well as finance and government directives."[6] In Ireland, too, the picture is one of gradual improvement but also considerable local variation. By the early twentieth century, standards of care across the country had improved, but workhouse hospitals remained poorly equipped and understaffed in comparison with county infirmaries and voluntary hospitals.

The difficulties and dilemmas facing Irish poor law medical officers in the mid-nineteenth century—parsimonious boards of guardians, poor pay and conditions, inadequate facilities, and untrained nursing staff—would have been all too familiar to their English colleagues.[7] Less familiar would have been the administrative structures within which they worked. Under the Irish Poor Relief Act of 1838, the country was divided into 130 poor law unions, each with a workhouse where the destitute could seek relief. Workhouses were provided with an infirmary under the control of a medical officer appointed by the local board of guardians. The duties of the medical officer were to attend the workhouse daily and when sent for by the master, matron, or porter; to examine paupers on admission to the workhouse and also patients in the sick wards; to give directions regarding the diet, classification, and treatment of the sick, children, and those of unsound mind; to report on defects in diet, drainage, and ventilation; and to record deaths on a weekly basis.[8]

During the late 1840s and early 1850s the poor law system was extended to meet the challenge of the Great Famine and its aftermath. A network of fever hospitals supported from the poor rates was established, outdoor relief was introduced, the number of poor law unions was increased, and a national dispensary system was created. Under the latter, the 163 poor law unions were divided into 723 dispensary districts, with at least one dispensary in each district staffed by a doctor.[9] There was also provision for the appointment of an apothecary and midwife. Any poor person unable to afford the fees charged by Irish physicians and surgeons was entitled to free medical treatment at the local dispensary. Since the normal fee was one guinea, the number of people who fell within this category was considerable. Once in full operation, the dispensary system was providing for the treatment on average of 754,243 cases a year from 1853 to 1862, increasing to 793,213 from 1863 to 1872. In subsequent decades the annual total declined somewhat, leveling out at around 600,000 cases in the 1880s and 1890s.[10]

The introduction of the dispensary system was followed in 1862 by the opening up of workhouse infirmaries to nondestitute patients. The poor law commissioners had originally hoped to create a comprehensive publicly funded medical service with county infirmaries, as well as dispensaries being brought within the poor law system. Leading figures within the Irish medical profession were strongly opposed to such a plan, since it would place them under the control of the poor law commissioners, and they fought a well organized and ultimately successful campaign to keep county infirmaries outside the poor law system. Not all members of the profession were hostile to the commissioners' plans for expansion. In the seventeenth and eighteenth centuries medicine was one of the few professions in Ireland open to Catholics. Control of the key regulatory bodies, the Royal College of Physicians of Ireland and the Royal College of Surgeons in Ireland, remained in the hands of Protestants, however, so that well into the nineteenth century Catholics found it difficult to obtain appointments within the majority of Irish hospitals. As a result Catholic doctors, in contrast to their Protestant colleagues, tended to welcome the expansion of poor law medical services as a way of opening up the profession.[11]

The creation of what were in effect general hospitals within the workhouse, accessible to both the poor and paying customers, was a second-best solution as far as the poor law commissioners were concerned, but they took satisfaction in what had been achieved. There was, they noted in 1863, "probably no country which possesses a more comprehensive and better organized system of intern and extern medical relief, established and secured by law, than Ireland."[12] By the later part of the 1860s, Ireland possessed what Ronald Cassell has described as "a rationally administered, nationwide system providing the Irish poor with the most comprehensive free medical care available in the British Isles." Furthermore, by forcing the different categories of medical practitioners to cooperate with one another, the poor law "played a central role in driving the doctors toward a professional framework from within which they could advance their case most successfully."[13] For others, the weaknesses inherent in the poor law system, particularly with regard to hospital provision, outweighed the strengths. The development of Irish hospitals "along twin or parallel lines" with workhouse infirmaries operating separately from county infirmaries, Laurence Geary has argued, was a fundamental flaw in the system.[14] Moreover, the stigma associated with poor law institutions is widely believed to have deterred many people from seeking treatment. The majority of sick poor, it has been claimed, "preferred to die at home rather than enter an institution."[15]

The decades after 1860 saw major changes in the way the poor relief system operated. Levels of outdoor relief rose progressively so that, by the early 1880s, the average daily number in receipt of outdoor relief exceeded the average daily number in workhouses. In the first five years of the twentieth century, the average daily number in receipt of outdoor relief fluctuated between 56,672 and 57,875, while the daily average in workhouses was between 40,120 and 42,228.[16] Regulations governing outdoor relief in Ireland were more restrictive than those operating in England and Wales, with the result that sickness and disability featured even more prominently in the decision-making process. Under normal circumstances only people falling within the following categories were eligible: destitute poor persons permanently disabled from labor by age or infirmity, those temporarily disabled by sickness or accident, and destitute widows with two or more legitimate children. Generally speaking, around one-third of cases relieved fell into the first category and between one-half and two-thirds into the second. In many unions, a medical certificate was a prerequisite for outdoor relief, placing considerable extra pressure on medical officers. Relief could be given in kind, in cash, or as medical assistance. Guardians could pay for poor people to be nursed in their own home, for example, if they were too ill to be moved to the workhouse hospital.

By the end of the nineteenth century large numbers of sick people (or people certified to be sick) were receiving assistance funded from the poor rates in their own homes. One consequence of this was a decline in the proportion of sick admissions to workhouses. The proportion fell from 36 percent of total admissions in 1860, to 27 percent in 1870, and 23.5 percent in 1890. Workhouse registers similarly record fewer people entering with medical complaints. The proportion of admissions to the Kinsale workhouse in County Cork noted to have some form or sickness of disability declined from 46 percent in 1871 to 28 percent in 1891.[17] An even sharper decline is evident in the registers of the North Dublin Union workhouse, where sick admissions fell from 63 percent in 1861 to 23 percent in 1891.[18] It is important to note, however, that this may be a result of less rigorous record keeping in addition to lower levels of sickness. In 1861 the NDU registers contain reference to a wide variety of illnesses and medical complaints. In 1891 such detail is largely missing, concealed beneath generic terms such as "sick" or "hospital treatment." This makes it impossible to draw meaningful conclusions about change over time with regard to the precise number admitted sick or the type of medical complaints suffered by workhouse inmates. Where detailed information is available, it is evident that the majority of complaints fall into two main categories, those such as chest and lung diseases and eye and skin conditions, which can be linked directly to poor diet and bad housing, and those such as broken or sore limbs, where the complaint was such as to prevent the person from working.

The decline in sick admissions can be accounted for in two ways. The health of the population was improving due to rising living standards and the availability of medical relief, and outdoor relief meant that fewer people were being forced to seek assistance in the workhouse. Within the workhouse, however, the proportion of sick and infirm inmates was increasing. The percentage of able-bodied inmates on the first Saturday in the year dropped from 17 percent of the total in 1870 to 13 percent in 1900, while the number in the hospital rose from 31 to 44 percent.[19] Within individual workhouses a similar trend is apparent. In the Tralee workhouse in County Kerry, the proportion of inmates in the hospital increased from 22 percent in 1871 to 39 percent in 1891, while in Kilmallock in County Limerick it rose from 20 percent in 1871 to 36 percent in 1891.[20] Large city workhouses housed more able-bodied inmates and thus recorded lower proportions in the hospital. In the North Dublin Union workhouse, for example, 26 percent of inmates were in the hospital in 1881, 27 percent in 1891, and 28 percent in 1911. However, while the proportion in hospitals was relatively small compared to rural workhouses, this should not be taken to mean that the majority of NDU inmates were healthy. In 1881, in addition to those in hospitals, 40 percent of inmates were classified as infirm under medical treatment and a further 5 percent were on a hospital diet. In all, 71 percent of NDU inmates in 1881 were on a hospital diet, and 62 percent in 1891.[21] In the majority of workhouses, the sick and infirm together made up between one-half and two-thirds of inmates in the decades after 1870.

With the able-bodied increasingly being relieved outside the workhouse and a corresponding increase in the proportion of sick and infirm among workhouse inmates, the function of the institution changed. As one workhouse medical officer noted in 1872, the operation of outdoor relief "gave the option to them of that class who were able to leave the house, to do so," leaving "none but those incapacitated by bodily infirmity to remain."[22] In 1879 Local Government Board inspectors were directed to pay particular attention to the treatment of the elderly and the sick in workhouses, since "much of the space which was formerly occupied by the able-bodied and healthy inmates has now been allocated to the aged and infirm and the sick."[23] The growing importance of medical matters in workhouse administration was given official recognition in 1885, when the central poor law authorities decided to reorganize their inspectorate and to separate the medical work from the general poor law administration.[24] Central inspection was a key element in poor law administration and inspections increasingly focused on medical treatment and facilities. The poor law commissioners and, subsequently, the Local Government Board placed considerable emphasis on maintaining and, where possible, improving the condition of medical facilities, but they were realistic about what could be achieved with limited resources. While anxious to promote improvements that would "tend to lengthen the lives of the aged poor and add to the comforts of the sick"; they were, they explained in 1896, bound "to keep the difficulties [boards of guardians] encounter in their financial administration constantly before us."[25]

The belief that the stigma of the workhouse prevented poor people from seeking treatment was, and is, widely held. The sick poor, Geary states, "were reluctant to avail of these hospitals' services because of their association with the workhouses and with pauperism. Hospital inmates had to endure the same conditions as paupers in the workhouse." But while it is true that they had to wear workhouse clothing and abide by "the same restrictive rules and regulations," hospital inmates were not required to work, they were allowed more visitors, and they received a better diet.[26] These privileges distinguished hospital inmates from ordinary paupers and were valued as such. In 1871 John Lyne, an inmate of the Tralee workhouse, was punished for abusing the medical officer of the workhouse and threatening "to fix him if he continued to refuse him a tea diet."[27] Indeed, many guardians worried about conditions in hospitals being so attractive that people were entering the workhouse to take advantage of them. A member of the Cork Board of Guardians, for example, complained in 1885 that people were coming into the workhouse knowing that they would be better fed and clothed there "than the honest and decent people that remained struggling and striving outside."[28]

Many of those involved in the administration of workhouse infirmaries believed popular attitudes to be rooted in sentiment, not rationality. Dr. J. Lynass, a medical officer at the Belfast workhouse, told the viceregal commission on poor law reform in 1905 that there was "a sentimental repugnance to a workhouse institution" that deterred the respectable poor from entering.[29] Popular prejudice against the workhouse was not based on sentiment alone, however. Reports of inadequate facilities and poor levels of care emerging from within the Irish medical profession in the 1890s prompted the *British Medical Journal* to send the trained nurse and experienced hospital administrator, Catherine Wood, to investigate the state of workhouse infirmaries in 1895.[30] Having visited twenty-eight poor law unions across the country, she concluded that the vast majority of workhouse infirmaries were not fit for purpose. They were generally too small, resulting in serious overcrowding. It was not uncommon, she found, for patients to be accommodated two to a bed. Buildings were often badly designed, with common problems being damp walls, inadequate ventilation, drainage and sanitation, and insufficient and untrained staff. A typical example was the infirmary at Cootehill in County Cavan. In the infirmary wards, she found walls of "undressed stone, colour washed, the roof open to the slates, small windows facing north, in heavy iron frames, badly fitted, draughty and leaking. . . . A rusty grate, a chimney, a bench, a bucket chair, a few arm chairs and a small table completes the picture of a country workhouse ward." Sanitary appliances were of "the most elementary kind," with none inside. Many infirmaries had no provision for hot water. Wood's report recommended the employment of trained nurses in every workhouse infirmary; the employment of night nurses; the introduction of efficient sanitary systems, including the provision of an adequate water supply and efficient methods for disposing of excreta; and the provision of day rooms and, where possible, gardens.[31]

The official response to the British Medical Association report and ongoing campaign to reform the workhouse system was to stress that workhouse infirmaries were regularly inspected and did meet basic standards of hygiene and care and that the responsibility for improvement lay with local boards of guardians rather than the central government. In 1896 the Local Government Board noted that during the past year their inspectors had reported "important improvements" in the condition and management of workhouses, including the appointment of a number of assistant nurses for night duty, which had "added materially to the comfort of inmates." At the same time, however, the financial condition of many poorer unions precluded the guardians "from placing the workhouses and hospitals under their charge upon the same level as regards comfort and equipment as the modern hospitals with which they have been to their disadvantage so frequently contrasted."[32] As in England, nursing was originally provided by untrained pauper attendants, but whereas in England poor law regulations defined the duties and responsibilities of the workhouse nurse, the Irish regulations made no reference to nursing except in relation to the duties of the workhouse matron, who was required to "take care, with the assistance of the nurses, of the children and sick paupers; and to provide the proper diet for the children and sick paupers, and to furnish them with such changes of clothes and linen as may be necessary."[33] From 1882 boards of guardians were required to appoint "such assistants as the Board of Guardians, with the consent of the Local Government Board, shall deem necessary" for the efficient performance of the duties of the medical officer and matron; all appointments were to be advertised and advance notice given in the minutes.[34]

Raising standards in workhouse infirmaries appears to have been an even slower and more protracted process in Ireland than in England. Poor law boards were reluctant to incur additional costs and regarded many of the circulars issued from the center as unwarranted and unnecessary. At the same time, the growing presence of nuns in Irish workhouses made it easier for boards of guardians to resist pressure to appoint trained nurses on the grounds that they were not needed. Nuns could be employed on lower salaries than trained nurses and were of impeccable moral standing.[35] During the 1870s and 1880s many workhouse infirmaries came under the control of nuns, although boards of guardians continued to rely on pauper assistants for general duties and night nursing. In 1881 the Cork workhouse infirmary, which accommodated an average of 961 patients, was attended by 15 paid nurses (9 nuns and 6 lay nurses) and 178 pauper nurses who received extra rations, including a daily allowance of porter. In 1877 the guardians had offered to replace the latter with a weekly cash allowance that could be claimed on leaving the workhouse. This offer was rejected and the pauper nurses stopped work until the allowance of porter was reintroduced.[36]

Throughout the 1890s the Local Government Board strove to convince boards of guardians of the importance of appointing nurses with training and experience. A circular issued in 1890 described nursing as "crucial to successful recovery. The highest skill and attention on the part of the medical officer, may be neutralized by the ignorance and incapacity of the nurse charged with the duty of carrying out his instructions." When filling vacancies, therefore, boards should offer such salaries as would persuade qualified persons to apply.[37] Exhortation having proved ineffective, the Local Government Board finally took a more proactive approach. In 1897 the board prohibited the appointment of any workhouse inmate as nurse and defined the latter's duties as superintending and controlling all the other nurses, assistant nurses, and attendants "subject to the directions of the Medical Officer in matters of treatment and to the directions of the master or matron in all other matters." Paupers could still act as attendants but only if "approved by the Medical Officer for the purpose, and . . . under the immediate supervision of a paid officer of the Guardians."[38]

Following the Local Government Act of 1898 the regulations regarding workhouse nursing were tightened further and the qualifications required of trained nurses clarified. A trained nurse was stated to mean anyone with a certificate of proficiency in nursing and two years of clinical or hospital experience. A qualified nurse was defined as a person who had obtained a certificate of proficiency in nursing from a public general hospital, a workhouse infirmary or fever hospital, or a nursing institution. Attendants were to be "at least 21 years of age" and "of good health and character." The nurse of the workhouse was responsible for nursing and feeding the sick, supervising the nursing staff, and maintaining proper order and discipline in the sick wards. She was "to carry out all reasonable directions of the medical officer, to whom and to the Board of Guardians only . . . she shall be subordinate, save as regards the general disciplinary control of the Master of the Workhouse." In an emergency, the master was directed to employ fit persons to act as temporary nurses if it appeared to the medical officer that this was "requisite for the proper treatment of any patient or patients" until the next meeting of the guardians.[39] Empowering the master to act directly on the advice of the medical officer significantly enhanced the latter's authority and was intended to prevent boards of guardians from repeatedly ignoring requests for additional nursing assistance. After 1898 the Local Government Board refused to sanction the appointment of any untrained or uncertified person as a nurse or assistant nurse in a workhouse infirmary, even in a temporary capacity. Guardians were not required to remove those already in place, however. By 1913 the total number of trained nurses employed in Irish workhouses had reached 268, together with 248 qualified nurses and 357 nursing sisters, but there were still twelve workhouses without a trained nurse.[40]

The efficiency of any workhouse hospital depended on the medical officer and his relationship with the board of guardians. "The benefit conferred on the poor by the hospital," one observer noted in 1867, "will depend partly on the professional character of the medical officer in charge, partly on the degree of independence which he may be able to maintain towards the guardians, partly on the certainty with which he can calculate on his orders being carried out by the subordinate officers of the house."[41] Where medical officers came into conflict with boards of guardians it was generally over money. They were spending too much on medicines, or they were making too many recommendations that involved extra expenditure, whether with regard to providing hot rather than cold water baths for new admissions or improvements in the diet or the necessity of boarding out orphan and deserted children. As the chair of the Cork guardians remarked in frustration to his colleagues in 1876, they had a simple choice, either "get rid of your doctors or be guided by them."[42] The competing demands made on medical officers are evident in the response of the medical officer of the Mountmellick workhouse, Dr. Joseph Clarke, to an order from the board of guardians in 1871 to explain "the cause of the great increase of stimulants for the last year, as compared with 1860." Clarke acknowledged that there had been a considerable increase in the amount of stimulants prescribed despite their being "no great difference in the numbers admitted into the hospital": 724 in 1860 and 722 in 1870. The explanation lay in the type of cases treated. Those in 1860 were generally of a mild form. They were chiefly children and did not require stimulants. In 1870, however,

the cases admitted were more adults, many suffering from very exhaustive diseases. Amongst them I had to treat 84 cases of ophthalmia. . . . Cases of this kind require stimulants, tonics and nutritious diet. They cause the greatest anxiety to the medical attendant, as the lapse of a few hours may be the loss of vision of one or both eyes. It would be false economy to withhold anything that might be the means of preventing blindness and consequently causing a permanent charge on the Union.

Furthermore, the type of fever prevalent in 1860 was milder than that he had been treating over the past year when he had to contend against the worst form of fever I have seen since the famine. I had 99 cases admitted to hospital, some of them heads of large, helpless families and again I am happy to say I was equally successful in restoring them to their homes. I have never spared the means allowed . . . for the preservation of life or health, and never shall. . . . I also beg to state that there is a great increase in the number of infirm since 1860, the average numbers being in that year 91, and in the present year 156, all very delicate, particularly those in the female departments and they have very often required stimulants.[43]

In justifying his actions, Clarke was careful to stress not only his professional competence, diligence, and care for his patients but also his concern to protect the financial interests of the union.

When assessing developments in workhouse medicine, there is an important distinction to be drawn between workhouse hospitals in the major urban unions, which treated large numbers of patients and were relatively well staffed and equipped, and those in rural unions, which could accommodate only a small number of patients often under very primitive conditions. The former were often seriously overcrowded, and the staff operated under constant pressure. In 1879, for example, the poor law authorities found it necessary to restrict admissions to the Belfast Union Infirmary due to the extent of overcrowding that was putting patients' lives at risk. An inspector's report in May 1879 noted that there were

at present 272 patients more than [there] should be. The medical officers have repeatedly reported on the state of the Infirmary and state that the recovery of their patients is retarded by it; that ulcers will not heal, that they dread to perform an operation lest erysipelas or some other disease attending on overcrowding would attack the patients. They add that on many occasions they found it necessary to discharge patients before a cure had been accomplished as they had observed that the illness came either to a standstill or retrograded.[44]

Overcrowding remained a problem, but by the early twentieth century the infirmary had developed into an important training hospital that treated large numbers of surgical cases and provided an array of specialist services.[45] The board of guardians had voted in favor of opening the workhouse wards to medical and surgical students from Queen's College, Belfast, in 1877, and a program for nurse training was established in the early 1900s. From 1901 all candidates for the position of probationer nurse in the Belfast workhouse were required to pass a preliminary qualifying examination in arithmetic, writing, and spelling. They then embarked on a three-year training program, at the end of which they were examined. Successful candidates received a certificate of training that qualified them to be registered as trained nurses by the Local Government Board.[46]

Situated in the grounds of the workhouse on Lisburn Road, the infirmary was by far the largest hospital in the city, containing 1,500 beds in 1909. This was more than all the voluntary hospitals put together. In 1911 the two major voluntary hospitals, the Royal Victoria and the Mater Infirmorum, had 234 and 200 beds respectively. Specialist institutions such as the Ophthalmic Hospital, Royal Maternity Hospital, and Forster Green Hospital for Consumption and Chest Diseases were considerably smaller.[47] The wards of the infirmary were open to medical students in the final year of their training, the "lock wards" providing what were described as "unrivalled opportunities for the study of venereal disease." There was a maternity department in which around 300 confinements were attended every year, and a children's block accommodating 200 patients had recently been opened. A fever hospital with a capacity of 100 beds was attached to the union, and a special hospital and sanatorium had been opened in Whiteabbey in the north of the city, where 265 consumptive cases were under treatment.[48]

In rural unions the most pressing problems facing workhouse medical officers were lack of facilities and nursing staff. In the mid-1890s the medical officer of Ballycastle Union made repeated requests for the appointment of a trained night nurse and for structural improvements such as the provision of a bathroom, "as the want of such a sanitary arrangement retards the treatment of disease and adds much to the labour of nursing." The guardians were unconvinced, noting that they had recently, "on the recommendation of the medical officer, procured two portable baths for the infirmary which are at present in use and found to be very convenient and satisfactory. . . . From frequent examinations of the infirmary etc. the guardians are satisfied that all necessary attendance etc. is provided for the patients and that any further expense in this direction would be only a waste of the poor rates."[49] It was only when the Local Government Board threatened to dissolve the board of guardians "if the guardians do not take the necessary steps to appoint a competent trained night nurse" that the board finally resolved to advertise for a trained nurse at a salary of twenty pounds per year.[50] Here, too, conditions did improve, but the Ballycastle guardians remained wary of unnecessary expenditure. They reacted most indignantly to an inspector's report in 1901 drawing attention to the lack of an operating room: "This subject is becoming a 'hardy annual' with your official. He returns to it again and again with a faithful persistence. The need is not a pressing one; since 1896 there have been only five, or five serious, operations and these were all on paying patients." While "not averse" to providing an operating room, the guardians claimed to be more concerned about improving the sewerage of the fever hospital on which they were spending £150, even though the "inspector never discovered the need. It escaped his eagle eye. He never reported on it." The guardians also rejected the inspector's critical comments regarding the nursing staff:

He is of opinion the nursing arrangements are not adequate. About ten years ago one woman, aged and unqualified, acted as a nurse. Now we have two nurses and a ward servant and yet like Oliver Twist your inspector wants more. Both our nurses are trained and are so recognized by your Board. One of them possesses your own diploma certifying she is a trained nurse within the meaning of the Local Government Act of 1898. . . . In addition to our infirmary staff being trained nurses, we have a nurse in the fever hospital also ranking as a trained nurse and did the act of 1898 permit two "trained nurses" she would qualify as she is also recognized by you. There is scarcely a union in Ulster can excel this and yet this is only a small and poor union which however believes in doing things well.[51]

Here, the guardians were seeking to demonstrate their superior understanding of local needs and interests, as well as their superior knowledge of the state of the workhouse.

The chief obstacles to improving standards of medical care were inertia on the part of boards of guardians and lack of finance. With no specific income set aside to support sick inmates or meet hospital expenses, guardians had neither incentive nor designated funds to initiate improvements.[52] Local government reorganization in 1898 provided an opportunity to remove these obstacles, at least in part. The Local Government Act made it easier for local authorities to borrow money for capital projects, and, under the financial regulations that accompanied the act, central government undertook to meet half the cost of officers' salaries. This included the salary of the workhouse nurse, but only if she was a qualified nurse. The act thus gave boards of guardians a direct financial incentive to appoint a trained nurse. It also empowered them to convert the union hospital into a district hospital providing, among other things, for the accommodation of paying patients. The aim was to create a new framework for poor law medicine that would further lessen the link between pauperism and health care. Few, if any, boards appear to have utilized the district hospital provision, and the full impact of the changes was lost in the political upheaval that followed the Easter Rising, but a significant number of boards did take out loans to undertake building works and other improvements.[53]

In 1905 the viceregal commission on poor law reform in Ireland circulated a questionnaire to workhouse medical officers regarding nursing arrangements and conditions in hospitals. In some unions little appeared to have changed since Wood had toured the country in 1895. The medical officer of the Enniskillen workhouse described his hospital as "far from what I would consider satisfactory. It is a relic [of] the barbarous past. . . . The guardians won't do anything." But others referred to recent improvements. All the wards in the Mount Bellew workhouse were reported to be "airy and well-lighted, and each has a lavatory erected within the last few years, and having all the latest sanitary accommodation." In Trim Union, the medical officer reported that the hospital was "taken advantage of by large numbers of the poor of the union, and in my opinion, the prejudices which existed in the minds of the poor as to entering the workhouse infirmary do not prevail amongst them at present. Many respectable people avail themselves of the advantages which the hospital affords." Significant progress had been made with regard to nursing; 125 out of 159 workhouse medical officers reported that nursing arrangements were satisfactory or better.[54]

By the end of the nineteenth century, the permanent population of work-houses in Ireland included a sizable proportion of elderly, infirm, and sick inmates. Their care occupied the time and attention of boards of guardians and their officers to an ever-increasing degree. The resulting pressures strained relations between boards of guardians and medical officers and between local and central authorities. Medical officers complained of poor conditions and inadequate facilities and pushed for more and better-trained nursing staff; boards of guardians grumbled about the cost of medicines and salaries; central government issued directives and sought to mediate between medical officers and guardians. As with other aspects of poor law administration, there was considerable local variation in the nature and quality of medical services provided. In far too many unions, poor law guardians found it impossible to reconcile their desire to keep rates low and adhere to the principle of less eligibility with the requirement to provide efficient and effective medical services.

But there were some in which medical officers were able to ensure that patients received effective treatment and were well cared for in reasonably comfortable surroundings. The workhouse doctor was described in 1895 as the Irish pauper's "only friend."[55] This is too simplistic a judgment. It fails to acknowledge the churchmen and philanthropists who lobbied for reform both individually and through organizations such as the Irish Workhouse Association. It also fails to acknowledge the role of the poor law authorities or those guardians who were prepared to follow their medical officer's advice. The tensions inherent in the relationship between medical officer and board of guardians have frequently been noted, but there was a third party in this relationship: the central authorities. While they were too tolerant of outdated facilities and poor quality care, they did consistently promote improvements and encourage more professional nursing provision. Additional research is needed before we can make a more comprehensive assessment of the practice of medicine within the workhouse and the standards to which this was expected to adhere. One thing is clear; only when we have a more complete understanding of how poor law medical services operated will it possible to evaluate either the evolution of medical care in Ireland or the complex relationship between health professionals, the public, and the state.

Notes

Research for this chapter was funded by an Economic and Social Research Council award for "Welfare Regimes under the Irish Poor Law, 1850–1921." I am grateful to project researcher Dr. Georgina Laragy for extracting the medical information from the North Dublin and Thurles Union admission registers and for her comments on an earlier draft. I am also grateful to Angela Negrine and Alistair Ritch for information and insights on workhouse nursing.

1. R. J. Kinkead, *The Guide for Irish Medical Practitioners* (Dublin: Falconer, 1889), v–vi.

2. Catherine Cox, "Medical Dispensary Service in Nineteenth-Century Ireland: Access, Transport and Distance," in *Cultures of Care in Irish Medical History, 1750–1970*, ed. Catherine Cox and Maria Luddy (Basingstoke, UK: Palgrave Macmillan, 2010), 57–78; Laurence M. Geary, "The Medical Profession, Health Care and the Poor Law in Nineteenth-Century Ireland," in *Poverty and Welfare in Ireland, 1838–1948*, ed. Virginia Crossman and Peter Gray (Dublin: Irish Academic Press, 2011), 189–206.

3. David Green, "Medical Relief and the New Poor Law in London," in *Health Care and Poor Relief in 18th and 19th Century Northern Europe*, ed. Ole P. Grell, Andrew Cunningham, and Robert Jütte (Aldershot, UK: Ashgate, 2002), 235.

4. See, for example, Michael W. Flinn, "Medical Services under the New Poor Law," in *The New Poor Law in the Nineteenth Century*, ed. Derek Fraser (London: Macmillan, 1976), 45–66; Margaret Anne Crowther, "Health Care and Poor Relief in Provincial England," in Grell, Cunningham, and Jütte, *Health Care and Poor Relief*, 203–19.

5. Margaret Anne Crowther, "Paupers or Patients? Obstacles to Professionalization in the Poor Law Medical Service before 1914," *Journal of the History of Medicine and Allied Sciences* 39 (1984): 33–55; Lynn Hollen Lees, *The Solidarities of Strangers: The English Poor Laws and the People, 1700–1948* (Cambridge: Cambridge University Press, 1998), 278–79.

6. Alysa Levene, "Between Less Eligibility and the NHS: The Changing Place of Poor Law Hospitals in England and Wales, 1929–39," *Twentieth Century British History* 20 (2009): 325. This point is confirmed by local studies, such as those by Angela Negrine, "Medicine and Poverty: A Study of the Poor Law Medical Services of the Leicester Union, 1867–1914" (PhD diss., University of Leicester, 2008); and Alistair E. S. Ritch, "Sick, Aged and Infirm: Adults in the New Birmingham Workhouse, 1852–1912" (MPhil diss., University of Birmingham, 2010).

7. For England, see Crowther, "Health Care," 214–16; Flinn, "Medical Services," 53.

8. General Order dated February 5, 1849, for Regulating the Management of Workhouses and the Duties of Workhouse Officers, article 68.

9. Virginia Crossman, *The Poor Law in Ireland, 1838–1948* (Dundalk: Irish Economic and Social History Society, 2006), 19–29, 38–43; Geary, "Medical

Profession," 190–91. From 1867 half the cost of the dispensary doctor's wages was met by the central government.

10. Figures for the number of cases of medical relief afforded under the Medical Charities Act extracted from the annual reports of the commissioners for administering the laws for the relief of the poor in Ireland and the Local Government Board for Ireland.

11. Laurence M. Geary, *Medicine and Charity in Ireland, 1718–1851* (Dublin: University College Dublin Press, 2004), 155–80; Geary, "'The Most Illiberal and Monopolising Corporation in Existence': The Royal College of Surgeons in Ireland and Professional Appointments to Irish County Infirmaries," in *Borderlands: Essays on Medicine and Literature in Honour of J. B. Lyons,* ed. Davis Coakley and Mary O'Doherty (Dublin: Royal College of Surgeons in Ireland, 2002), 106–14.

12. *Annual Report of the Commissioners for Administering the Laws for Relief of the Poor in Ireland . . .*, Parliamentary Papers (hereafter PP), 1863 (3135), xxii, 353.

13. Ronald D. Cassell, *The Irish Dispensary System and the Poor Law, 1836–1872* (Woodbridge: Boydell, 1997), 164.

14. Geary, *Medicine and Charity,* 215.

15. John F. Fleetwood, *The History of Medicine in Ireland* (Dublin: Skelling, 1983), 168.

16. *Annual Reports of the Local Government Board for Ireland,* PP, 1900 (Cd. 338); 1902 (Cd. 1259); 1903 (Cd. 1606); 1904 (Cd. 2012); 1904 (Cd. 2213); 1905 (Cd. 2320).

17. There were 311 sick people out of 618 admissions in 1871, and 291 out of 911 admissions in 1891, including those noted to be infirm (26 in 1871 and 47 in 1891). Cork County and City Archives, Kinsale Poor Law Union, indoor relief registers, BG/108/G.

18. Sick admissions were 2,599 out of 4,112 in 1861, and 796 out of 3,440 in 1891. National Archives of Ireland (hereafter NAI), North Dublin Union, indoor relief registers, BG/78/G. A similar trend is evident in the admission registers of the Thurles workhouse in County Tipperary, where the proportion of sick admissions declined from 38 percent (258 of 671 admissions) in 1871 to 12 percent (264 of 2,237 admissions) in 1889. County Tipperary, Thurles, Tipperary Local Studies Library, Thurles Poor Law Union, indoor relief registers.

19. The classified return of the number of inmates in workhouses on the first Saturday of January is from the *Local Government Board,* PP, 1900 (Cd. 338), xviii.

20. The average number remaining in the Tralee workhouse at the end of the week was 410 in 1871 and 417 in 1891; the average number in the hospital was 90 in 1871 and 158 in 1891. For Kilmallock the figures were 554 and 460 remaining, and 112 and 166 in the hospital. Kerry County Library, Tralee Board of Guardians Minute Books; Limerick County Library, Kilmallock Board of Guardians Minute Books, BG/106/A.

21. In 1881 the average number remaining was 2,343; in the hospital, 619; infirm under medical treatment, 940; and on a hospital diet, 1,665. In 1891 the average number remaining was 2,651; in the hospital, 714; and on a hospital diet, 1,651. NAI, North Dublin Board of Guardians Minute Books, BG/78/A.

22. Laois County Library, Portlaoise, Mountmellick Board of Guardians Minute Books, Medical Officer's Report, March 16, 1872.

23. General Instructional Circular to Inspectors, August 25, 1879, *Local Government Board,* PP, 1880 (C2603), xxviii, 58.

24. Following the introduction of the dispensary system in 1851, five medical inspectors had been appointed to oversee the administration of the system and provide regular reports on the facilities, medicines, and treatment provided in dispensaries, fever hospitals, and workhouse infirmaries. During the 1860s, partly in an effort to save money and partly to provide more flexibility, the poor law commissioners had merged the two separate inspectorates, allowing medical inspectors to conduct general inspections and general inspectors to report on medical facilities. In 1885, however, it was decided to revert to the previous arrangement "with a view to the better supervision of the administration of the Medical Charities and Public Health Acts and the inspection of the sanitary and dispensary districts throughout Ireland." *Local Government Board*, PP, 1885 (C4400), xxxiv, 43.

25. *Local Government Board*, PP, 1896 (C8153), xxxviii, 16.

26. Geary, "Medical Profession," 198.

27. Kerry County Library, Tralee Board of Guardians Minute Books, September 2, 1871.

28. Cited in Colman O'Mahony, *Cork's Poor Law Palace: Workhouse Life, 1838–90* (Cork: Rosmathun, 2005), 214.

29. *Poor Law Reform Commission (Ireland): Report of the Vice-regal Commission on Poor Law Reform in Ireland*, PP, 1906 (C3202), li, 385.

30. See, for example, Austin Meldon and Arthur Benson of the Irish Medical Association to the editor of the *Irish Times*, July 19, 1895. As in England, much of the pressure for reform came from the medical profession supported by social activists and philanthropists.

31. "Reports on the Nursing and Administration of the Irish Workhouse Infirmaries," *The British Medical Association Reports of the Poor-Law Medical System in Ireland, the Case of Irish Dispensary Doctors, and the Nursing and Administration of Irish Workhouse Infirmaries* (reprinted from the *British Medical Journal*) (London, 1904), 50, 60; Geary, "Medical Profession," 199–201.

32. *Local Government Board*, PP, 1896 (C8153), xxxviii, 16.

33. General Order, For Regulating the Management of Workhouses and the Duties of Workhouse Officers, February 5, 1849, art. 65, no. 11. For a discussion of developments in workhouse nursing in England, see Angela Negrine, "Nursing Paupers: A Case Study of Nursing at the Leicester Workhouse Infirmary, 1850–1905," unpublished paper. I am most grateful to Angela Negrine for providing me with a copy of this paper.

34. General Order, For Regulating the Meetings and Proceedings of Boards of Guardians in Ireland and the Appointment and Duties of Union Officers, December 18, 1882, arts. 24, 28.

35. For a discussion of the role of nuns as workhouse nurses, see Maria Luddy, "'Angels of Mercy': Nuns as Workhouse Nurses, 1861–1898," in *Medicine, Disease and the State in Ireland, 1650–1940*, ed. Greta Jones and Elizabeth Malcolm (Cork: Cork University Press, 1999), 102–17.

36. O'Mahony, *Cork's Poor Law Palace*, 204, 230.

37. *Local Government Board*, PP, 1896 (C8153), xxxviii, 16, 99–101.

38. Workhouse Rules: Nursing of the Sick, *Local Government Board*, PP, 1898 (C8958), 67–68.

39. Workhouse Hospital Trained Nurse, January 12, 1899, *Local Government Board*, PP, 1899 (C9480), 741; Order Amending General Regulations, July 5, 1901, *Local Government Board*, PP, 1903 (Cd. 1606), 68–72.

40. *Local Government Board*, PP, 1913 (Cd. 6978), xvi.

41. Rev. William Anderson, "Workhouse Hospitals in the West of Ireland," *Transactions of the National Association for the Promotion of Social Science* (London, 1868), 515.

42. Cited in O'Mahony, *Cork's Poor Law Palace*, 229.

43. Laois County Library, Mountmellick Board of Guardians Minute Books, September 23, 1871.

44. Public Record Office of Northern Ireland (hereafter PRONI), Belfast Board of Guardians Correspondence, Inspector's report, BG/7/BC/1, May 23, 1879.

45. In the half year to December 1900, thirty operations under chloroform were performed as well as a large number of minor operations. PRONI, Belfast Board of Guardians Minutes, BG/7/A, February 26, 1901.

46. PRONI, Belfast Board of Guardians Minutes, BG/7/A/42, BG/7/A/67, December 26, 1877, July 2, 1901.

47. Voluntary Hospitals Database, accessed November 7, 2012, http://www.hospitalsdatabase.lshtm.ac.uk/.

48. Robert J. Johnstone, *Handbook and Guide to Belfast and North-East Ireland* (Belfast: British Medical Association, 1909), 77–78.

49. PRONI, Ballycastle Board of Guardians Minute Books, Medical Officer's report, BG/3/A/3, August 17, 1895; Minutes, August 31, 1895.

50. PRONI, Ballycastle Board of Guardians Minute Books, Letter from Local Government Board, BG/3/A/5, November 1, 1895; Minutes, November 2, 1895.

51. PRONI, Ballycastle Board of Guardians Minute Books, BG/3/A/13, July 20, 1901.

52. Separate funding was provided under the Medical Charities Act to fund the dispensary system. For the Local Government Board's use of "economic incentives" to promote the expansion of medical services in England, see Keir Waddington, "Paying for the Sick Poor: Financing Medicine under the Victorian Poor Law; The Case of the Whitechapel Union, 1850–1900," in *Financing Medicine: The British Experience since 1750*, ed. Martin Gorsky and Sally Sheard (London: Routledge, 2006), 95–111.

53. See, for example, Workhouse Loans, *Local Government Board*, PP (Cd. 1606), 183.

54. Replies of Workhouse Medical Officers to Queries Respecting Their Hospitals Put by the Commission, *Poor Law Reform Commission (Ireland). Appendix to the Report of the Vice-regal Commission on Poor Law Reform in Ireland*, vol. 2, PP, 1906 (Cd. 3203), 83–101.

55. "Nursing and Administration," 61.

Chapter Seven

Exploring Medical Care in the Nineteenth-Century Provincial Workhouse

A View from Birmingham

JONATHAN REINARZ AND ALISTAIR RITCH

Addressing Workhouse Infirmaries

The history of medical institutions has been central to the emergence of medical history as a field in British and other national contexts. Hospitals and medical schools, for example, have attracted considerable attention from historians, and published histories began to appear after the first anniversaries of these institutions were publicly memorialized in the nineteenth and twentieth centuries. A catalog of these celebrated institutions is literally too long to reproduce here but is confirmed by the most cursory glance at any history of medicine collection. Compared to the history of voluntary hospitals and medical faculties, however, other institutions have received minimal attention from historians. Workhouse infirmaries in particular continue to be neglected, appearing as second-rate institutions to the venerable voluntary hospitals, contrasting in particular with hospitals that achieved official teaching status.

Few workhouse infirmaries have been the subject of detailed, book-length histories. Exceptions in the British literature are few in number, including a history of the Battle workhouse in Reading, as well as a history of Dudley Road Hospital in Birmingham.[1] The former study covers the history of a Berkshire institution from its inception as a union workhouse into a municipal hospital until its closure in 2005. George Hearn's history of Birmingham's workhouse infirmary concentrates on a midlands institution and its evolution from the late nineteenth century throughout much of the next century. Both volumes can be described as traditional institutional histories, documenting staff changes, administrative highlights, and gradual institutional growth. A number of general histories of workhouses also contain chapters on sick and old inmates, medical treatment, and the lame and blind, but most draw on evidence from a wide geographic area and therefore do not discuss change in medical provisions in a workhouse infirmary in a particular place over time.[2] A regional approach to provincial workhouses seems particularly justified given the preference for local control demonstrated by guardians historically.[3] In any case, additional bounded studies are clearly wanted and have been encouraged but have yet to appear. Knowledge of workhouses and their infirmaries therefore remains patchy.

This chapter is an effort to address the poverty of literature in this area. It offers a regional study of medicine at the Birmingham workhouse from 1733, when it was first erected in the town, to the end of the nineteenth century, when a new workhouse infirmary was built and renamed Dudley Road Hospital in 1912. It is roughly divided into two parts, the first section covering the foundation of a workhouse, the establishment of a separate workhouse infirmary, and its eventual move to a larger site on Dudley Road, to the northwest of the town center. The second half more explicitly addresses the medical staff and patients of the institution, focusing primarily on the second half of the nineteenth century, given the neglect of this period in the existing history of the Birmingham workhouse infirmary. It commences with an examination of the careers of the medical officers who served the institution between 1850 and 1900. It is important to focus on some of the medical successes reported in the archives since the quality of poor law institutional medical care is a controversial topic among historians. Poor law medical officers have been depicted as third-rate doctors who neglected the needs of sick paupers and did little to prevent guardians from denying inmates new forms of treatment.[4] The chapter also concentrates on the dismissal of staff and other local scandals, events that are often far better documented than ordinary day-to-day work but often offer many important insights to workhouse life; it does not concentrate on nursing, which is a chapter on its own and deserving of additional study.[5] Equal attention is paid to the patients, documenting not only provision in terms of numbers, space, and specialist wards but also the treatment they were offered by medical officers, as well as some glimpses of their experiences. In particular, the chapter addresses four distinct categories of the workhouse population, at least in Birmingham: children, venereal cases, and inmates in the epileptic wards, as well as the institution's older patients.

Establishment and Evolution, 1733–1852

The Birmingham workhouse was originally constructed in 1733, following the passage of a private act of Parliament in 1731. The original institution on Lichfield Street, originally said to resemble "a gentleman's house," was built at a cost of £1,173 at a time when the population of Birmingham was just over twenty thousand.[6] Minutes of the board of guardians reveal 369 inmates in May 1785 and 442 at Easter 1812.[7] At the end of the eighteenth century, 300 children were residing in placements throughout Warwickshire because of lack of accommodation in the workhouse.[8] An Asylum for the Infant Poor was therefore erected on Summer Lane in 1797 to bring them under one roof within Birmingham. The number of inmates in the workhouse itself did not surpass 500 until after 1847. Before 1733 the parish guardians had annually dispersed between £500 and £1,000 annually to the poor and presumably convinced many taxpayers that this was a reasonable investment. At the time it opened in 1734, and for decades thereafter, all sick pauper inmates would have been mixed with healthy residents in an institution famously referred to as a "prison."

By 1766, in a decision that would more clearly emphasize the institution's health care role, an infirmary wing was first constructed at a cost of £400 and a workshop wing was also added in 1779, allowing the workhouse to accommodate around 400 inmates.[9] The capacity of the infirmary is uncertain, but only 37 adult patients were being cared for in May 1785.[10] Four years later the accommodation for sick paupers was felt to be so inadequate that a detached building was eventually erected in 1793, as the "Town Infirmary" at a cost of £1,475.[11] By August 1818, a total of 94 patients were being treated in the infirmary, the number increasing steadily to reach about 233 by 1847.[12] New buildings were also erected in 1835 as the "Lunatic Branch of the Town Infirmary." In April that year, the new buildings accommodated 36 "idiotic cases" and patients suffering "mental aberration," who would otherwise have been transferred to a lunatic asylum, but 25 insane women remained in the old apartments. As the workhouse's role in the treatment of mental illness became more important, the number of patients had increased to 78 by 1847.[13] This contrasts with another huge provincial urban workhouse in Manchester, which in 1841 housed 1,261 paupers with 268 in sick wards, but only 10 lunatics. Debates about relocating the institution to the healthier, more airy site of Birmingham Heath emerged before the end of the eighteenth century.[14] There is evidence of some reconstruction and patching up in these years, but few records document the medical work that was undertaken by staff at the time.

The most valuable resource that discusses medical work in Birmingham in these years, including that undertaken at the workhouse, is *Medical Miscellany*, a publication by a Birmingham surgeon, Thomas Tomlinson. One of the first provincial practitioners to deliver a series of anatomical lectures, Tomlinson published his reflections on medical practice in the midlands, as well as many other views and reviews, in a volume he wrote while performing the duties of workhouse surgeon.[15] Born in Warwickshire in

1734, Tomlinson trained at St. George's in London before returning to the midlands and successfully obtaining the post of surgeon to the Birmingham workhouse in 1760.[16] Besides publishing a synopsis of his anatomy lectures, Tomlinson discussed the health of Birmingham's population in *Medical Miscellany*, suggesting that epidemics were in fact rare in the town during the 1760s. According to Tomlinson, in 1766 the town's sole medical institution, the workhouse infirmary, relieved 1,022 "sick objects": 270 inpatients and 752 outpatients. Over the next two years, patient numbers even declined. Presumably, all medical cases were seen by Tomlinson and his apprentice, who commenced his seven-year training in 1764. In general, Tomlinson argued that the diseases of paupers he treated tended to be the result of bad diet, uncleanliness, close crowded rooms, and intemperance rather than real want. According to the outspoken house surgeon, the "Pharmacopeia Pauperum," or items regularly dispensed to the workhouse inmates, contained few medicines. "Remove the sick to the infirmary, allow clean linen and good beds, with gruel and suitable nourishment, and they soon recover."[17] In general, this tended to suggest that conditions in the workhouse in these early years were better than most poor laborers would have enjoyed outside the institution.

The town's second medical institution did not appear until 1779, when the General Hospital, a charity originally founded in 1765, was finally completed and opened to patients.[18] It is evident from the early records of this voluntary hospital that paupers and "the deserving poor" were not always directed to their appropriate institutions. Over many decades numerous paupers continued to gain access to the new voluntary hospital and presumably entered other medical charities, which emerged in Birmingham during the late eighteenth and early nineteenth centuries.[19] These included a dispensary (1792), as well as orthopedic (1817) and eye charities (1823), all of which initially treated only outpatients.[20] This may have lowered attendance at the parish infirmary, as admission figures at the workhouse for 1831 totaled only 740, while annual costs increased more dramatically, reaching five thousand pounds.[21] A new workhouse was again discussed in 1835, following the introduction of the New Poor Law. In general, very little construction of medical institutions took place nationally in these years, though Birmingham did, unusually, gain a second general hospital in 1841.[22] By 1852, however, pressure on facilities finally led to the establishment of a new workhouse and infirmary at Birmingham Heath, approximately a mile to the northwest of the town center and first identified as a suitable location for such an institution in the 1780s.[23]

From its earliest incarnation, the workhouse appears to have had an identified educational role. Though not clearly defined, medical posts appear to have been used to support education, and the institution was clearly valued for the educational opportunities it offered, both in terms of the cases available to staff and the provision of bodies or simply body parts for the purpose of anatomical instruction. Workhouse surgeons, before and after Tomlinson, would regularly take their apprentices into the workhouse for training. Access to clinical material would almost certainly have justified Tomlinson's decision to charge his apprentice a higher than average eighty-pound premium, especially after a medical wing was constructed at the Birmingham institution in 1766.[24] The medical school that grew out of a series of lectures first held in 1825, and the proper school built in 1828, also relied on a good working relationship with the guardians.[25] This was especially important given the school's founder's poor relations with staff at the town's General Hospital. Though many pupils presumably accompanied their masters into the workhouse in these years, and possibly assisted on rounds, this has not been formally recorded in the archives. The one exception was Murray Burgess, who was allowed to attend the lying-in ward for six months in 1843 as the pupil of Charles Gem, one of the infirmary's six surgeons.[26]

Despite these developments, by the mid-nineteenth century, the educational role of the workhouse had become almost insignificant, in part due to opposition from the central authority. A request in 1852 by John Humphrey, workhouse medical officer, to appoint an articled pupil to assist him, due to "an extensive increase in duties," was initially agreed to by the guardians. The Poor Law Board, however, did not approve on the grounds that they had "no legal authority" to allow anyone to reside in the workhouse who was not directly responsible to the guardians through the master.[27] In the last decades of the century, the institution's minimal teaching role first led a prominent local surgeon, Lawson Tait, to suggest it be used more effectively for its valuable teaching material.[28] Tait's views, which were published in the local newspapers, may have been prompted by a decision to advertise the workhouse as a clinical teaching site in the prospectus of the medical school in 1887, when, in reality, few students entered the institution. In the late 1860s Louisa Twining had already recommended that Parliament open all infirmaries to medical students.[29] Although workhouse infirmaries were officially opened to medical students in 1867, students were again banished in 1869, given concerns that "the peculiar dependency of sick paupers would make them vulnerable to medical experimentation." Despite calls from the British Medical Association and Poor Law Medical Officers' Association to open infirmaries for the purposes of medical education, resistance to granting the workhouse infirmary official teaching status in towns such as Birmingham was clearly great and changed only when the medical school faced a potential crisis in the early twentieth century when clinical material was in limited supply.[30]

Unable to offer all its students access to sufficient maternity cases to satisfy the recommendations of the General Medical Council regarding midwifery training, the medical faculty at the University of Birmingham finally permitted students to access workhouse beds, which outnumbered the city's voluntary hospital beds by a ratio of two to one.[31] Despite the other possible advantages of improving access to patients, students in this case were limited to maternity cases. Though the workhouse infirmary was recognized as a teaching institution in 1921, relations between the institutions improved only slowly, despite the city's two workhouse infirmaries taking in more than 1,700 voluntary cases due to a lack of space at charity hospitals.[32] Interestingly, Thomas McKeown, Birmingham's first professor of social medicine, argued along lines reminiscent of Tait in the 1970s when he suggested a broader range of medical cases be offered to Birmingham's medical students, who were seeing only a select group of cases in the city's voluntary hospitals.[33]

In terms of the workhouse's education role, much previous research has concentrated on these institutions as suppliers of corpses for dissection and anatomy classes.[34] Besides taking his own apprentice into the workhouse, Tomlinson also relied on access to human material from the workhouse to organize his anatomical lectures in the 1760s. Interestingly, Tomlinson referred to the difficulty of acquiring entire bodies but obtained many body parts, presumably following amputations and operations, thereby allowing him to run his dissection classes.[35] So important was the workhouse to Sands Cox's early medical school that he was eventually dubbed the institution's "seventh surgeon."[36] This informal title emphasized that, while there were only six official medical men attached to the institution by the 1820s and 1830s, Cox spent as many, if not more, hours at the institution to identify interesting cases, attend operations, and, most important, obtain the bodies of the dead. Clearly, his strategy worked. The 1834 Select Committee on Medical Education indicates that the small school at Birmingham had managed to procure forty-three bodies in the 1833–34 school year.[37] This compared well with other provincial schools, which acquired a fraction of this number, and in the case of Nottingham and Hull, none at all. In return for their generosity, Cox granted the guardians access to the school's newly constructed museum free of charge in 1838.[38] By the 1850s he was still corresponding with the guardians to ensure a healthy supply of cadavers at the medical school.[39] The relationship remained successful for at least the next thirty years, as the school received twenty-one bodies from the 624 deaths that took place in the workhouse in the year ending Lady Day, 1886.[40]

By this time, Birmingham workhouse had transformed dramatically. In 1852 the institution was rebuilt at a cost of £44,476.[41] Though it was a major building project, descriptions of the institution are still relatively sparse compared with voluntary hospitals that opened with much fanfare, usually closer to the town center, during these years.[42] Nevertheless, the infirmary was described as "one of the finest in the country." The workhouse had a total of 1,603 beds, and 310 of these were reserved for sick inmates. Built in the corridor style on an extensive site, its ventilation system attracted particular attention at the time.[43] Medical cases were also divided among a number of separate wards, including those for common cases, convalescent patients, "idiots," and epileptics. Detached buildings were similarly provided for fever, infectious, and maternity cases.[44]

Though the workhouse was only recently completed, four years later, in 1856, additional plans were presented to add another 274 beds to the institution. When the Cape Hill School opened with 200 places for boys in 1864, this alleviated some pressure on the institution, allowing the old school to be converted into an epileptic ward the following year. A more elaborate extension that same year added a further 340 places to the infirmary.[45] In keeping with most workhouses at that time, the erection of extra accommodation was necessitated by overcrowding, as a result of Birmingham parish's population increasing by over one-fifth throughout the 1850s. Although there was no clear vision of the workhouse as a "place of healing" until the 1860s, illness was an important factor, giving rise to the need for extended facilities. In 1867 isolation wards were augmented when a shed was converted into a smallpox ward, and new wards for two hundred elderly women opened the following year.[46] By 1871 the workhouse possessed six infectious wards and three years later, in 1874, separate wards were leased to the town council to establish an isolation hospital on the same site.[47] Within the next years many infectious cases, previously admitted to other local hospitals, including the Children's Hospital, were admitted to the new hospital for infectious diseases. Hosting the workhouse, isolation hospital, an asylum, and a prison, Birmingham Heath had become a blighted area, ideally suited to prisoners, the sick, and the destitute.

Medical Work at the Workhouse Infirmary

In 1823, when the guardians appointed Thomas Green as the first resident house surgeon to the workhouse infirmary at an annual salary of fifty pounds plus accommodation, six visiting surgeons and a "House Apothecary" were already contracted to provide medical care to paupers in the workhouse, at the dispensary, and in their own homes.[48] An additional dispenser was appointed in 1835 and by 1847 sixteen nonresident surgeons were being employed.[49] Ruth Hodgkinson praises this system of medical relief as being unique and "more progressive than those of Poor Law Unions."[50] As Birmingham guardians had been set up under a local act, they were able to be more liberal in the provision of medical relief. However, as the degree of control by the central authority increased, the surgeons were reduced in number and confined to outdoor medical care in 1850. As a result, the house surgeon lost the support of his more senior colleagues.

Table 7.1. Workhouse medical officers in the Birmingham workhouse, 1850–1914

Name	Date appointed	Annual salary (£)	Date terminated	Reason for termination
John Humphrey	March 1850	150–175	April 1855	Appointed to civil hospital
William Fernie	May 1855	150	April 1857	Resigned
John Wilmshurst	May 1857	150	May 1858	Resigned
John Redfern Davies	June 1858	150–200	October 1861	Resigned at request of guardians
Edmund Robinson	October 1861	200–350	January 1869	Appointed public vaccinator
Edmund Whitcombe	February 1869	200	July 1870	Appointed to Borough Lunatic Asylum
Adam Simpson	August 1870	200–350	August 1886	Removed from office by Local Government Board
Charles Mitchell	August 1886 (acting) January 1889	207	January 1890	Resigned
Edmund Corder	February 1890	150–200	February 1890	Resigned
Ebenezer Teichelmann	February 1890	150–200	September 1891	Resigned
George Ferraby	October 1891	150	October 1894	Appointed district medical officer
George Barber	November 1894	?	May 1895	Resigned
Alexander McDougall	May 1895	150–200	March 1899	Appointed district medical officer

Source: BCLA, BBG, GP/B/2/1/6-67, January 1850 to September 1899.

In the sixteen years following Thomas Green's appointment, three other house surgeons held the post until the appointment of Charles Smith in 1839.[51] He did not apply for the post when it was advertised as part of the new medical arrangements, creating the division between workhouse and district medical officers. Between 1850 and 1899 thirteen medical officers held the office of resident surgeon, serving for periods varying from one month to sixteen years, with an average just short of four years (see table 7.1). With only three medical officers spending more than five years in office, there was little continuity of medical care, which varied according to the practices of the individual officer.[52] This is similar to the situation at the town's General Hospital, where the resident medical officers between 1857 and 1875 had an average length of service of approximately three years. However, some degree of continuity was provided by eight honorary physicians and surgeons, whose periods in office ranged from eight to thirty-seven years.[53] A similar situation was not initiated at the workhouse until 1882, when a visiting physician was appointed, followed by a visiting surgeon five years later.

This is not to say, however, that there was no continuity among staff at other workhouses. At the Battle workhouse in Reading, three medical officers served the institution during its first sixty years, making for a twenty-year average period of service, and none of the officers worked for fewer than twelve years.[54] Leicester Union similarly required only three medical officers for the workhouse over a period of fifty-seven years from 1857.[55] The medical officers to these workhouses were appointed part-time and could continue in private practice in the town, explaining their long lengths of service, while limiting their attendance at the institution to a short period in the day. Full-time employment within workhouses was a controversial issue, opposed by the *Lancet* and Dr. Edward Smith, medical officer to the Poor Law Board.[56] Joseph Rogers, a reformer and workhouse medical officer in the 1860s, was instrumental in getting the requirement for the infirmaries in London to have resident medical officers supervised by visiting physicians included in the Metropolitan Poor Act of 1867.[57] Over the following four years, the number of workhouse medical officers who were resident in the capital increased from three out of a total of twelve to seven out of thirteen.[58] Although full-time contracts became more usual from the 1870s, a full 93 percent of the 625 unions in England and Wales still had no resident medical officer in 1900.[59]

In the provinces resident workhouse medical officers were most likely to be appointed in large urban workhouses, such as Liverpool, Nottingham, and Manchester.[60] In Birmingham, from the 1850s, they continued to be given full-time duties in the workhouse, where they were required to be residents and so private practice was not permitted. Starting salaries rose from £150 per annum plus board, lodgings, and a personal servant to £200 per annum in 1861, but returned to the previous level in 1890 after the new infirmary opened.[61] Medical officers during these decades resigned for a variety of reasons. For example, in 1855, John Humphrey took up an appointment at a new civil hospital near Constantinople. George Barber left because of ill health, and William Fernie resigned due to the heavy workload. A few were appointed to public posts locally, for instance as public vaccinator in 1869 and two as district medical officers in the 1890s. Edmund Whitcombe, who resigned in 1870 to take up his appointment as assistant medical superintendent at the Borough Lunatic Asylum, was later to be appointed to a chair of mental health at the University of Birmingham (see table 7.1).[62] In general, there were few workhouse medical officers in Birmingham who left public service and entered posts at the local voluntary hospitals. Such movement between institutions was more common in the first century of the workhouse's existence and almost certainly in the first years following the establishment of a voluntary hospital locally. In fact, during the second half of the nineteenth century, few applicants for the post of medical officer were local men. This contrasts with events elsewhere. In the case of the Battle workhouse, assistant surgeons from the Royal Berkshire Hospital often applied for the post of medical officer to the workhouse.[63]

Despite the low standing of poor law medical officers within the medical profession and the limited contact between Birmingham's officers and staff at the local teaching hospitals, some of those employed at the town's workhouse did attempt to introduce advances in medical care. In general, innovations tended to be based in areas where one would expect the medical officer's clinical experience to have surpassed that of practitioners at voluntary institutions. In 1857, for example, John Wilmshurst introduced a new treatment from Belgium for "itch," an affliction that was particularly prevalent at poor law institutions.[64] It consisted of a single application of a lime and sulfur dressing. Not only would this be more effective for scabies, but Wilmshurst also emphasized that the adoption of this measure would immediately create more space in the infirmary for more urgent cases.[65] The sulfur and lime solution was used in preference to sulfur ointment, as it did not spoil bed linen and allowed patients to be dressed while being treated. Wilmshurst introduced it to Birmingham ten years before it became the standard treatment in other workhouses.[66]

Wilmshurst resigned in 1858 and was succeeded by John Redfern Davies, the son of the eminent local physician and coroner, John Birt Davies. Through his attempts to promote surgery within the workhouse infirmary, Davies came into conflict with the guardians, who preferred that inmates requiring "capital operations" be transferred to the local voluntary hospitals because of the "practiced skill and combined judgment of medical men usually connected with such establishments."[67] Despite these instructions,

Davies amputated the leg of Edward Waite in June the following year, assisted by Oliver Pemberton, surgeon to the General Hospital, without the guardians' permission. He eventually had to concede that he would perform surgery in the workhouse only in cases of emergency and when transfer to hospital was not possible.[68] The situation at other workhouse infirmaries was the same, operating theaters being a notable absence from workhouse plans. For this reason, guardians often subscribed to other local medical charities where such operations were undertaken. The guardians of the Battle workhouse in Reading, for example, increased their subscription to the Royal Berkshire Hospital in 1868 from six guineas to ten guineas, which enabled five of their patients to be sent to the hospital as inpatients each year.[69] Davies published the results of other procedures in the *British Medical Journal*, one of which involved the removal of a glandular enlargement in the neck of an eight-year-old boy, as the growth was pressing on the trachea and interfering with his breathing. The other was a newly introduced, radical cure by metallic seton to treat a hydrocele.[70] Following an accident in December 1860, Davies was observed to be taking frequent daily absences from the workhouse and tendered his resignation at the request of the guardians. Operative treatment gradually became more common within workhouse infirmaries and by 1882, about six capital operations per week were being undertaken in Liverpool, whose workhouse was of a similar size to that in Birmingham.[71]

More notoriety surrounded the longest serving medical officer, Adam Simpson, who worked from 1870 to 1886. One possible reason for his long length of service may have been the appointment of an assistant medical officer in January 1876 following a local government inspector's report, which argued that medical staffing at the institution was insufficient. When an additional officer was appointed in December 1878, the two assistants shared the basic care of the inmates, and Simpson took on what could be described as a supervisory role. When Cornelius Suckling was appointed visiting physician in 1882 with responsibility for the medical portion of the workhouse, Simpson's work was further limited to the surgical wards.[72] Another reason may have been his dedication to the poor law medical service. He played a prominent role in the Poor Law Medical Officers' Association and has been praised for his interest in the management of lunatic patients.[73]

During Simpson's career at the workhouse, three Local Government Board inquiries were held to investigate his conduct. At the first, in 1877, he was found to have been guilty of grave neglect of duty regarding the death of an inmate but was not required to resign as he received the support of the guardians. In general, all complaints against doctors at this time were centered on neglect rather than malpractice, and medical officers were rarely punished even in clear cases of neglect.[74] The second incident, five years later, concerned his use of the padded room as an instrument of punishment. Although Simpson escaped the censure of the board, it considered that he had committed a grave error of judgment. The final inquiry, in 1886, related to his conduct during an outbreak of puerperal fever, during which he had attended infected women. Simpson was found to have disobeyed an important order by the guardians not to attend the lying-in wards subsequent to this contact. When he failed to tender his resignation, the central authority removed him from office.[75] Kim Price is of the opinion that his dismissal had more to do with his poor law reforming activities than the performance of his duties.[76]

Young, Venereal, Epileptic, and Older Patients

While patients in the old workhouse numbered 160 in 1847, the detached infirmary in the new workhouse could accommodate 310 sick paupers. Yet in January 1855 the workhouse medical officer reported that the "daily average of patients in the Infirmary is 318."[77] Numbers could fluctuate quickly in this period. For example, Tomlinson's emphasis on the relative healthiness of the population in the 1760s was reflected in as few as 37 patients in the sick wards, constituting only 10 percent of the workhouse population in May 1785. Thirty-three years later, their proportion had grown to 17 percent, with 94 patients. Although at times, as in the summer of 1822, the proportion of sick inmates would return quickly to 10 percent, the general trend was a gradual increase to 46 percent (194 patients) by October 1846.[78] Given the limited number of staff, these figures would have kept the medical officers busy in this period. Unfortunately, during most years, very little additional evidence about the patients at the workhouse, other than their number, is included in the guardians' minutes.

Though workhouse medical cases are rarely broken down in the sort of detail contained in even the annual reports of voluntary hospitals, some evidence describes the variety of patients seen by Birmingham's workhouse medical officers in these years. A report by the poor law inspector on July 13, 1866, for example, recorded 566 cases under the supervision of the medical officer and divided these into the following categories:

Bedridden	147
Epileptic	64
Harmless lunatic idiots	64
Ulcered legs	38
Minor ailments	30
Syphilitic	42
Under special medical treatment	181[79]

Two years later, on September 4, the master recorded 651 patients in the infirmary, representing 32 percent of the total inmates. This was less than the 39 percent who were classed as requiring medical care in London work-houses in 1869, although imbeciles were not included in the Birmingham figure. However, it was similar to most of the larger urban provincial work-houses examined in a national inquiry at that time, including Liverpool, Leeds, and Sheffield. By contrast, in the large rural workhouses of Norwich and Portsea only 19 percent and 13 percent of inmates were sick.[80] Although additional building had taken place, the dining room was being used to accommodate 110 inmates by day and 70 at night.[81] A further dou-bling of the number of patients in the infirmary had taken place by the early 1880s. The Infirmary Sub-Committee kept detailed records of the number of patients, which continued to rise from 1,045 in September 1881 to 1,232 in September 1884, representing 55 percent of the workhouse population.[82]

The new detached workhouse infirmary opened in Birmingham in 1889 with accommodation for 1,300 patients. Only 990 of these spaces were in the new pavilion-style building, while the remainder were in some of the old infirmary wards. By March the following year, the new building was almost fully utilized, with 1,286 patients accommodated.[83] Given that the records of medical officers at workhouses have often not survived, existing archives usually offer only glimpses of the work undertaken at these insti-tutions.[84] In the remainder of this section, four specific constituencies will be discussed, including children, venereal cases, epileptics, and the institu-tion's older patients.

As indicated by the poor law inspector's report of 1866 discussed earlier, workhouses had separate wards for sick inmates from the middle of the nine-teenth century. Though offering very specialized treatment in the case of venereal disease, mental illness, and even ulcerous legs, most institutions did not have a separate ward for sick children, which probably meant that young inmates shared these wards with adult paupers.[85] If anything, the guardians had traditionally attempted to remove children from the workhouse entirely. This had led Birmingham's guardians to decide in 1797 to create a separate Infant Poor Asylum, largely to reduce some of the pressure on the main insti-tution. When the workhouse was rebuilt on Birmingham Heath, however, many children returned to the main institution. Of 674 children in the care of the poor law at the time, 240 resided in the new buildings.

It has been estimated that 30 percent of the sick in English workhouses were children.[86] In general, children inside the workhouse were less likely to suffer accidents than those who resided outside the institution. Unfortunately, tables detailing conditions among the youngest workhouse inmates do not survive, but it would be safe to conclude that they included those diseases and ailments common at children's hospitals, which increased in number in the late nineteenth century. The most common conditions seen at children's hospitals in these years were skin affections, rickets, and infectious diseases.[87] During epidemics, the number of ill could increase rapidly and occasionally necessitated emptying other wards, such as those for vagrants, to accommodate children requiring isolation.[88] However, infectious diseases were also easily isolated at the workhouse, and from midcentury all children were vaccinated by the resident surgeon.[89] Very few sick children were lunatics, as these would often be kept by relatives, who were paid outdoor relief to maintain them.[90]

In general, many children were removed to schools when they were old enough. As a result, approximately 200 workhouse children were attending the Cape Hill School in 1864. Nevertheless, additional accommodation was being provided for 100 infants in 1865. In general, children would not have required as much medical attention as those who lived with their families. Most underwent an examination to be certified medically fit before beginning an apprenticeship, a regulation that remained in force until after 1871.[91] By 1880 new facilities were built at Marston Green, where 420 children were placed in fourteen cottage homes. The site was self-sufficient, possessing, for example, a separate infirmary. In other localities children were similarly removed from the workhouse and placed in some system of "scattered homes," where they were taught a marketable skill.[92] Concern with the "pauper taint" in many unions led to similar late nineteenth-century initiatives aimed specifically to separate children from adult workhouse inmates.[93]

Venereal disease, while occasionally seen among the younger inmates, tended to afflict the adult workhouse inmates.[94] As noted in the previous list, syphilitic cases constituted more than 7 percent of sick cases at the Birmingham workhouse infirmary in 1866. However, venereal disease had begun to concern the guardians a decade earlier. In 1857 they expressed concern over the large increase in syphilitic cases and overcrowding on the venereal wards. The medical officer, John Wilmshurst, explained that these patients were "neglected in many Unions, dosed with salt and senna and discharged cured," whereas "it is not surprising they come where they can get some specific medical treatment in wards set apart for the care of these complaints." His claim was supported by a statement from Emma Rose, a twenty-three-year-old inmate suffering from venereal disease. She had not been satisfied with the treatment she had received in the Kidderminster workhouse and had sought admission to Birmingham on the grounds, saying, "if I came to Birmingham Workhouse, I should be sure to get cured."[95] She had been influenced by a fellow inmate at Kidderminster, Elizabeth Edwards, who claimed that she "had more good done to her in six weeks" in the Birmingham workhouse than in two years in Kidderminster.[96] The actions of these two venereal patients illustrate how some sections of the poor, such as prostitutes, viewed workhouses as places to obtain medical treatment and how such treatment was considered of poor standard in many of them. Nevertheless, one of the major roles of the poor law medical services was the management of venereal disease.[97] Whatever the nature of Wilmshurst's explanation, or even his treatment, the numbers in the venereal wards had decreased from sixty-four, when he took up his appointment, to twenty-three only three months later.[98] Interestingly, venereal patients increased again after his departure, so that in July 1866 there were forty-two "syphilitic" cases. Two years later, in June 1868, this had risen to sixty-seven cases, but, in addition, there were a further sixty-four of the "hereditary form."[99] Although Birmingham had a greater proportion of patients with venereal disease (7 percent) at this time than most unions, overcrowding was never subsequently recorded as a problem.[100] Indeed, the number of women with venereal disease was so small in the early 1890s that the guardians had hoped to transfer them to the local lock hospital, but this did not prove possible due to the high demand on its one dozen beds.[101]

In contrast, there was a continual problem of too many patients than accommodation in the epileptic wards permitted (see table 7.2). The lunatic wards in the old workhouse were renamed "epileptic wards" in the new one but continued to accommodate both lunatics and epileptic patients, as they both required similar methods of management and levels of supervision. Frequently, these inmates were placed in other parts of the infirmary, such as the venereal ward and within the body of the workhouse. This was one factor leading to the unsatisfactory condition of the wards, as exemplified by the report of the Commissioner in Lunacy in November 1855: "the rooms are overcrowded, several sleep in double beds . . . some of the straw beds scantily filled and several wet." Among the commissioner's suggestions were that the practice of placing two patients in one bed should be discontinued and instruments of restraint be removed from the wards. However, two years later he reported that women were still being "habitually restrained." The master's defense was that it was due to the helpless physical condition of the patients, which required protection against falling out of bed, and he therefore suggested that "it is not restraint."[102] Conditions improved and, in April 1891 the medical officer could report that no case of mechanical restraint had been used in the epileptic wards during the previous quarter.[103]

Other examples of improved conditions on the wards and in the management of the patients are to be found in the last two decades of the century. In 1884 the guardians received a letter from the vice-consul for Sweden and Norway, expressing his appreciation for the "extreme kindness" with which one of his countrymen had been treated while a patient in the epileptic wards.[104] Eleven years later, some patients were being taken for a walk each day outside the workhouse grounds.[105] In July 1899 a Mrs. George Albright was thanked by the guardians for arranging for 70 women to go for a drive and have tea, despite the medical officers' concerns that the vehicles used for the outing may have been unsafe for epileptic patients.[106]

Table 7.2. Number of beds and inmates in selected wards of the Birmingham
workhouse infirmary on May 6, 1873

Department	Number of beds	Number of inmates	Excess/shortfall of inmates compared with beds
Male infirmary	66	69	+3
Female infirmary	73	77	+4
Bad leg ward	33	30	-3
Fever ward	38	24	-14
Smallpox	103	15	-88
Male epileptic	102	115	+13
Female epileptic	101	110	+9
Male venereal	31	24	-7
Female venereal	35	38	+3

Source: BCLA, HSC, GP/B/2/3/3/3, June 3, 1873.

The early overcrowding in the epileptic wards of the new workhouse, for
example, 87 patients with accommodation for only 64, prompted the building of new epileptic wards to hold 100 patients in 1865. Within a few months
these too proved insufficient for the 133 patients present. Over the following twenty years, increasing numbers of inmates were admitted to the epileptic wards, reaching 323 in 1885 and constituting the largest single group
(23.9 percent) of those classed as sick.[107] Despite this situation the guardians, four years later, were considering reducing the number of attendants
for the male ward and requested a report on the frequency of fits on the
ward. As a result of this request, the visiting physician recorded the number
of men having fits per week over a nine-week period as 36 to 39. The number of fits per week varied from 89 to 168. In addition, one man had 150 fits
during one of the weeks. The outcome was the appointment of four paid
assistant attendants to replace two pauper assistants in these wards.[108]

Detailed information on epileptic patients in workhouses is difficult to
find in the literature and references to them are usually included in sections
on lunatics and imbeciles.[109] From the beginning of the nineteenth century, epileptics were confined with the insane in asylums and workhouses.[110]
Whether workhouse wards were labeled "lunatic" or "epileptic," it was rarely
possible to identify one group of patients from the other. One opportunity
arose in the medical officer's report of the admissions to the lunatic wards
of the old workhouse in Birmingham. In 1845 he recorded 42 patients out

of 143 admissions as suffering from epilepsy, but only 9 of these patients had a mental illness or disability.[111] A national survey in 1869 revealed that epileptic patients constituted greater than 5 percent of sick inmates in only 139 unions, being most numerous in Wolverhampton at 43 percent of sick inmates, in Salford at 30 percent, and Stockport at 21 percent. Birmingham, with 9 percent, had the seventh largest number and the 65 patients at that time were of similar proportion within the epileptic wards to that recorded in 1845.[112] Perhaps it is because they were a significant group in only a small number of workhouses, and shunned by society in general, that we know so little about them.

Another group even more difficult to identify within the workhouse is that of older patients, namely those both old and sick. Christoph Conrad has argued that the health needs of elderly people were marginalized in the second half of the nineteenth and early part of twentieth century, and Michael Denham considers that this amounted to medical neglect with regard to chronic sick and elderly patients. According to Pat Thane, interest in the ill health of older people was of little interest to medical specialists.[113] A further difficulty in identifying older patients lay in the lack of definition within the classification of paupers by the Poor Law Board.[114] The category of "aged and infirm" was the only alternative to able-bodied adults, and no guidance was provided on placing older patients within the institution. In consequence, some were dealt with on the basis of age, while others were classified according to their state of health.[115] Furthermore, older people as a group were not clearly identified within the workhouse population, even though the studies of Nigel Goose and Andrew Hinde and Fiona Turnbull have shown that inmates aged sixty years and over constituted between 20 percent and 32 percent of inmates in the mid-nineteenth century.[116] Although the central authority never defined the age beyond which an inmate was regarded as no longer able-bodied, guardians generally accepted sixty years as the commencement of old age in terms of applying for relief.[117]

Birmingham's wards for inmates who were not able-bodied were designated "old and infirm" and for "bedridden cases." During the first quarter of 1859 to the same period in 1866, the numbers of those classed as old and infirm rose from 377 to 614, although the proportion of total inmates was similar at 32 percent and 30 percent respectively.[118] However, there was no disproportionate increase in the admission of older people. The proportion of older inmates in Birmingham was similar to that in London workhouses in 1851 for those aged over sixty-five years, but greater than the national figure of 20 percent and the provincial figure of 14 percent.[119] A similar increase in the number of patients occurred in the bedridden wards, from 146 in 1865 to 288 in 1888. Not all these patients were totally confined to beds, as one-third of these cases were recorded as able to leave their beds and their rooms in 1866.[120] Furthermore, not all severely disabled patients were placed in these wards, since 20 percent of women in the epileptic wards were confined to beds.[121]

When considering the size of the new infirmary and which patients would require transfer from the workhouse, the guardians felt that those in the bedridden wards should not be classed under the heading of sick, as they required mainly good nursing. However, the medical officer decided that half should be designated acute cases requiring medical treatment and were appropriate for transfer to the new infirmary.[122] Older patients were not the only ones considered unsuitable for initial transfer to the new infirmary, as this also applied to those with venereal disease. Subsequently, there were difficulties regarding the transfer of patients between the infirmary and the workhouse, with reports of patients going back and forth between the two, occasionally several times on the same day.[123] The infirmary developed a more selective policy toward admissions, preferring patients with acute short-term illness, emulating the practice of the voluntary hospitals. Its role began to change toward that of an acute hospital, and in 1948 it was recognized as a general hospital and renamed Dudley Road Hospital. This left the workhouse to care for those disabled by chronic illness, and after the establishment of the National Health Service it became a geriatric hospital, with the name of Summerfield Hospital. As was the case with older patients, much of the medical work carried out in the workhouse remains hidden and difficult to trace in the history of the sick in poor law institutions.

The Role of the Workhouse in British Health Care

Within the historiography of poor law institutions, workhouses and their infirmaries in the large, provincial cities of England have been a neglected subject of research. Birmingham's rapidly expanding population in the nineteenth century due to industrialization created a severe problem of increasing admissions to the workhouse, requiring frequent expansion of accommodation. This was exacerbated by its gradual adoption of an important medical role within the local community. Lunatics and epileptic patients formed one of the largest groups of sick inmates and were the most severely affected by the subsequent overcrowding, despite the provision of additional wards. Conditions for these patients improved after the new infirmary was built and trips out of the workhouse were arranged. However, conditions in these specialist wards must have remained unpleasant, as about 120 epileptic fits occurred in each ward per week.

This chapter has also attempted to shed some light on older patients and has demonstrated how difficult it is to identify them within the workhouse, compared with epileptic cases, children, and sufferers of venereal disease.

Although the number of older inmates increased toward the latter part of the nineteenth century, this was commensurate with the overall increase in admissions of paupers of all ages. Many suffered from chronic disability and were admitted to the bedridden wards. There was considerable disagreement between the guardians and the medical officers over the acuteness of their conditions and the degree to which they required skilled nursing.

While many other workhouses were populated with similar types of poor patients, there appears to have been greater variation in the organization of medical staff. Birmingham guardians were unusual in appointing full-time, resident medical officers. This brought the advantage of having them on-site and able to attend to patients quickly at any time of night or day, although the number of patients in the infirmary was so large that medical staff continued to suffer from overwork. These two factors may have contributed to the relative short length of service of most of them, with the resultant lack of continuity of care when compared with other workhouses. Despite this, there is evidence that some medical officers, such as Wilmshurst and Davies, did introduce new treatments and techniques to the benefit of patients.

Innovative work of this nature and an abundance of clinical teaching material, however, did not ensure that workhouses would secure a place in formal medical education during these years. The admission of students to Birmingham's workhouse for instruction purposes was very much a twentieth-century occurrence, despite a very early recognition, by Tomlinson and others, of the institution's educational value. Surprisingly, arguments in favor of its pedagogical uses never gained impetus even when Birmingham, like many other workhouses, had by the 1860s effectively become "'asylums and infirmaries' by default."[124] Although the first surgeon at the workhouse in Birmingham may have brought his apprentices into the infirmary wing, and other local practitioners eagerly collected the cadavers of unclaimed paupers and brought them into medical schools, suggestions that medical students should be brought into workhouse infirmaries as part of their formal instruction appears to have fallen on deaf ears. The institution's second-class status, reinforced, if not determined, by its second-class inmates, clearly determined its place in local educational hierarchies. Ultimately, these views also effectively secured the workhouse's secondary place in the historiography of British health care.

Notes

1. Margaret Railton and Marshall Barr, *Battle Workhouse and Hospital, 1867–2005* (Reading: Berkshire Medical Heritage Centre, 2005); George W. Hearn, *Dudley Road Hospital, 1887–1987* (Birmingham: Postgraduate Centre, Dudley Road Hospital, 1987).

2. Norman Longmate, *The Workhouse: A Social History* (London: Temple Smith, 1974), 136–55, 194–220; Anne Digby, *Pauper Palaces* (London: Routledge and Kegan Paul, 1978), 161–79; Margaret Anne Crowther, *The Workhouse System, 1834–1929: The History of an English Social Institution* (London, Methuen, 1983), 156–90; Frank Crompton, *Workhouse Children: Infant and Child Paupers under the Worcestershire Poor Law, 1780–1871* (Stroud: Sutton, 1997), 73–105; Simon Fowler, *The Workhouse: The People, the Places, the Life behind Doors* (Richmond, Surrey: National Archives, 2007), 149–81; Kathryn Morrison, *The Workhouse: A Study of Poor Law Buildings in England* (Swindon: English Heritage, 1999), 155–78.

3. Felix Driver, *Power and Pauperism: The Workhouse System, 1834–1884* (Cambridge: Cambridge University Press, 1993), 70.

4. Crowther, *Workhouse System*, 167, 181; Margaret Anne Crowther, "Paupers or Patients? Obstacles to Professionalization in the Poor Law Medical Service before 1914," *Journal of the History of Medicine and Allied Sciences* 39 (1984): 33–35, 53; Joan Lane, *A Social History of Medicine: Health, Healing and Disease in England, 1750–1950* (London: Routledge, 2001), 63; Alan Kidd, *State, Society and the Poor in Nineteenth-Century England* (Basingstoke, UK: Palgrave Macmillan, 1999), 41; Kim P. Price, "A Regional, Quantitative and Qualitative Study of the Employment, Disciplining and Discharging of Workhouse Medical Officers of the New Poor Law throughout Nineteenth-Century England and Wales" (PhD diss., Oxford Brookes University, 2008), 336.

5. While touched on in a number of workhouse histories, including Crowther, *Workhouse System*, one of the few histories of poor law nursing is Rosemary White, *Social Change and the Development of the Nursing Profession* (London: Kimpton, 1978).

6. William Hutton, *An History of Birmingham* (Birmingham: Pearson and Rollason, 1783), 216. The first and second editions of Hutton's *History* record the workhouse as being the home of four hundred paupers, whereas later editions state six hundred paupers. In light of the number of inmates recorded in the minutes of the board of guardians in the 1780s, the lower figure appears the more appropriate.

7. Birmingham Central Library Archives (hereafter BCLA), Birmingham Board of Guardians, Minute Books (hereafter BBG), GP/B/2/1/1, May 30, 1785; GP/B/2/1/2, March 2, 1813.

8. BCLA, BBG, GP/B/2/1/1, March 30, 1796.

9. Hutton, *History of Birmingham*, 366, 216–17.

10. BCLA, BBG, GP/B/2/1/1, June 6, 1785.

11. BCLA, BBG, GP/B/2/1/1, March 23, 1879, June 3, 1793.

12. BCLA, BBG, GP/B/2/1/2, August 11, 1818; GP/B/2/1/5, October 12, 1847.

13. BCLA, BBG, GP/B/2/1/3, April 7, 1835, November 15, 1837; GP/B/2/1/5, April 20, 1847.

14. John V. Pickstone, *Medicine and Industrial Society: A History of Hospital Development in Manchester and Its Region, 1752–1946* (Manchester: Manchester University Press, 1985), 86–87, 302.

15. Jonathan Reinarz, "The Transformation of Medical Education in Eighteenth-Century England: International Developments and the West Midlands," *History of Education* 37, no. 4 (2008): 549–66.

16. Joan Lane, "Medical Education in the Provinces in Eighteenth-Century England," *Bulletin of the Society for the Social History of Medicine* 41 (1987): 30.

17. Thomas Tomlinson, *Medical Miscellany* (London: Pearson and Aris, 1769), 203–4, 205.

18. Jonathan Reinarz, *The Birth of a Provincial Hospital: The Early Years of the General Hospital, Birmingham, 1765–1790* (Stratford-upon-Avon: Dugdale Society, 2003).

19. BCLA, General Hospital, Birmingham, General Committee Minute Book, 1766–84, GH/1/2/4.

20. Jonathan Reinarz, *Health Care in Birmingham: The Birmingham Teaching Hospitals, 1779–1939* (Woodbridge: Boydell, 2009), 5.

21. Birmingham Central Library, Local Studies (hereafter BCLLS), Birmingham Poor Law and Workhouse, Miscellaneous Documents, vol. 3, Poor Law Amendment Act, 1830, BCOL 41.11.

22. Reinarz, *Health Care in Birmingham*, 56–66.

23. Hearn, *Dudley Road Hospital*, 8.

24. Reinarz, "Transformation of Medical Education," 558.

25. Reinarz, *Health Care in Birmingham*, 52.

26. BCLA, House Committee, GP/B/2/3/1/1, March 28, 1843.

27. BCLA, Visiting and General Purposes Committee (hereafter VGPC), GP/B/2/8/1/1, December 31, 1852; BBG, GP/B/2/1/12, January 5 to February 5, 1853.

28. Hearn, *Dudley Road Hospital*, 18.

29. Ruth G. Hodgkinson, *The Origins of the National Health Service: The Medical Services of the New Poor Law, 1834–1871* (London: Wellcome Trust Historical Medical Library, 1967), 539.

30. Crowther, *Workhouse System*, 162, 169.

31. University of Birmingham Special Collections (hereafter UBSC), University of Birmingham Medical School, Faculty Minute Book, 1921–24.

32. BCLLS, Birmingham Poor Law and Workhouse, Miscellaneous Documents, vol. 1, BCOL 41.11.

33. Thomas McKeown, *The Role of Medicine: Dream, Mirage or Nemesis* (Oxford: Basil Blackwell, 1979), 136–37 and 150–53.

34. Ruth Richardson, *Death, Dissection and the Destitute* (London: Routledge and Kegan Paul, 1987); Elizabeth T. Hurren, *Protesting about Pauperism: Poverty, Politics and Poor Relief in Late-Victorian England, 1870–1900* (Woodbridge: Boydell, 2007); Hurren, *Dying for Victorian Medicine: English Anatomy and Its Trade in the Dead Poor, c. 1834–1929* (Basingstoke, UK: Palgrave Macmillan, 2012).

35. Tomlinson, *Medical Miscellany*, 208.

36. Laurence Nagley, "A History of Summerfield Hospital," *Midland Medical Review* 10 (1975): 11.

37. *Report of the Select Committee on Medical Education*, Parliamentary Papers, 1834 (13), 71–72.

38. UBSC, Birmingham Medical School, Minute Book, 1831.

39. BCLA, Aston Union Minute Books, GP/AS/2/1/7, November 11, 1857.

40. BCLA, Incident Book, GP/B (ACC 2009/109), box 5.

41. John A. Langford, *Modern Birmingham and Its Institutions* (Birmingham: Downing, 1871), 383.

42. Reinarz, *Health Care in Birmingham*, 58, 64.

43. Hodgkinson, *National Health Service*, 539, 530–31.

44. Langford, *Modern Birmingham*, 383.

45. BCLA, VGPC, GP/B/2/8/1/4, January 1, December 16, 1864; GP/B/2/8/1/5, November 10, 1865.

46. Pickstone, *Medicine and Industrial Society*, 123; GP/B/2/8/1/5, July 27 and August 10, 1866.

47. BCLA, BBG, GP/B/2/1/43, August 19, 1874.

48. BCLA, BBG, GP/B/2/1/1, March 11, July 1, 1823.

49. BCLA, BBG, GP/B/2/1/3, January 4, 1835; GP/B/2/1/5, March 15, 1847.

50. Hodgkinson, *National Health Service*, 190–91.

51. BCLA, BBG, GP/B/2/1/4, July 8, 1839.

52. BCLA, BBG, GP/B/2/1/6-68, January 1850 to December 1899.

53. BCLA, General Hospital, Birmingham, Annual Reports, 1857–75.

54. Railton and Barr, *Battle Workhouse and Hospital*, 17, 64, 90–91.

55. Angela Negrine, "Medicine and Poverty: A Study of the Poor Law Medical Services of the Leicester Union, 1867–1914" (PhD diss., University of Leicester, 2008), 53.

56. A detailed discussion of the two sides of the argument appears in Ruth G. Hodgkinson, "Poor Law Medical Officers of England, 1834–1871." *Journal of the History of Medicine and Allied Sciences* 11 (1956): 317–19.

57. James E. Thorold Rogers, ed., *Joseph Rogers, MD: Reminiscences of the Workhouse Medical Officer* (London: Unwin, 1889), xviii–xix, 60–61.

58. Hodgkinson, *National Health Service*, 399–401.

59. Sidney Webb and Beatrice Webb, *State and the Doctor* (London: Longman, Green, 1910), 100n1.

60. Hodgkinson, "Poor Law Medical Officers," 319–20; BCLA, Returns, GP/B/18/2/1, October 15, 1856.

61. In the 1860s the starting salary of the medical officer at the Battle workhouse was £120; see Railton and Barr, *Battle Workhouse and Hospital*, 16.

62. BCLA, BBG, GP/B/2/1/15, April 4, 1855; GP/B/2/1/39, August 10, 1870.

63. Railton and Barr, *Battle Workhouse and Hospital*, 64, 90.

64. Hodgkinson, *National Health Service*, 528; Crompton, *Workhouse Children*, 92–93; Railton and Barr, *Battle Workhouse and Hospital*, 10, 271; Fowler, *Workhouse*, 57.

65. BCLA, BBG, GP/B/2/1/19, June 24, 1857.

66. Hodgkinson, *National Health Service*, 528; British Parliamentary Paper, *Provincial Workhouses*, HC 1867–68 (4), 8.

67. BCLA, BBG, GP/B/2/1/22, February 9, 1858.

68. BCLA, BBG, GP/B/2/1/23, June 8, 22, 1859; VGPC, GP/B/2/8/1/3, June 3, 24, 1859.

69. Railton and Barr, *Battle Workhouse and Hospital*, 44.

70. BCLA, BBG, GP/B/2/1/23, June 8, 1859; R. Redfern Davies, "Birmingham Workhouse Infirmary," *British Medical Journal* 2 (1858): 677; and 2 (1859): 284.

71. BCLA, House Sub-Committee (hereafter HSC), GP/2/3/3/8, July 4, 1882.

72. BCLA, VGPC, GP/B/2/8/1/6, July 2, November 29, 1875; BBG, GP/B/2/1/50, November 1, 1882.

73. Price, "Quantitative and Qualitative Study," 33.

74. Hodgkinson, *National Health Service*, 420; Crompton, *Workhouse Children*, 101.

75. British Parliamentary Paper, *Copies "of Evidence Taken by Inspectors of the Local Government Board at Sworn Inquiry,"* HC19, 1886; BCLA, BBG, GP/B/2/1/54, August 4, 1886; BCLA, Local Government Board, Orders, GP/B/1/1/4, August 2, 1886.

76. Price, "Quantitative and Qualitative Study," 32.

77. Langford, *Modern Birmingham*, 381–83; BCLA, BBG, GP/B/2/1/15, January 9, 1855.

78. BCLA, BBG, GP/B/2/1/1, May 30, 1785; GP/B/2/1/2, August 11, 1818, June 25, 1822; GP/B/2/1/5, October 13, 1846.

79. BCLA, BBG, GP/B/2/1/33, July 18, 1866.

80. British Parliamentary Paper, *Provincial Workhouses*, 104, 113, 123, 130, 139.

81. BCLA, HSC, GP/B/2/3/3/1, January 7, September 16, 1868; Hodgkinson, *National Health Service*, 466.

82. BCLA, Infirmary Sub-Committee, GP/B/2/4/1/1–2, July 10, 1882, to March 20, 1885; BBG, GP/B/2/1/34, November 25, 1885.

83. BCLA, BBG, GP/B/2/1/59, May 7, 1890.

84. Railton and Barr, *Battle Workhouse and Hospital*, 64–65.

85. Crompton, *Workhouse Children*, 77.

86. Ibid., 81.

87. Elizabeth Lomax, *Small and Special: The Development of Hospitals for Children in Victorian Britain* (London: Wellcome Trust, 1996), 94–95.

88. Crompton, *Workhouse Children*, 82.

89. BCLLS, *Birmingham Poor Law and Workhouse, Miscellaneous Documents*, vol. 2, "Rules and Regulations of the Guardians of the Poor, of the Parish of Birmingham, 1841," BCOL 41.11.

90. Crompton, *Workhouse Children*, 85.

91. Ibid., 80–81.

92. Railton and Barr, *Battle Workhouse and Hospital*, 114.

93. Driver, *Power and Pauperism*, 158–59.

94. Crompton, *Workhouse Children*, 43, 44.

95. BCLA, BBG, GP/B/2/1/20, November 18, 1857.

96. BCLA, BBG, GP/2/1/20, December 2, 1857.

97. Hodgkinson, *National Health Service*, 300–302.

98. BCLA, VGPC, GP/B/2/8/1/2, August 7, 1857.

99. "Prevention of Contagious Diseases," *Lancet*, March 20, 1869, 414–15.

100. British Parliamentary Paper, *Poor Relief*, 468-I, 1870.

101. BCLA, HSC, GP/B/2/3/3/14, June 21, October 11, 1892.

102. BCLA, VGPC, GP/B/2/8/1/2, November 30, 1855; November 9, 1855; April 3, 1857.

103. BCLA, Workhouse Infirmary Management Committee (hereafter WIMC), GP/B/2/4/4/2, April 10, 1891.

104. BCLA, VGPC, GP/B/2/8/1/9, September 26, 1884.

105. BCLA, WIMC, GP/B/2/4/4/2, January 25, 1895.

106. BCLA, Infirmary House Sub-Committee, GP/B/2/4/5/1, July 24, 1899.

107. BCLA, VGPC, GP/B/2/8/1/2, November 30, 1855; GP/B/2/8/1/4, May 22, 1865; GP/B/2/8/1/9, August 14, 1885.

108. BCLA, WIMC, GP/B/2/4/4/1, February 6, 18, 1889.

109. Michelle Higgs, *Life in the Victorian and Edwardian Workhouse* (Stroud: Tempus, 2007), 78–81, is one of the few to include a specific section on epileptics, but the coverage is brief. Negrine, "Medicine and Poverty," includes a more extensive discussion, but the number of epileptic patients in the Leicester workhouse was small, for example, twenty-eight patients in 1881. A number of the other sources cited in this chapter contain no reference to these patients.

110. Owsei Temkin, *The Falling Sickness: A History of Epilepsy from the Greeks to the Beginning of Modern Neurology* (Baltimore: Johns Hopkins University Press, 1971), 255–56.

111. BCLA, Register of Insane, MH/344/12/1, 1845.

112. British Parliamentary Paper, *Poor Relief*, 468-I, 1870; BCLA, HSC, GP/B/2/3/3/2, October 25, 1870.

113. Christoph Conrad, "Old Age and the Health Care System in the Nineteenth and Twentieth Centuries," in *Old Age from Antiquity to Post-Modernity*, ed. Paul Johnson and Pat Thane (London: Routledge, 1998), 132; Michael J. Denham, "The History of Geriatric Medicine and Hospital Care of the Elderly between 1929 and the 1970s" (PhD diss, University College London, 2004); Pat Thane, *Old Age in English History: Past Experiences, Present Issues* (Oxford: Oxford University Press, 2000), 436.

114. Digby, *Pauper Palaces*, 144; Mary MacKinnon, "The Use and Misuse of Poor Law Statistics, 1857 to 1912," *Historical Methods* 21 (1988): 6.

115. These issues are discussed in Digby, *Pauper Palaces*, 163; Peter Townsend, *The Last Refuge* (London: Routledge and Kegan Paul, 1962), 23; they were also recognized in *The Minority Report of the Poor Law Commission* (1909; repr. Clifton, New Jersey: A. M. Kelley, 1974), 361.

116. Nigel Goose, "Workhouse Populations in Mid-Nineteenth Century: The Case of Hertfordshire," *Local Population Studies* 62 (1999): 57; Andrew Hinde and Fiona Turnbull, "The Populations of Two Hampshire Workhouses, 1851–1861," *Local Population Studies* 61 (1998): 42.

117. George R. Boyer and Timothy P. Schmidle, "Poverty among the Elderly in Late Victorian England," *Economic History Review* 62 (2009): 253; Parliamentary Papers, 895 (C7684), xii; Thane, *Old Age*, 167.

118. BCLA, BBG, GP/B/2/1/33, July 18, 1866.

119. David Thomson, "Workhouse to Nursing Home: Residential Care of Elderly People in England since 1840," *Ageing and Society* 3 (1983): 47; Karel Williams, *From Pauperism to Poverty* (London: Routledge and Kegan Paul, 1981), 205.

120. BCLA, VGPC, GP/B/2/8/1/4, May 22, 1865; GP/B/2/8/1/9, August 14, 1885; BBG, GP/B/2/1/33, July 18, 1866.

121. BCLA, Local Government Board Letters, GP/B/1/2/1/1, February 18, 1871.

122. BCLA, VGPC, GP/B/2/8/1/9, August 14, 1885.

123. BCLA, WIMC, GP/B/2/4/4/2, November 24, 1893.

124. Driver, *Power and Pauperism*, 69.

Chapter Eight

"Immediate Death or a Life of Torture Are the Consequences of the System"

The Bridgwater Union Scandal and Policy Change

SAMANTHA SHAVE

That the Poor Law Amendment Act (1834) was a controversial piece of legislation is a historical given. Through the creation of union workhouses, it removed the long-held rights of the poor to obtain outdoor relief, and through the establishment of a centralized welfare authority the Poor Law Commission weakened the powers of local parish officers and magistrates in the administration of relief. The transition from Old to New Poor Law was not a smooth one, and even "compliant" localities faced a number a problems with the new system—especially so in relation to medical relief. In the early years of the operation of the Bridgwater Union, established in 1836, several medical claimants had either died or suffered long-term ailments in consequence of delayed medical treatment. This chapter examines how this one event escalated into a "scandal," how those who witnessed the scandal influenced policy development, and the repercussions of new medical policies on relief claimants and administrators alike. It is influenced by an understanding of the "policy process," a concept developed in the social sciences to understand policy. Also known as the "policy life-cycle," the concept analyzes policy at a series of stages: the identification of a problem, policy making, policy implementation, policy evaluation, and the further development or creation of new policies.[1] This chapter offers a new perspective on the role of welfare scandals in poor law studies, locating them at the center of New Poor Law policy development.

The anti–New Poor Law movement sought to expose flaws in the operation of the new relief system, with zealous activities bringing local problems in the administration of relief to a national stage. The print media played an important role in this movement, reporting true, exaggerated, and false cases of neglect and abuse toward relief claimants. David Roberts's analysis of such reports in the *Times* between 1837 and 1842 uncovered reports of sixteen wife and husband separations, thirty-two accounts of punishments, fourteen cases of overcrowding, twenty-four cases of inadequate diets, ten cases of diseased conditions, and seven workhouse-based murders. Outside of the workhouse, there were forty-two reported cases of inadequate out-door relief to the aged and infirm and thirty-three cases where emergency relief was refused. This seemingly systematic cataloging of abuse, Roberts argues, demonstrates the effectiveness of the anti–New Poor Law movement in securing publicity and bringing news of maltreatment and maladministra-tion to a wider audience.[2] This interpretation prompted a response from Ursula Henriques, who believed that the reports illustrated "a climate of opinion in which abuses were more likely to occur," a "climate" effectively of the Poor Law Commission's making.[3]

A further study by Peter Dunkley took a different approach, suggesting that cases of abuse occurred before 1834, but that because the New Poor Law was organized on a centralized basis, local problems now assumed national importance.[4] Whatever the case, evidence of abuse and how it was reported and responded to not only provides us with an important understanding of the role of crises in the development of the New Poor Law but also gives us a unique lens on the negotiations between local and national relief authorities. Such an approach has already helped to modify our understanding of several aspects of poor law administration post-1834. Using correspondence between the commission and the board of guard-ians regarding the death of Henry Williams in Llantrisant, John Stewart and Steven King have revealed the complexities faced both in Wales and in Somerset House when implementing the Amendment Act.[5] Others, notably Norman McCord on Tyneside and Roger Wells on east Hampshire, have also examined local-center relations through the correspondence created in similar periods of turmoil.[6]

While the abuses at the center of these studies all garnered significant public attention, few cases escalated into "welfare scandals." As Ian Butler and Mark Drakeford have contended, scandals are produced through "the process whereby everyday tragedies are transformed into something extraor-dinary; the process whereby events that are local and personal become national and public; the process whereby the specific comes to stand for the general."[7] Indeed, while all scandals necessarily developed from "every-day tragedies," not all everyday tragedies escalated into scandals. Indeed, although everyday tragedies and scandals during the early years of the New Poor Law *have* caught the attention of poor law historians, hitherto no explicit distinction has been drawn between the two. Nor did all scandals in the early years of the New Poor Law lead to policy change.

Regardless of the number of scandals that emerged in the first years of centralized welfare provision, the only scandal invariably acknowledged in more generalized studies of the New Poor Law is the Andover Union Scandal of the 1840s.[8] Here, malnourished paupers gnawed on the bones they were supposed to crush for the guardians to sell as fertilizer.[9] Andover's powerful legacy has endured for two key reasons. First, the Andover scandal has been mobilized as a graphic example of maladministration, evoking a clear "grim symbolic feature" of life behind the workhouse doors.[10] Second, the Andover scandal is also believed to have put the final nail in the coffin of the commission, it being left to expire without renewal by Parliament in 1847 and duly replaced by the Poor Law Board.[11]

This chapter shifts our focus from the totemic Andover scandal, to consider instead the impact of scandals on the policy decisions made by the commission. It does this by tracing the consequences of death and long-term afflictions caused by delayed medical treatments in the New Poor Law Union of Bridgwater, Somerset, formed in 1836. In November 1837 a group of local medical men published a pamphlet detailing their cases. Their avowed intention was to bring "these and other equally horrible circumstances" to "the public attention," though, unsurprisingly, theirs was a more complex agenda than just highlighting abuse.[12] The publicity that followed amplified the cases into a national scandal. This chapter traces how the events in one union had long-lasting repercussions, focusing in particular on how this scandal informed national medical policy making, culminating in the General Medical Order of 1842. This perspective on the role of New Poor Law scandals is inspired by Butler and Drakeford, who conceptualized scandals as important feedback mechanisms between the policy implementation and policy-making stages of the policy process mentioned earlier. Scandals can make central welfare authorities review their policies and the way in which policy has been implemented. In consequence, authorities can revoke or change their policies or create new ones altogether.

Not all scandals produced in the early years of the New Poor Law caused such direct policy change, however. Butler and Drakeford note, "to have an impact an individual scandal needs to take place at a time of policy strain . . . to be capable of catching a tide that is already beginning to run in a fresh policy direction."[13] It is important that, before I examine the events at Bridgwater and the repercussions, an outline of the area of "policy strain" is provided. Medical relief practices were not explicitly stipulated before the General Medical Order of 1842, an omission that led to a number of conventions and tensions between the passage of the Amendment Act and 1842. In addition, as social scientists and historians alike remind us, just because a policy is released does not mean it is successful in resolving the problem it sought to address. Building on the findings of others, the final section underlines the problems faced by unions in the implementation of the new medical relief policy, casting some doubt

over its usefulness beyond its place in history of the first statutory acknowl-
edgment of the poor's right to medical relief.

Medical Relief Provision

The founding Old Poor Law legislation, the Act of Forty-Third Elizabeth,
did not make any explicit reference to medical relief. Subsequent legislation was also silent on the provision of medical relief, besides a couple
of statutes passed during the early years of George III, which permitted
justices to order medical relief for indoor poor. As such, the provision of
medical relief was not compulsory, relief being driven by custom rather
than stipulation. While, by the early nineteenth century, some parishes
employed medical men, according to George Cornewall Lewis, appointed
as a poor law commissioner from 1839, such provision was not universal.
Medical relief, he asserted, "did not extend beyond the counties in the
south, and east, and the centre of England."[14] Because there were no
legally stipulated minimum standards, the actual standard of care varied
from parish to parish. This meant that the provision of medical relief varied from both place to place and over time. In addition, parish-stipulated
entitlement to medical relief varied. As the analysis of pauper letters shows,
individual claimants detailed their ailments in different ways to secure a
modicum of assistance in a context of "uncertain and uneven entitlement
to relief and medical intervention."[15]

Medical relief was little alluded to in the 1834 report of the Royal
Commission. The report simply concluded that medical relief was "ade-
quately supplied, and economically, if we consider only the price and
amount of attendance."[16] Unsurprisingly then, the Poor Law Amendment
Act contained only one reference to medical relief: section 54, which
empowered magistrates to order medical attendance in an emergency.[17] To
Michael Flinn, this is suggestive of the fact that medical relief under the New
Poor Law was built on the "foundations inherited" from what went before.[18]
The poor law commissioners soon acknowledged the long-held traditions of
parish relief, noting in their first annual report the "deficiencies" of medical
relief under the Old Poor Law.[19] The parish doctor had been employed at
a small sum per year, on the "condition that he should be allowed to make
whatever charges he pleased for his attendance," while medicines were supplied "at the highest rates." Consequently, large profits, especially in more
"populous parishes," were being accrued by medical men and apothecaries.
There were other "evils" too. People in remote parishes "had no adequate
protection," and any individual could be supplied with "medicines considerably beyond what is required."[20] Regardless of the ambiguous position on
medical relief created by the Royal Commission, the poor law commissioners

immediately believed that not only would medical relief continue under the New Poor Law but that it would be improved.

Although no statute directly stipulated that medical relief should be provided, two further sections of the Amendment Act allowed boards of guardians to appoint medical men. Section 46 permitted boards to appoint paid officers and section 109 noted that a medical officer could be used to denote "any . . . Person duly licensed to practice as a Medical Man."[21] Medical officers were appointed under these powers upon the establishment of unions throughout England and Wales. For instance, at the first meeting of the Fareham Union, Hampshire, the guardians, in the presence of an assistant commissioner, divided the union into two medical districts. The acreage and population of each district, taken by the guardians from the 1831 census, were unequal.[22] A medical officer was then allocated to each district. The administrative aspects of medical relief were, therefore, forged under the guidance of the commission. The lack of medical relief stipulations and guidance beyond this point, however, resulted in numerous difficulties. These centered on several fundamental, albeit interrelated, themes: the qualifications and wages of medical officers, to whom and what medical relief should be allocated, and the size of medical districts. It is worth outlining these issues before providing an account of the Bridgwater scandal.

The position of medical officer could be given only to an individual "duly licensed" to act as a medical man, although the Poor Law Commission did not stipulate what qualifications or level of experience such a medical man should have. The quality of medical relief could, therefore, vary greatly depending on whom boards of guardians appointed. In their first annual report, the Poor Law Commission was glad to announce that, as a check to the "expense of medical relief," they "generally required that medical services should be retained by contract and open tender."[23] Medical men were paid on a case-by-case basis or, as the commissioners implied, in a lump sum or at a rate per head of the population of the medical district set before the commencement of their appointment. Competitive agreements were difficult to engineer in the latter case. In May 1836 the attention of assistant commissioner William Henry Toovey Hawley was brought to the "troublesome medical contracts" in his Hampshire unions. Of particular concern to Hawley was the offer of eight shillings per head of the population offered to the Hartley Wintney guardians by the local medical men, a sum he thought was too high.[24] The board of guardians of newly established Bridgwater Union had similar problems, which had far-reaching consequences. As Anne Digby notes, the financial preoccupations of the welfare authorities meant that "cost rather than adequate qualification became the driving force" for medical officers' appointments.[25]

Financial considerations also impacted entitlement to medical relief. Writing in 1836, the commissioners had already received queries from boards of guardians, asking to whom medical relief could be issued. Their response was that "actual necessity or destitution is the condition on which all applications for relief, medical or otherwise, are to be decided." Those in the workhouse had "passed" the workhouse test and therefore were deemed to be sufficiently eligible for medical assistance. For those outside the workhouse, the situation was less clear-cut. Although individuals on the "list" would have been entitled to medical relief, those who were not on the list may have been told to pay for their own medical assistance. The commission also encouraged the formation of "independent" sick clubs.[26] Even when an individual was "entitled" to medical relief, judgments had to be made regarding what treatment would be offered. Medicines were expected to be supplied from the medical officers' own funds, while food, primarily consisting of meat and alcohol, was commonly allocated to the sick poor from union funds. It was unclear whether medical men should have to deliver children and undertake surgery, however, and they would often bargain for additional payments for such services. In practice, it was often the decision of the workhouse master and matron or the relieving officer as to whether these procedures were required from a medical officer. Besides, other individuals, such as nurses and midwives, would often perform such tasks for lower wages.[27]

Another source of contention was the size of the medical districts. Doctors, who had previously served just one or two parishes, were now required to attend many parishes. This was problematic in rural unions, where large medical districts would "make it insuperably difficult for even the most conscientious medical officer to operate efficiently."[28] The medical officer would undertake rounds, visiting parishes on a regular basis. When medical relief was required outside of these times, the poor had to search for their medical officer. In addition, it was assumed by the commission that medical officers would secure the consent of a relieving officer before providing an individual with medical relief. This generated conflict. Medical officers thought that relieving officers were not capable of judging individuals' medical needs, and the relieving officers believed that medical officers were taking "little account of the many moral and economic factors" surrounding relief provision.[29] This meant that the poor would have to obtain the attention of two officers, sometimes in different places. In the early years of the New Poor Law, much correspondence passed between the guardians and the commission containing details of those who had traveled vast distances to obtain assistance. Henry Williams's walk of "several miles" to obtain outdoor relief within the confines of the Llantrisant Union, as detailed by Stewart and King, was far from unique. As Digby suggests, the outdoor poor, compared to those in the workhouse, suffered from a "deterioration in the quality of care."[30] Such problems were only brought to wider attention through a series of high profile medical relief "scandals" that exposed these deficiencies of medical provision.

The Bridgwater Scandal

The problems at the Bridgwater Union surfaced immediately after its formation by assistant commissioner Robert Weale in April 1836 (for a timeline of events, see table 8.1). The union encompassed forty parishes in the northwest of Somerset covering parts of Exmoor and the Quantocks and had a low population density. The interests of all parishes were represented at the largest board of guardians in Somerset, made up of forty-eight elected members and fifteen ex-officio members.[31] Immediately after the formation of a union, it was a common practice to select existing workhouses to temporarily house the poor until a more substantial union workhouse was built. The Bridgwater and North Petherton houses were selected, with adults going into the former house and children into the latter. Both soon became overcrowded.[32] In the winter of 1836–37, one-third of the inmates had died from enteric infection, deaths mainly occurring in the Bridgwater parish workhouse, which accommodated 105 paupers during the winter.[33] While overcrowding and unsanitary conditions were likely to have been the main cause of the deaths, the workhouse diet also received some blame. The guardians chose to adopt dietary table number three, one of six dietaries designed by the commission for implementation in every union workhouse. This table, akin to three other commission-designed tables, contained the controversial foodstuff gruel, which Abraham King, the workhouse medical officer, thought the main cause of the sickness.[34]

Although rumors had spread among the guardians about the overcrowding and sickness, it was not general public knowledge until the following year. Still, guardian William Baker, who had been appointed to the Visiting Committee, visited the Bridgwater poorhouse and advised the guardians to change the inmates' diet and to stop sending paupers to the institution. He had little success.[35] John Bowen, Baker's friend and colleague, then intervened.[36] Bowen was a Tory and heavily involved in Bridgwater borough's politics.[37] He was a fierce opponent of the New Poor Law and frequently corresponded with the editor of the *Times*. In one such letter, Bowen expressed a dislike of the design of the new Bridgwater Union workhouse, which contained windows six feet above the ground. He claimed that the commission-supported architect Sampson Kempthorne had "shut out . . . all enjoyment of the light of heaven" from the poor. The editor agreed, calling the building "a nest of Kempthorne dungeons."[38] After becoming aware of the article, Weale wrote to the commission, explaining that the parish workhouse that Bowen had claimed to be a "palace" was, in fact, "ten thousand times more worthy of the name of dungeon."[39]

Table 8.1. Medical relief policy and the Bridgwater scandal timeline

Local		National
Deaths in the poorhouses of the Bridgwater Union	1836	John Bowen contacts the editor of the *Times*
John Bowen is elected to the board of guardians of the Bridgwater Union	1837	Bowen publishes his notes regarding the operation of the Bridgwater Union in the *Times*
Guardians decide to change medical arrangements		
Guardians negotiate with the medical men (Bridgwater Medical Association) and organize temporary medical relief arrangements		Commission directs assistant Robert Weale to advise the Bridgwater Union board
Guardians pay medical men's bills		
William Lakin Caswell, medical man, commits suicide		Bridgwater Medical Association publishes pamphlet outlining events in the union; subsequently reprinted in the *Times*
John Rodney Ward, medical man, is tried at Assizes	1838	Lord Wharncliffe moves that several cases should be investigated by the House of Lords
Many individuals involved in the Bridgwater Union scandal interviewed		Lords Select Committee commences (March–July)
Jonathan Toogood (chair of Bridgwater Medical Association) is interviewed		Commons Select Committee begins "Medical Inquiry" (July)
Problems in unions reach the commission	1839	Commission directs assistants to undertake detailed survey of medical relief
British Medical Association refers to cases of maladministration and incompetency (including Bridgwater)		Commission meets with a deputation of the Bridgwater Medical Association, and George Webster presents ideas
		Summaries of commission's medical relief investigations published

(continued)

Table 8.1. Medical relief policy and the Bridgwater scandal timeline—*(concluded)*

Local		National
Guardians do not react to the commission's letter	1840	Commission issues circular letter to all unions to call attention to the publication
	1841	Pressure stems from the medical associations to release policies
	1842	General Medical Order is released by commission
	1843	Stipulations of the General Medical Order take effect

Regardless of the tension evident between Bowen and the commission, Bowen wanted to become a member of the Bridgwater board of guardians. It was not his intention, though, to help administer the New Poor Law; on the contrary, he wanted access to information that would prove the board's negligence. Bowen was elected in May 1837, and having the previous month visited the Bridgwater poorhouse and inspected the report book of the Visiting Committee, he immediately asked for a change of diet and better handling of the inmates. He was ignored.[40] In July 1837 Bowen resigned and duly sent his notes to the *Times.*

While the union evidently had problems caring for their indoor poor, their outdoor poor also suffered from a lack of adequate attention. Many of the medical-relief problems derived from the board's desire to reduce associated costs. In the year before the formation of the union, medical salaries for the parishes totaled £577 per annum. After the formation of the union, seven large medical districts were created and seven medical officers were appointed to attend to the poor. Their wages came to £363 per annum. The medical men in the Bridgwater area resented the reduction, but the chair of the board stressed that the first year was one of "probation," implying that their wages would increase the following year.[41] When the year ended in May 1837, the board decided to discontinue the previous year's arrangements and proposed the creation of twelve medical districts, including one specifically for the attendance of the workhouse. Details of these districts were circulated to the medical officers in the hope that they would respond to the proposal positively. By the following week, five of the medical men had replied. Although their comments cannot be found in the archive, their opinions clearly vexed the board and discussion was adjourned. On May 18 a specially arranged meeting of the board called for another "fresh Division of the Union," deciding to carve the union into nine medical districts, including one for the attendance of the union workhouse.[42] The salaries proposed varied greatly because they were calculated on the basis of the population of each district. The medical men were then invited by the board to state their offers, which ranged from three pence and four pence per head in certain districts and a flat rate of fifty pounds for the workhouse district. Although, cumulatively, these salaries were fifty pounds below the preunion medical costs, their proposal was once again rejected by the board.[43]

The election of the medical officers to districts was to proceed on June 16, 1837, and the new allocations were to start a fortnight later. In the meantime some members of the board were concerned that this would attract unskilled medical men to the union and argued that those appointed had to possess specific medical qualifications. Anxious that *no* medical men would apply for the positions, the motion was rejected. By early June the medical men were still in disagreement with the guardians, writing a collective letter expressing that "they cannot with justice to the Poor, the Guardians, and themselves, continue their charge at the salaries proposed."[44] The letter was written during a meeting of the Bridgwater Medical Association, formed of medical men from Bridgwater and the surrounding area, many of whom had previously acted as medical officers. By September 1838 it was documented as a branch of the Provincial Medical and Surgical Association (PMSA), one of the largest medical associations in Britain.[45] It was at such meetings that the medical men discussed their grievances and continued to exert pressure on the guardians for fairer wages. Indeed, by June 1837 the medical men resorted to printing a handbill detailing their demands.[46] The public protest caused no material alteration in the views of the guardians who, while acknowledging the men's concern for the poor, were adamant that no change should occur to the proposed districts and salaries until the second election day.[47]

Locked in a stalemate with the medical men, the board decided to contact Somerset House to request the commissioners to recommend "a candidate or two."[48] The commission, realizing the magnitude of the problem, directed Weale to attend the next meeting of the Bridgwater board.[49] Weale offered little advice, simply agreeing with the board that the wages demanded by the medical men "were more than adequate remuneration for their services and that they be not accepted."[50] The board also decided that there should be only six districts, each covering a vast area of land. In consequence, just two of the medical men were allocated to districts, with the remaining vacancies advertised in the local and London press. One of the forthcoming candidates was unfamiliar with the area, while three local men took the remaining districts at the low rates offered by the board.[51] One of these individuals was apprehensive about taking such an expansive district, ten miles long and eight miles wide, containing fourteen parishes.[52] After raising his concerns, he took the district alongside another local medical man. Overall, of the seven medical men appointed for the first year of the union, just four had been reemployed, on terms they found unsatisfactory.

During these extended negotiations and discussions, the old medical arrangements—in operation from May 1836 to May 1837—had expired and a temporary medical service was established. Thinking on their feet, board members directed their medical officers to continue their services into July but "to attend the poor on the same terms as they did their private patients." Mindful of the potential cost, the guardians instructed the relieving officers "to be sparing in their orders for medical relief."[53] John Stagg, relieving officer for the Huntspill District, informed the medical officer of the district, William Lakin Caswell, that "I am directed by the Board of Guardians to inform you that you are to discontinue your attendance on the under mentioned Paupers in Woollavington."[54] A further four letters were sent to Caswell, directing him to stop attending four other paupers.[55] Caswell conformed to these orders reluctantly. On July 2 Caswell wrote in his notebook, "in consequence of the Order of Mr. Stagg I have this Day been *reluctantly compelled* to refuse Medicine to George Reynold's Child, Kesia Coles, and Nancy Millard." On July 6 Caswell wrote a letter to the board of guardians, arguing that they should not stop his attendance of the poor.[56]

For some of his patients, Caswell's protest was too late. Several paupers had been left without medical attendance, with devastating consequences. One case was that of thirty-one-year-old Charlotte Allen, who lodged with Jane Fenn and Richard and Mary Date, a nurse, in the small parish of Nether Stowey.[57] A month before giving birth on June 30, 1837, Charlotte fell ill. She had no savings and was not able to draw on alternative sources of support.[58] As she approached motherhood, Charlotte received one shilling and sixpence and a loaf of bread every week from her relieving officer, James Franklin Waites. Thereafter, there was some confusion over who was going to deliver her child. Mary Date informed the relieving officer that Charlotte wanted Kitty Walker (Mary's sister) to act as her midwife, even though Charlotte had made no such request.[59] Mary Date had obviously abused her position and exploited the vulnerability of Charlotte to obtain her sister employment. Nevertheless, Kitty Walker was a trained midwife with nine years' experience.[60] The birth of Charlotte's child was, however, difficult. Charlotte suffered from a laceration of the perineum during "the violent Efforts of Labour," leading to a prolapsed womb.[61]

From this point, Charlotte should have been attended by a medical officer. Kitty thought there was nothing unusual with Charlotte's injuries and gave her castor oil, senna tea, and some hot towels to aid her recovery. Charlotte was certain she should be seen by the medical officer and tried to relay her message to another person, Betty Woolley, who was going to see Waites for some bread.[62] Betty failed to pass on the details of Charlotte's illness, and Waites subsequently claimed it would be "indelicate for me to ask Questions." Waites suggested that Betty went to his wife to explain, after which Mary Waites and Betty went to see Charlotte.[63] In the meantime, Kitty had spoken to Mr. Waites, which reinforced her opinion that nothing was especially wrong with Charlotte. Mr. Waites did not, therefore, send for a surgeon. Several days later, Charlotte sent another message from her bed, and a medical man, Richard Beadon Ruddock from Stowey, was finally sent. Ruddock visited Charlotte that Wednesday night, but he did not examine her until the following morning. It was only on this examination that Charlotte was told the extent of her injuries. Ruddock then notified Abraham King, another medical man, and from then on visited her regularly. This was because the womb needed to be constantly "replaced," as it "protruded by some little Exertion on her part."[64] The type of injury sustained by Charlotte was fairly common, although it was rare for this injury to be so bad on the birth of a woman's first child. According to Charles Locock, another medical man, Charlotte was "for many Months [after the birth] . . . constantly in pain, suffering from very distressing and painful Sensations."[65]

While Charlotte had developed a lifelong, but not life-threatening, illness, there were two fatalities in the union. One of the four paupers Caswell was instructed not to attend, George Reynold's child, died.[66] Little information has been found about the circumstances surrounding his death; however, the fatality of young John Cook is well detailed. John lived at Pig Cross and had been suffering from croup. One morning Lucretia Cook was anxious about her child's health and left the house to obtain an order. James Newman asked her about her circumstances, presumably to gauge her need for medical relief, and Lucretia explained that although her husband was a shoemaker, he did not always have work. Lucretia later stated, "I recollect telling him. . . . I was very poor, and in great Distress, and not able to pay a Doctor; and that I had before been attended by a Parish Doctor." Newman informed her that she must pay for private medical assistance. Lucretia immediately pawned her son's jacket (for three shillings) and found King, who was not at home, only to hear that he charged five shillings for a week's worth of attendance. Lucretia rushed to pawn a gun (for four shillings). At eleven o'clock, she saw James Coles Parker, a local medical man, and asked him to see her son. Parker gave her medicine, free of charge, and asked her to pass a note onto Newman.[67] The letter stressed that John was "*literally dying for want of surgical assistance.*"[68] Newman took the note to the board of guardians and told Lucretia to visit him half an hour afterward. After Newman had attended the board, Mrs. Ware (Lucretia's neighbor) went to the "Hall" (supposedly where the board had met) and obtained a note for Lucretia stating that King would attend John.[69] King finally arrived that afternoon and visited on several occasions. During this time John's illness had advanced, and he died that evening.[70]

The board's desire to keep the union purse strings tight had fatal consequences for the medical officers as well as medical relief claimants. After the medical officers had worked, temporarily, for the union for three weeks, their bills were sent into the board. The guardians decided not to keep to their word by paying the medical officers on a case-by-case basis as had been agreed. On Friday, October 27, the board voted, by a majority of one, to pay a proportion of the bills based on their previous salaries, working out the cost of three weeks' pay.[71] It transpired that a very small proportion of Caswell's bill had been reimbursed.[72] Some of the guardians had anticipated the consequences of their actions and immediately declared that they would defend any legal actions brought against the board. The following week, Caswell was "in a State of the greatest Excitement," believing that "the Guardians had taken advantage of his Poverty."[73] He could not afford to take legal action against the guardians, being nearly bankrupt from attending more poor than he had intended to, a function of the size of his district, and also having worn out two horses in the process. Caswell committed suicide; his body was found on November 4.[74]

Caswell's suicide did not mark the end of the problems within the Bridgwater Union. A medical man appointed to attend the poor of the Bridgwater workhouse from July 1837, John Rodney Ward, had lied about his qualifications. He claimed he had obtained a qualification in the Netherlands at Leiden University, but it transpired that he left before the course finished.[75] Unsurprisingly, in 1838 he was convicted at the Wells Assizes Court for botching a surgical procedure.[76] There was a similar trial in the Kingston Union, in Surrey, but, according to Ruth Hodgkinson, such cases were rare, medical men usually being only reprimanded by the guardians.[77] That the Bridgwater Medical Association was hostile toward Ward may have been a factor in Ward's prosecution.[78] However, after the trial, Ward was, astonishingly, reappointed for a second year. When a "more moderate" set of guardians was elected in 1839, his contract was not renewed again.[79]

Inquiries and Impacts

The events at Bridgwater highlighted many of the fundamental problems with medical relief provision under the early New Poor Law. The competitive tendering desired by the guardians and permitted by the assistant commissioners meant that a medical man's willingness to accept low wages, rather than his skills, was a prerequisite to his employment. This drive for economy led to temporary case-by-case payments, the hiring of unsuitable people to act as medical officers, the founding of large medical districts, and, ultimately, the retrenchment of medical relief. As Butler and Drakeford have demonstrated, a scandal could not simply derive from such policy stipulations. A scandal *develops* from "unanticipated exposure, followed by disapproval," after events created by policy decisions.[80] The events at Bridgwater were brought to light in a range of publications. In November 1837 the Bridgwater Medical Association wrote a pamphlet summarizing their negotiations with the board of guardians and their subsequent broken promises. The medical men emphasized their inadequate pay, the temporary measures orchestrated by the board, and the sufferings of the claimants: "It is to such heart rendering cases as Charlotte Allen's, & Reynold's and Cook's, where the very bed clothes of the dying are stripped off and pawned to obtain relief, where immediate death or a life of torture are the consequences of the system acted on by the Board of Guardians."[81] They detailed Charlotte's case, although the facts were exaggerated. Indeed, the pamphlet states that she was suffering from puerperal fever, although Charlotte herself did not acknowledge that she had suffered from the disease.[82] Just nine days after the pamphlet was published, it was reprinted in the *Times*.[83] News of the medical relief problems, combined with earlier news of overcrowding in the Bridgwater workhouse, had led to greater awareness of Bridgwater as a troubled union.[84]

In March 1838 the Bridgwater guardians sent a petition to the government expressing their support for the New Poor Law. Although this action was commended by the Poor Law Commission, it was unable to stop public curiosity.[85] The same month Lord Wharncliffe, a Tory, felt that it was time to investigate what he thought were unfounded allegations about the maladministration of the Amendment Act. There were several cases that had caught his attention, for which he thought papers should be requested and pursued. First, accusations had been made by General Johnson, a magistrate and ex-officio guardian, about the operation of the New Poor Law in the Bourne Union, Lincolnshire. Wharncliffe was angered that Johnson had "take[n] facts on mere hearsay, and not to institute anything like a sufficient investigation." Second, in the West Riding of Yorkshire, where there had been much "violence and outrage," Clergyman G. S. Bull had spoken at public meetings with stories of great cruelty resulting from the new welfare system. While these two cases were not, as far as he was concerned, based on fact, Wharncliffe thought there were several other cases from which he "did not think the working of the Poor-law was altogether satisfactory" and perhaps "some alteration should be made in the Act." It was in this context that knowledge of the events at Bridgwater reached Parliament. According to Wharncliffe, two issues needed investigation: sickness in the poorhouse and the allocation of medical officers. Bowen and his writings were also mentioned. After the Poor Law Commission completed their own investigations, Wharncliffe thought that "it was his duty to move their Lordships for a Committee to inquire into all those transactions," as both the circumstances of the Bridgwater Union and actions of the commissioners appeared unsatisfactory. Last, he brought forward the case of a family who wanted to place their children in the Hungerford Union workhouse in Berkshire. Somerset House did not allow such an arrangement, as it was tantamount to relief in aid of wages, a position that Wharncliffe thought was most inflexible.

While Prime Minister Viscount Melbourne thought this an overreaction to several operational problems, and others saw this as a chance to push for the repeal of the Amendment Act itself, the lords agreed for the papers to be requested. The Earl of Radnor moved for the papers relating to the sickness and dietary in the Dudley Union to be examined, showing further support for the inquiries. This did not mean that the other House was not proceeding with its own investigations. A Commons Select Committee was already underway, to "Inquire into the Administration of the Relief of the Poor," but, according to Wharncliffe, it had done little more than collect minutes of evidence from the poor law commissioners themselves.[86]

By the following May, a Select Committee was appointed in the House of Lords with Wharncliffe as chair, commencing its investigations in March 1838. Regardless of the fact that the inquiry was triggered by many cases of maladministration, the majority of the committee's time was occupied with examining the events at Bridgwater. A full 787 pages of the 1,312-page report consisted of minutes of evidence taken from those involved in the Bridgwater scandal alone. Key individuals, including Weale and Bowen, in addition to medical and relieving officers and relief claimants from the Bridgwater Union, were interviewed at length. It was only during these investigations that the full extent and state of medical administration in the union had been revealed.[87] At the end of the investigations, the committee found the evidence to be inconclusive and did not allocate blame to any one party. Yet this did not mean the contents were of little importance.

Bridgwater also featured within the 1837–38 Commons Select Committee, the committee about which Wharncliffe had previously been critical. Although this committee had initially interviewed each assistant on the implementation of the new welfare regime, it moved on to explore a number of policy themes.[88] According to the poor law commissioners, medical relief was "one of the most important subjects considered."[89] The committee's "Medical Inquiry," as they called it, began in July 1838, overlapping with the lords' investigations into Bridgwater.[90] To gauge the opinions of those who had experience and knowledge relating to providing medical relief, the committee interviewed "several gentlemen connected with that profession."[91] These included the secretary of the PMSA, Henry Wyldbore Rumsey, and the president of the British Medical Association (BMA) and long-standing editor of the *Lancet*, Dr. George Webster. Ten other men, who either represented medical men in local medical associations or had acted as medical officers, were also selected. It was no coincidence then that

Jonathan Toogood, the chair of the Bridgwater Medical Association, was called on to give evidence. Toogood was considered by the committee to be a man of "great experience."[92] He had been a surgeon all his professional life and had spent twenty-five years working in the Bridgwater Infirmary. He was also employed as a parish doctor prior to the formation of the Bridgwater Union. His opinions on the organization and current state of medical relief were unsurprising, considering the recent events at Bridgwater. Toogood thought that allocating large medical districts was problematic.[93] He suggested that medical officers should reside near, or in, their districts and that medical officers should be familiar with the neighborhood in which they practiced. He also believed there should be "a fixed salary for the fixed paupers" rather than any tendering or allowing payments "per case."[94] Toogood thus conveyed the views of the Bridgwater Medical Association at a national level. That they were similar to the national medical practitioners' associations, the PMSA and the BMA, must have helped his case. The national associations sent a joint petition to the Commons during the inquiry, asking for medical relief stipulations. The committee agreed with their analysis, positing that there were two main deficiencies in the administration of relief: "that the medical districts, in some instances, seem to be inconveniently large . . . and that the remuneration should be such as to insure the proper attention and the best medicines."[95] Although the committee did not stipulate any particular policies, "the introduction of these and other alterations" was left "to the discretion of the Poor Law Commissioners."[96] Instead of making immediate, rash decisions over the medical policy, the commission wanted to gather further information about the ways in which guardians provided medical relief.

The following year the commission instructed the assistant poor law commissioners to make detailed reports about medical relief provision in their districts. The assistants were directed to document how the medical officers were selected, whether they tendered for positions, how medical officers were paid, the size of each district, whether any dissatisfaction had arisen relating to medical relief, and what types of individuals or families were being provided with medical relief.[97] Bridgwater, unsurprisingly, did not receive a sparkling report. Bridgwater's new assistant commissioner, Daniel Goodson Adey, had already written to the commission, explaining, "the business of this Union appears to be done in a less satisfactory manner than *any* I've visited."[98] Adey's district contained thirty-five unions, so clearly Bridgwater's medical relief provision was still flawed. This did not mean that everything was ticking over nicely in every other place under his superintendence. In ten of Adey's unions, medical officers were unhappy with the size of their medical districts, and the medical men of fourteen unions were dissatisfied with their salaries. In addition, the guardians of three unions and the poor of two were not satisfied with the attendance or efficiency of the medical officers.[99]

Before a deputation of men from the BMA had met with the commission, similar reports were being drafted by the other assistant commissioners across England and Wales. The commissioners gave the men a copy of the survey recently issued to their assistant commissioners and asked them for any further thoughts they had on medical relief beyond those discovered in the "Medical Inquiry."[100] The following month another deputation of the association met with the commissioners, this time to specifically complain that the system of tendering had continued. The commission decided not to issue any immediate policies.[101] A couple of days later, the BMA president, Webster, presented a comprehensive "Report and Plans for an Amended System of Parochial Medical Relief," which was soon to be discussed between the deputation, the commissioners, and the home secretary.[102] The recent medical relief problems, however, could not be forgotten by the commission. During their meeting, members of the BMA drew on examples of bad practice from all over England and Wales to argue their points. Bridgwater featured at least twice. In relation to the objectionable practice of tendering and how, specifically, the lowest tender was taken in opposition to "character, personal qualification, and residence," they referred to cases of maladministration at "Aylesbury, Wallingford, Eastry, Hambledon, Ongar, Penshurst, Wheatenhurst, Leighton Buzzard, the Bridgewater [sic] and other Unions." In relation to the inadequate skills possessed by men appointed by the boards of guardians, the deputation made reference to the cases in the "Bridgwater and Kingston Union[s], as evinced by actions at law and verdicts of juries."[103]

Notwithstanding that summaries of the assistants' reports were published at the end of 1839 in the commission's *Report on the Further Amendment of the Poor Laws*, it took another two years for any policy stipulations to be enforced.[104] This delay was not in any way related to being unable to make policies but was rather an anxiety of the commission not to dictate over the localities. In March 1840 the commission issued a circular letter to guardians, calling for "their suggestions in this Report [*on the Further Amendment*]" to be considered.[105] The commission, in their seventh annual report, pessimistically admitted that "no extensive change in the existing [medical relief] arrangements were likely to originate with the Boards of Guardians."[106] Much "dissatisfaction continued to prevail amongst many members of the medical profession" and pressure on the commission for reforms continued to be exerted.[107]

The commission finally released compulsory and legally binding policies on March 12, 1842. Known as the General Medical Order, it took effect from March 1843. There were seven main sections to the order, each on different aspects of medical administration. The first addressed the problems of setting salaries but made it unlawful for boards of guardians to invite tenders.

Rather, if a vacancy arose for a medical officer in a union, the board had to specify the salary he would receive alongside a list of the places he would have to visit. Any salary given to an officer in an alternative manner would be disallowed in the union accounts and the guardians would personally become responsible for the cost. The order also stipulated that the medical officers should have both medical and surgical qualifications. By Lady Day 1843 medical officers were not permitted to attend districts larger than fifteen thousand acres in size or containing populations of more than fifteen thousand. A fourth theme in the order set out a list of payments per case, but only for particular procedures. Medical officers could claim five pounds, in addition to their normal salary, for several types of operation, such as amputations. Medical officers would also receive an extra three pounds per case for the treatment of simple fractures of the thigh or leg and just one pound for a fracture of the arm. For each case of midwifery, medical officers were to receive between ten and twenty shillings, and two pounds for difficult deliveries.[108]

The next section of the General Medical Order ensured that a union could check whether a patient had been visited and also that someone was always present to attend the sick within each district. Every officer was instructed to keep a weekly return, which should include the date of visits to paupers and their names. In addition, within twenty-one days of a new officer's appointment, he should provide the guardians with the name of a substitute who would act on his behalf during absence or illness. Guardians were instructed to create a list of "permanent paupers" every six months, including "all such aged and infirm persons, and persons permanently sick or disabled, as may be actually receiving [outdoor] relief." With a ticket these poor were allowed to see a medical officer without gaining the prior permission of a relieving officer. The final theme of the order related to the continuance of medical officers, indicating that they should lose their duties only if they resigned, became disqualified by the commission, or died.[109]

As Hodgkinson suggests, the policies closely follow the ideas of the medical men, and in particular Webster's report presented to the commission in 1839.[110] The policies were inspired by and developed out of the medical relief problems experienced at the local level, including the events that culminated in the Bridgwater scandal. These stipulations were evidently important in the development of medical relief during the New Poor Law, but adherence to the order was another matter.

The Implementation of the General Medical Order

The fact that the order had been issued did not mean that the practices altered instantaneously. Issued on March 12, 1842, the order was supposed to take effect by Lady Day the following year, the commission factoring in ample time to advise boards of guardians about its contents.[111] The commissioners used the boards' 1842 sanction requests to warn the guardians of the new policies. For instance, in 1841 the Dulverton guardians in Somerset divided their union into only two medical districts. By the following year the union was redivided into three districts, but although these districts had very small populations they had far exceeded the maximum acreage stipulated in the order.[112] The commission therefore requested that the guardians again redivide their union.[113] While all unions had already received the documents containing the order itself in 1842, the commission was making sure that the stipulations of the order had been read.

Although plenty of time had been allowed for the unions to adjust their practices, the General Medical Order had been applied with great difficulty and "guardians from all over the country demanded its suspension for their own Unions on one or several grounds." According to Hodgkinson, between twenty and thirty unions obtained a suspension within the first year of the order's implementation. Hodgkinson, drawing on the case of several northern towns and cities, thought that limiting the areas or population for the attendance of each medical officer was problematic, as there was ample charitable provision, including voluntary hospitals and dispensaries, to meet the needs of the poor. In addition, in such urban areas there was no point in limiting the population allocated to each officer because they "resided so close to the poor." The system of extras for surgical or midwifery cases was also ignored. Hodgkinson believed that the guardians thought it had given medical relief recipients an unfair advantage over the independent laborer, deterring them from obtaining their own surgery and midwifery attendance. Sometimes there was simply a lack of resident medical officers, making the reduction of districts impossible. The ticket system did not work either. Referring to the Stepney Union, Hodgkinson argued that some unions did not adopt the practice because there were simply "numerous claims constantly being made for urgent and pressing cases." In addition, ticket distribution gave individuals an entitlement to medical relief that apparently encouraged applications for help.[114]

There appear to have been three main problems with implementing the order in rural unions. First, many unions had a low population density, meaning that the restriction of each medical district to 15,000 acres was problematic. The result would be a great number of medical officers, each one with a small wage, which was both unpopular with the medical men and inefficient for a union to administer. Some unions also contained vast expanses of unpopulated land, including woodlands and forests. The Wimborne and Cranborne Union in Dorset, for example, contained a segment of Cranborne Chase. The total acreage of the union was 78,358, with a population of 15,793. Although the union was divided into four districts, each one exceeded the maximum acreage stipulated in the general order. So eager were the guardians to conform to the order that they corresponded with their eastwardly neighboring unions, Ringwood and Fordingbridge, asking whether they could take charge of medical attendance on the Chase.[115]

As Hodgkinson suggests, there was an increase in the number of medical officers "by a few hundred every year" after 1843, which indicated "the desired effect of diminishing the size of medical districts."[116] Yet a lack of medical men in rural locations meant that large medical districts *had* to be accepted. One medical district in the Mere Union (consisting of parishes from Wiltshire, Dorset, and Somerset), which had covered parts of the Wiltshire Downs, was large simply because there were no other resident medical men.[117] The commission simply had to accept that, even if the district was divided in two, no one could fill the vacancy.[118] And, even if medical men were in residence, they were sometimes deemed unsuitable to perform the role of a medical officer. In 1844 the commission heard how one medical officer, appointed by the South Stoneham Union, had practiced for three years with just one of the two required qualifications.[119] The second problem with implementing the order, therefore, was a lack of medical men, either in the right place or with suitable qualifications, to take up the positions available. Third, the "ticket" system did not always work because, rather than there being a plethora of cases to attend, there were too few. For instance, the Kingsclere guardians, Hampshire, reported that, as "all the paupers here were known to the medical officers," so the provision of tickets was futile.[120]

Although the commission wanted all unions to follow the stipulations of the order, they used their discretionary powers to sanction deviations where implementing the stipulations proved difficult. Whether these deviations were detrimental to the health of the medical claimants within these unions is, however, open to question. Nevertheless, for the first time in poor law history, medical relief standards had been set.

Scandal and Policy under the New Poor Law

Welfare scandals do not just provide us with insights into the maltreatment and neglect suffered by the vulnerable or with examples from which we can judge how cruel a system of welfare was. The Bridgwater case tells us that the early welfare scandals impacted policy development and, because of the centralization of poor relief from 1834, formed an early and essential feedback mechanism by which experiences of policy could become general knowledge and acted on. Of course, this was not a clear-cut or straightforward process, but neither was the control and management of the New Poor Law in the first instance.

As Butler and Drakeford suggest, welfare scandals have all the makings of a novel: "All contain stock heroes and villains and many descend . . . to little more than morality plays."[121] In the process whereby these everyday tragedies were constructed into a scandal, the commission and Bridgwater board of guardians remained remarkably silent. Indeed, why would welfare authorities draw attention to cases of cruelty and neglect when it was not within their best interests to do so? Rather, there was another level, confined neither to the local or center, of key actors and stakeholders who brought events to wider public attention. Without John Bowen's investigative reporting, news of Bridgwater's inept board of guardians would neither have reached the press nor the House of Lords. Key actors working at the national level, however, had more power than those working between the national and local levels. It was the decision of lords and members of Parliament whether to instigate an inquiry into these local events or not. Indeed, Bowen's views on the problems at Bridgwater had caught the eye of Lord Wharncliffe. He wanted the government to ask, "were those stories of neglect true, or false?"[122]

Social policy analysts have viewed the policy-making process "as an inescapably *political* activity into which the perceptions and interests of individual actors enter all stages."[123] Stakeholders were also part of this political activity—united together to represent their own shared "perceptions and interests." This been illustrated in the events that culminated after the neglect of medical relief claimants at Bridgwater. The Bridgwater Medical Association produced a pamphlet that was subsequently published in the *Times*, evidence that Lord Wharncliffe was able to utilize in a House of Lords investigation. The House of Commons, aware of the problems faced by members of the local medical association, also interviewed their chair to obtain an idea of what they thought were the deficiencies of medical relief policy. Thereafter, the BMA and PMSA were in constant contact with the Poor Law Commission, allowing them to showcase their policy ideas and exert pressure for change. Thus, by inviting a representation of medical men to Somerset House and corresponding with the national associations in a cordial manner, commission members showed their ability to negotiate with stakeholders.

Although the case highlights the processes through which policies were generated and issued during the early years of the New Poor Law, it also demonstrates the different ways in which scandals impacted this process. The Bridgwater scandal fed into a wider understanding that medical relief policies were inadequate. Medical relief policies were undeveloped in the Amendment Act, and, as a consequence, individuals and stakeholders demanded—and set—minimum standards. "Policy strain" is, therefore, a catch-all term that can be used to encapsulate policy areas at a time before they are reviewed and changed.

The policies developed from scandals were not easily implemented. The General Medical Order was released a year before it was to come into force, informing boards and guardians across England and Wales that they should adhere to its stipulations the next time the medical officers' contracts were set. Yet in the long-term the order was implemented in piecemeal. Such policies may have established minimum medical relief standards, but there is no way of knowing how far this change in approach made a positive impact on the lives of relief claimants. Indeed, the General Medical Order simply reinforced district-based rather than parish-based medical relief provision, a system that may have better served the needs of medical claimants.

Notes

I would like to thank Carl J. Griffin, Bernard Harris, and John Mohan for their helpful comments on this work. This research was funded by an ESRC PhD Award (PTA-030-2005-00267), which I was very grateful to receive. A version of this paper was presented at the "Medicine and the Workhouse" conference in 2008.

1. See chapter 2, "The Implications of a 'Policy Process' Approach to Understanding the Poor Laws," in Samantha Shave, "Poor Law Reform and Policy Innovation in Rural Southern England, c. 1780–1850" (PhD diss., University of Southampton, 2010), 11–46. For examples of social science literature about the policy process, see Paul Spicker, *Policy Analysis for Practice: Applying Social Policy* (Bristol: Policy, 2006); and Catherine Bochel and Hugh M. Bochel, *The UK Social Policy Process* (Basingstoke, UK: Palgrave Macmillan, 2004).

2. David Roberts, "How Cruel Was the Victorian Poor Law?" *Historical Journal* 6 (1963): 98–99.

3. Reading of Henriques by Bernard Harris, *The Origins of the British Welfare State: Social Welfare in England and Wales, 1800–1945* (Basingstoke, UK: Palgrave Macmillan, 2004), 50; Ursula Henriques, "How Cruel Was the Victorian Poor Law?" *Historical Journal* 11 (1968): 365–71.

4. Peter Dunkley, "The 'Hungry Forties' and the New Poor Law: A Case Study," *Historical Journal* 17 (1974): 329–46.

5. John Stewart and Steven King, "Death in Llantrisant: Henry Williams and the New Poor Law in Wales," *Rural History* 15 (2004): 69–87.

6. Norman McCord, "The Implementation of the 1834 Poor Law Amendment Act on Tyneside," *International Review of Social History* 14 (1969): 104–7; Roger Wells, "Andover Antecedents? Hampshire New Poor-Law Scandals, 1834–1842," *Southern History* 24 (2002): 91–227.

7. Ian Butler and Mark Drakeford, *Scandal, Social Policy and Social Welfare* (Bristol: Policy, 2005), 1.

8. For instance, Anthony Brundage, *The English Poor Laws, 1700–1930* (Basingstoke, UK: Palgrave Macmillan, 2002), 87–88; Peter Wood, *Poverty and the Workhouse in Victorian Britain* (Stroud: Sutton, 1991), 100; David Roberts, *The Victorian Origins of the Welfare State* (Yale: Yale University Press, 1960), 120, 128.

9. Ian Anstruther, *The Scandal of the Andover Workhouse* (Stroud: Sutton, 1984).

10. Wells, "Andover Antecedents," 91.

11. Brundage, *English Poor Laws*, 88.

12. Medical Association, "Facts Connected with the Medical Relief of the Poor in the Bridgwater Union" (Bridgwater, November 13, 1837); a copy can be found in the National Archives (hereafter NA), Home Office (hereafter HO), 73/52/62, Correspondence and Documents Received by the Home Office.

13. Butler and Drakeford, *Scandal*, 238.

14. British Parliamentary Paper (hereafter BPP), 1844 (531) Report from the Select Committee on Medical Poor Relief, together with the minutes of evidence, appendix, and index, interview of George Cornewall Lewis, 1.

15. Steven King, "'Stop this Overwhelming Torment of Destiny': Negotiating Financial Aid at Times of Sickness under the English Old Poor Law, 1800–1840," *Bulletin of the History of Medicine* 79, no. 2 (2005): 234.

16. BPP, 1834 (44), Report from His Majesty's Commissioners for Inquiring into the Administration and Practical Operation of the Poor Laws, 146, cited in Michael W. Flinn, "Medical Services under the New Poor Law," in *The New Poor Law in the Nineteenth-Century*, ed. Derek Fraser (London: Macmillan, 1976), 48.

17. Poor Law Amendment Act, 1834, 5 & 6 Vict., c. 57, s. 54.

18. Flinn, "Medical Services," 48.

19. "Instructional Letter Respecting the Formation of Independent Medical Clubs," in *Second Annual Report of the Poor Law Commissioners* (London: HMSO, 1836), app. A.3, 50.

20. "To the Right Honorable Lord John Russell, His Majesty's Principal Secretary of State for the Home Department," Thomas Frankland Lewis, John George Shaw Lefevre, and George Nicholls to Lord John Russell, August 8, 1835, in *First Annual Report of the Poor Law Commissioners* (London: HMSO, 1835), 51–52.

21. Poor Law Amendment Act, 5 & 6 Vict. c. 57, s. 109.

22. Hampshire Record Office, Fareham Union, Minute Book, PL3/8/1, May 29, 1835.

23. "Lord John Russell," 52.

24. NA, Ministry of Health (hereafter MH), 32/38, Hawley (Hartford Bridge) to Lefevre, May 29, 1836.

25. Anne Digby, *Making a Medical Living: Doctors and Patients in the English Market for Medicine, 1720–1911* (Cambridge: Cambridge University Press, 1994), 244.

26. "Instructional Letter," app. A.3, 50.

27. Flinn, "Medical Services," 50.

28. Digby, *Making a Medical Living*, 244.

29. Flinn, "Medical Services," 49.

30. Stewart and King, "Death in Llantrisant," 74; Digby, *Making a Medical Living*, 244.

31. Somerset contained a population of 28,566 (in 1831) and was 10.5 miles in length and 15.5 miles in breadth. NA, MH, 32/85, Schedule A: Summary of the Unions Formed by Robert Weale Esq., Assistant Poor Law Commissioner, October 21, 1837. It was officially established on April 16, 1836.

32. Colin A. Buchanan, "John Bowen and the Bridgwater Scandal," *Proceedings of the Somerset Archaeological and Natural History Society* 131 (1987): 185.

33. "Report from the Select Committee of the House of Lords Appointed to Examine into the Several Cases Alluded to in Certain Papers Respecting the Operation of the Poor Law Amendment Act; and to Report Thereon," with the minutes of evidence taken before the committee, and an index thereto, hereafter BPP, 1837–38 (719), Bridgwater Inquiry, interview of William Baker, 967; Jonathan Toogood suggests that 40 percent of their paupers in the union had died, written 15 January, "To the Editor of the Times," *Times,* January 26, 1841.

34. Buchanan, "John Bowen," 186; dietaries reproduced in Peter Higgenbotham, *The Workhouse Cookbook* (Stroud: History, 2008), 53–55.

35. BPP, 1837–38 (719), Bridgwater Inquiry, interview of William Baker, 958, 965–66.

36. Baker had known Bowen for a number of years; they had also worked as overseers together in the town.

37. Buchanan, "John Bowen," 187.

38. John Bowen, written 9 September, "To the Board of Guardians of the Bridgewater [*sic*] Union," *Times,* October 12, 1836.

39. NA, MH, 32/85, Weale (Worcester) to Poor Law Commission (hereafter PLC), October 23, 1836.

40. Buchanan, "John Bowen," 187.

41. "Report of the Poor-Law Committee, 1840," *Provincial Medical and Surgical Journal* 1, no. 13 (1841): 212; Medical Association, "Medical Relief," 27.

42. Somerset Record Office (hereafter SRO), Bridgwater Union, Minute Book, D\G\BW/8a/1, May 15, 12, April 28, 1837.

43. "Poor-Law Committee," 212.

44. SRO, Bridgwater Union, Minute Book, D\G\BW/8a/1, May 18, 26, June 2, 1837.

45. BPP, 1837–38 (719), Bridgwater Inquiry, interview of Robert Young, 676–77, 688–89. The Provincial Medical and Surgical Association was founded in 1832; the members were Abraham King, William Lakin Caswell, Baruch Toogood, Joseph Addison, Horatio Nelson Tilsley, John Evered Poole and Richard Beadon Ruddock, and their chairman was Jonathan Toogood; SRO, Bridgwater Union, Minute Book, D\G\BW/8a/1, May 31, 1836; Medical Association, "Medical Relief," 4–5.

46. NA, MH, 12/10243, Handbill received by the PLC, June 6, 1837.

47. SRO, Bridgwater Union, Minute Book, D\G\BW/8a/1, June 9, 1837.

48. NA, MH, 12/10243, George Warry (Shapwick, Glastonbury) to PLC, June 17, 1837.

49. NA, MH, 12/10243, Underdown to PLC, June 16, 1837; NA, MH, 12/10243, Lefevre to Weale, June 22, 1837.

50. SRO, Bridgwater Union, Minute Book, D\G\BW/8a/1, June 23, 1837.

51. "Poor-Law Committee," 212–13.

52. Medical Association, "Medical Relief," 22.

53. Ibid., 22, 16.

54. Ibid., 18. This letter was written on July 1, 1837.

55. This time sent from an overseer, John Knight. NA, HO, 73/52/62, Correspondence and Documents, Copy of Letter from Caswell (Huntspill) to the Board of Guardians of Bridgwater, July 6, 1837, sent by Weale to the PLC, December 1837, 463–64.

56. BPP, 1837–38 (719), Bridgwater Inquiry, interview of Jonathan Toogood, 751–2.

57. Medical Association, "Medical Relief," 16.

58. There was an established Women's Friendly Society based at Stowey, but, at the subscription rate of twenty shillings a year, Charlotte could not afford to join; see BPP, 1834 (44), 31, Report from His Majesty's Commissioners for Inquiring into the Administration and Practical Operation of the Poor Laws, app. B 1, pt. 2, question 14, Nether Stowey (Somerset). The only possible alternative support for Charlotte was a small charity for regular church attendees, but this was unlikely to provide support to pregnant single women, Robert W. Dunning, ed., *The Victoria History of the Counties of England: History of the County of Somerset*, vol. 5 (Oxford: Oxford University Press for the Institute of Historical Research, 1985), 200.

59. NA, HO, 73/52/62, Correspondence and Documents, Weale to the PLC, December 1837; Evidence of Mary Date sent by Weale to the PLC, December 1837, 456; BPP, 1837–38 (719), Bridgwater Inquiry, interview of Mary Date, 855; BPP, 1837–38 (719), Bridgwater Inquiry, interview of Charlotte Allen, 941.

60. Kitty attended many members of the Stowey Female Friendly Society, NA, HO, 73/52/62, Correspondence and Documents, Evidence of James Franklin Waites and Kitty Walker sent by Weale to the PLC, December 1837, 443, 451.

61. BPP, 1837–38 (719), Bridgwater Inquiry, interview of Charles Locock MD (physician and accoucheur of Bridgwater), 981.

62. These were administered by her fellow lodger and nurse, Mary Date; NA, HO, 73/52/62, Correspondence and Documents, Weale to the PLC, December 1837; BPP, 1837–38 (719), Bridgwater Inquiry, interview of Charlotte Allen, 942; BPP, 1837–38 (719), Bridgwater Inquiry, interview of Mary Waites, 449; BPP, 1837–38 (719), Bridgwater Inquiry, interview of Kitty Walker, 451.

63. BPP, 1837–38 (719), Bridgwater Inquiry, interview of James Franklin Waites, 772; NA, HO, 73/52/62, Correspondence and Documents, Evidence of James Franklin Waites sent by Weale to the PLC, December 1837, 444.

64. BPP, 1837–38 (719), Bridgwater Inquiry, interview of Charles Locock, 980.

65. Charles Locock said that medical men and midwives have "met the same Accident" on the birth of a woman's first child, "though rarely to this Extent." BPP, 1837–38 (719), Bridgwater Inquiry, 981, 980.

66. Medical Association, "Medical Relief," 18; NA, HO, 73/52/62, Correspondence and Documents, Evidence of John Stagg, December 1, 1837, 457.

67. BPP, 1837–38 (719), Bridgwater Inquiry, copy of affidavit in interview of Jonathan Toogood, 761.

68. Medical Association, "Medical Relief," 10.

69. In the meantime, the relieving officer went into Cook's house, saw the child, and left without speaking to anyone, probably to assess John's need for medical relief. This illustrates the board of guardians' inability to trust Parker's opinion.

70. BPP, 1837–38 (719), Bridgwater Inquiry, copy of affidavit in interview of Jonathan Toogood, 761–62.

71. Medical Association, "Medical Relief," 24.

72. Caswell's bill was ninety-two pounds and his payment was forty pounds.

73. BPP, 1837–38 (719), Bridgwater Inquiry, interview of Jonathan Toogood, 750.

74. He was married and had three children. "Poor-Law Committee," 213.

75. BPP, 1837–38 (719), Bridgwater Inquiry, interview of John Rodney Ward, 1085–144. He was a licentiate of the Society of Apothecaries only.

76. "The case 'Webber versus Ward'" and "Western Circuit, Wells, Tuesday, August 7," *Times*, August 9, 1838, cited in Buchanan, "John Bowen," 188.

77. Ruth G. Hodgkinson, *The Origins of the National Health Service: The Medical Services of the New Poor Law, 1834–1871* (London: Wellcome Trust Historical Medical Library, 1967), 26.

78. BPP, 1837–38 (719), Bridgwater Inquiry, interview of Ward, 1101.

79. "Poor-Law Committee," 213.

80. Butler and Drakeford, *Scandal*, 223.

81. Medical Association, "Medical Relief," 27.

82. Puerperal fever "affected women within the first three days after childbirth and progressed rapidly, causing acute symptoms of severe abdominal pain, fever and debility." Christine Hallett, "The Attempt to Understand Puerperal Fever in the Eighteen and Early Nineteenth Centuries: The Influence of Inflammation Theory," *Medical History* 49 (2005): 1. Charlotte did not mention suffering from this disease in her Select Committee interview. She did, however, mention breast-feeding her child. It was uncommon for mothers suffering from the disease to breast-feed in case it passed onto the child. BPP, 1837–38 (719), Bridgwater Inquiry, interview of Charlotte Allen, 944.

83. "Facts Connected with the Medical Relief of the Poor in the Bridgewater [*sic*] Union," *Times*, November 22, 1837, reprinted in George Robert Wythen Baxter, *The Book of the Bastilles, or the History of the Working of the New Poor-Law* (London: John Stephens, 1841), 477–80.

84. In addition, a petition had been received by the House of Lords from the "Bridgwater Members of College of Surgeons," which was critical of the administration of medical relief to the poor. BPP, 1837–38 (719), Bridgwater Inquiry, app. 5 "Abstract of Petitions on the Poor Law Presented during Session 1837," see fifth division, 46.

85. SRO, Bridgwater Union, Minute Book, D\G\BW/8a/2, March 23, 1838; NA, MH, 12/10244, Clerk (Bridgwater Union) to PLC, cited in Buchanan, "John Bowen," 193.

86. Lord Wharncliffe, House of Lords, March 26, 1838, *Hansard's Parliamentary Debates* 41, cc 1217–18, 1224–25, 1248–49.

87. This was the view of Jonathan Toogood; written 15 January, "To the Editor of the Times," *Times*, January 26, 1841.

88. This Select Committee produced a total of forty-nine reports.

89. "Letter Accompanying General Medical Order," Poor Law Commission to Clerk of the Guardians of Unions, March 12, 1842, *Eighth Annual Report of the Poor Law Commissioners* (London: HMSO, 1842), app. A.6, 138.

90. The Bridgwater inquiry was held from March to July 1838; the medical inquiry was held from July 1838. British Parliamentary Papers (hereafter BPP), Forty-fourth, forty-fifth and forty-sixth reports from Select Committee on the Poor Law Amendment Act, with the minutes of evidence, and appendixes, 1837–38 (518), Medical Inquiry.

91. BPP, 1837–38 (518), Medical Inquiry, "Select Committee," 22.

92. Ibid., 23.

93. Districts of four or five miles in diameter were thought to be satisfactory by Jonathan. Toogood; BPP, 1837–38 (518), Medical Inquiry, interview of Jonathan Toogood, 367.

94. BPP, 1837–38 (518), Medical Inquiry, interview of Jonathan Toogood, 368–70.

95. BPP, 1837–38 (518), Medical Inquiry, "Select Committee," 25.

96. "Letter Accompanying General Medical Order," app. A.6, 138.

97. "Commissioners, Circular to Assistant Commissioners, Calling for Reports," Edwin Chadwick to Assistant Poor Law Commissioners, February, 21, 1839, app. B.6; *Report on the Further Amendment of the Poor Laws* (London: HMSO, 1839), 157.

98. NA, MH, 32/6, "Quarterly Summary of Unions Visited, &c. during the Quarter Ended 30th Day of December 1838" (emphasis mine). The visit was on November 16, 1838. In another quarterly report on July 30, 1839, Adey notes that Bridgwater is "still far from what is desirable," NA, MH, 32/6. For details about his district, see NA, MH, 32/6, Adey to PLC, October 4, 1838; "Medical Relief: Reports of the Arrangements of Affording Medical Relief," "Reports of Assistant Commissioners," "D. G. Adey, Esq.: Counties of Somerset, Gloucester, Wilts, Dorset," in *Further Amendment*, app. A.6, 158.

99. "D. G. Adey, Esq.," app. A.6, 159.

100. Edwin Chadwick, written 21 February, "British Medical Association," *Lancet*, March 9, 1839, 886.

101. "British Medical Association. Tuesday 26th March, 1839. Half-Yearly Meeting." *Lancet*, April 6, 1839, 90–91.

102. Article about the "British Medical Association. Tuesday, April 9th, 1839. Meeting of Council," *Lancet*, April 13, 1839, 120–21.

103. "Communications from a Deputation from the Council of the British Medical Association," Letter British Medical Association (Dulwich) to Poor Law Commission, April 1, 1839, in *Further Amendment*, app. B.6, 281, 283. In the piece the BMA referred the Commissioners to the evidence given at the Medical Inquiry, and on page 281 specifically a question answered by their President; BPP, 1837–38 (518), Medical Inquiry, interview of Henry Wyldbore Rumsey, 36.

104. *Further Amendment.*

105. "General Medical Order," app. A.6, 138, circular letter dated March 6, 1841.

106. Ibid., 139. Details of these responses can be found in "Seventh Annual Report to the Most Noble Marquess of Normandy, Her Majesty's Principal Secretary of State for the Home Department," John George Shaw Lefevre, George Nicholls, and George Cornewall Lewis, May 1, 1841, *Seventh Annual Report of the Poor Law Commissioners* (London: HMSO, 1841), 8–14.

107. "Letter Accompanying General Medical Order," app. A.6, 139; "Parochial Medical Relief," *Provincial Medical and Surgical Journal* 1, no. 22 (1841): 361. Also, an association sent another petition to the government and details of medical relief sagas, including the Bridgwater scandal, were published in the *PMSA Journal*, see "Report of the Poor-Law Committee, 1840" vol. 1, no. 10 (1840): 166–68; vol. 1, no. 11 (1840): 184–87; vol. 1, no. 12 (1841): 197–99; vol. 1, no. 13 (1841): 209–13; vol. 1, no. 14 (1841): 228–30.

108. "General Medical Order," app. A.5, *Eighth Annual Report of the Poor Law Commissioners* (London: HMSO, 1842), 129–35; for salaries to officers, see articles 1 and 2; for qualifications, see articles 3 and 4; for district sizes, see articles 6 and 7; for payments per case, see articles 10 to 13.

109. Ibid. For weekly returns and substitutes, see articles 14 and 15; for the list of "permanent paupers," see articles 16 and 17 (quote in 16); for the continuance of medical officers, see article 20.

110. Hodgkinson, *National Health Service*, 14.

111. The appointment of medical officers had to be sanctioned annually by the commission, usually after each Lady Day.

112. The districts were of 29,982 and 21,746 acres with populations of 2,805 and 2,222, respectively; NA, MH, 12/10346, Warren, Clerk (Dulverton Union) to PLC, May 9, 1842.

113. NA, MH, 12/10346, PLC to Warren, Clerk (Dulverton), June 3, 1842.

114. The towns and cities included Derby, Sheffield, Leeds, Manchester, and Liverpool; see Hodgkinson, *National Health Service*, 15, 14, 27.

115. NA, MH, 12/2913, Parker, Clerk (Wimborne and Cranborne Union) to PLC, July 26, 1843.

116. Hodgkinson, *National Health Service*, 15.

117. NA, MH, 12/13820, Snook, Clerk (Mere Union) to PLC, February 15, 1844.

118. NA, MH, 12/13820, PLC to Snook, Clerk (Mere Union), February 19, 1844.

119. Stephen Stranger had only a Royal College of Surgeons qualification, NA, MH, 12/11037, Patterson, Clerk (South Stoneham Union) to PLC, May 3, 1844. The union obviously trusted him in his duties but realized he had only one of the qualifications the commission desired, so the position was readvertised in local newspapers.

120. NA, MH, 12/10854, Holding, Clerk (Kingsclere Union) to PLC, February 4, 1845. The commission, however, stipulated that tickets must be issued; see NA, MH, 12/10854, PLC to Holding, Clerk (Kingsclere Union), February 12, 1845.

121. Bulter and Drakeford, *Scandal*, 4.

122. Lord Wharncliffe, *Hansard's Parliamentary Debates*, cc 1224.

123. Ian Gordon, Janet Lewis, and Ken Young, "Perspectives on Policy Analysis," in *The Policy Process: A Reader*, ed. Michael Hill (London: Harvester Wheatsheaf, 1993), 7.

Chapter Nine

Practitioners and Paupers

Medicine at the Leicester Union Workhouse, 1867–1905

Angela Negrine

The Status of Workhouse Medicine

In England and Wales the Poor Law Amendment Act (1834) required all unions to appoint a medical officer to attend the sick in the workhouse. The 1842 General Medical Order required poor law medical officers to be doubly qualified in both medicine and surgery, which often meant that they were better trained than other local private practitioners, who may have had only one qualification. The requirement to be doubly qualified did not, however, bestow a high status on the post, nor was it rewarded by a significant or even standard scale of remuneration.[1] Despite working in a profession that gradually rose in esteem during the nineteenth century and despite being the only trained and qualified workhouse officers, medical officers remained subservient to lay poor law guardians. Furthermore, medical relief orders for paupers were made by nonmedical relieving officers. As Irvine Loudon points out, the status of an individual general practitioner was dependent on his income and the class of patient he treated.[2] Consequently, the lack of medical autonomy experienced by workhouse medical officers, along with their acceptance of lowly paid posts and their willingness to treat the poorest patients, undermined their status among the medical profession, which was itself concerned to establish its authority within hospitals and society in general.

The poor law medical service was regarded by the contemporary medical profession as a second-class service since workhouse infirmaries did not have the same prestige as voluntary hospitals: they could not be used as teaching hospitals, which would have provided opportunities for career advancement; they did not have wealthy patrons or prestigious hospital consultants; and their patients were the destitute—elderly, disabled, imbecilic, and syphilitic—those considered to have "uninteresting" chronic diseases. Besides, workhouses had not been intended to act as hospitals for the pauper sick. Workhouse sick wards were originally provided simply for able-bodied inmates who became ill. However, the poor law rapidly became the main source of medical help for the poorest in the population since sickness was a primary cause of poverty. Workhouses, therefore, were soon filled with sick and disabled paupers rather than the able-bodied male at whom the legislation was aimed to deter claims for poor relief. Medical officers were required to detect suspected "malingers," which imposed a conflict between their professional medical ethos and their need to adhere to the deterrent principles of the poor law system to retain a post.[3]

Competition for posts was keen, however, as the medical profession was crowded and highly competitive. Young, newly qualified doctors needed to gain a local foothold and practical experience, while older, established practitioners wished to keep out competitors and supplement their income.[4] Hence, despite the unattractive work and conditions of service, posts were easily filled, and guardians could offer low rates of pay. Acceptance of such working conditions has undoubtedly contributed to workhouse medical officers being generally characterized in the historiography as apathetic, ineffectual, self-interested, and, accordingly, guilty of medical neglect by complying with the system.[5] Although workhouse and district medical officers complied with the system, they also frequently complained about their working conditions and the principles of the poor law system though the medical journals the *Lancet* and the *British Medical Journal.* The journals' editors robustly defended criticism of poor law medical officers and, instead, blamed the poor law system for the inadequacies of its medical service and its exploitation of medical officers and paupers alike.

The new poor law imposed a centralized standard policy; however, historians agree that its implementation was always differentiated locally.[6] Yet a surprising lack of detailed research since the work of the historians Ruth Hodgkinson, Jeanne Brand, Michael Flinn, and Margaret Anne Crowther has allowed simplistic generalizations about workhouse medical officers to persist.[7] The poor law medical officer was a vital person in the function of the medical service, therefore judgment of the service needs knowledge of his work and who he was. This chapter redresses the balance by providing a more nuanced picture of medicine practiced at a provincial workhouse. The first half of the chapter briefly describes the situation of the Leicester workhouse and then focuses primarily on two medical officers, Dr. Julius St. Thomas Clarke and Dr. Clement Frederick Bryan, who worked successively at the workhouse from 1867 until 1914. Their personal attributes and relationships and attitudes toward the guardians and patients are described and examples are given of the medical service they provided. Knowledge of the treatment of sick paupers in the workhouse is limited, and the remainder of the chapter gives some examples of the medical treatment received by different classes of workhouse patients. The chapter concludes by considering the quality of medical care provided at this workhouse and how insights gained from a microstudy of a workhouse can contribute toward a broad knowledge of workhouse medicine.

The Leicester Workhouse and Infirmary

In common with many other English towns in the nineteenth century, Leicester experienced a rapid population growth as it evolved from a small East Midlands market town into a large industrial town due to the development of the hosiery and boot and shoe industries and allied trades, which collectively encouraged migration into the town. Its prosperity fluctuated until the mid-nineteenth century but accelerated thereafter, although there were infrequent periods of unemployment when many families suffered ill health and poverty and had to resort to poor relief and the workhouse. The majority of paupers admitted to the workhouse were unskilled, such as laborers and charwomen, or children and the elderly, many being former framework knitters. Despite its growing prosperity, Leicester was reported to be one of the unhealthiest of the large English towns for much of the nineteenth century. Infant mortality from annual summer diarrhea was a major contributor to its high mortality figures. This was primarily caused by the inadequate sewage system serving the rapidly built back-to-back houses that provided overcrowded and unhealthy living conditions for the town's rising population.[8]

The workhouse built outside the town in 1838 was soon found to be inadequate for the number of paupers who required poor relief, particularly when the town suffered trade depressions in the winters of 1841–42 and 1847–48. In 1851 a replacement workhouse was built on the same site with space to accommodate up to a thousand inmates. The new workhouse incorporated an infirmary at the back of the main building with wards overlooking the railway line. There was a separate small building for fever and smallpox cases and two large lunacy wards in a wing of the main workhouse. By 1867 the infirmary had 147 beds, but overcrowding continually created difficulties for staff and discomfort for patients, even though more space was created when the children, who had initially been treated in the main workhouse infirmary, were removed to a detached workhouse school with its own sick wards. The guardians made piecemeal attempts to deal with the problems created by overcrowding, and many alterations and extensions were made to the workhouse building throughout the period. In 1884 the children were removed from the workhouse and thereafter accommodated in cottage homes several miles away, where they were attended by a resident nurse and a local medical officer, who was employed on a nonresident, part-time basis.[9]

The workhouse school was converted into extra infirmary wards, and by the 1890s the workhouse infirmary had expanded to contain 300 beds. The guardians' minute books show that, by then, they had accepted the need to build an entirely separate infirmary. Eventually, in 1905 the union opened a purpose-built hospital in a healthier location at North Evington, about a mile and a half from the workhouse. The majority of workhouse patients were transferred to the new infirmary, where they were treated by newly appointed, full-time resident medical officers. Until then, as in most unions, the Leicester medical officers were nonresident and worked part-time for the union while also practicing privately.[10]

The Workhouse Medical Officers

Dr. John Moore

In her study of the Leicester Union, Kate Thompson concluded that the early workhouse medical officers were mostly indifferent and inadequate and not as well qualified and committed as those in other unions.[11] Support for this assertion can be found by an incident that took place in the final months of John Moore's service at the Leicester workhouse. Moore, who was appointed in 1857, attended the workhouse daily, except on Sundays. He spent forty-five minutes visiting the patients and attended the lunatics three times a week. In addition to his workhouse post, and in common with many other workhouse medical officers who also held posts in other medical or public institutions, Moore worked part-time as the borough's medical officer of health, for which he was recorded as being "zealous, able and thoroughly efficient."[12]

By 1867 after ten years in post, Moore's own failing health caused him to become deficient and neglectful of his workhouse duties. One incident led to the death of a patient, when Moore found that he was incapable of setting her broken leg. Instead of calling for help, he apparently said there was no point in setting it and left the unfortunate patient untreated. The patient subsequently died from gangrene.[13] A complaint was made, but to avoid a scandal the guardians gave Moore leave of absence. However, two months later they asked him to resign. The register of appointments recorded that Moore resigned due to "ill health."[14] He died shortly afterward. It seems likely that Moore stayed in his post due to financial insecurity since a report to the Poor Law Board (PLB) in 1867 of a visit to the Leicester workhouse made in 1866 by Dr. Edward Smith recorded that Moore's salary was eighty pounds per annum. The report stated that "he finds all drugs at

a cost of about £20 per annum and dispenses them himself. He is satisfied
with his emoluments and does not care that the Guardians should provide
the drugs."[15] As Kim Price notes, without superannuation, medical officers
often clung on to poor law posts long after they were capable of carrying
out their duties.[16] Fortunately for the patients, the two successive medical
officers at the Leicester workhouse, Julius St. Thomas Clarke and Clement
Frederick Bryan, were of a rather different caliber to Moore and the earlier
medical officers.

Dr. Julius St. Thomas Clarke

Dr. Clarke, who had been Moore's deputy, was appointed as the new workhouse medical officer. He remained in the post from 1867 to 1880. The son
of a Leicester manufacturer of sewing cotton, Clarke began his medical education at the local voluntary hospital, the Leicester General Infirmary, after
training at Guy's Hospital in London, where he gained a gold medal in anatomy and physiology at the University of London and also gold in clinical
surgery at Guy's Hospital. He was thirty years old when he became the workhouse medical officer, and he was evidently a very busy and successful man
with many other public commitments in addition to his workhouse duties.
He became a magistrate and had a seat on the borough council. In addition, he was an honorary medical officer to the Institution for the Blind, the
Leicester Borough Asylum, and the Leicester Trained Nurses' Institution.[17]
Clarke's reputation earned him an obituary in the *Lancet*, which stated that
he became "an eminent surgeon."[18] As for his personal qualities, the *Leicester
Guardian* newspaper praised him for being a keen advocate of the temper-
ance cause, by stating that "he was a total abstainer and his whole life was
one of great asceticism and a single-minded devotion to duty was the key-
stone of his life." The newspaper also commented that "throughout the
whole of his medical career, Dr. Clarke took the most earnest interest in the
science of medicine and its daily development."[19]

A fascinating example of this interest is shown by entries that Clarke
made in his medical report book in 1872, where he stated that he had carried out skin-grafting operations on some twenty-five workhouse patients
with ulcerated legs who he said he had managed to "induce" to "voluntarily
undergo a newly-introduced operation of skin-grafting."[20] The *Lancet* had
published an article in 1870 on skin grafting, under the heading "The healing of wounds by transplantation."[21] The article reported that the procedure had been developed by a Monsieur Reverdin in Paris in 1869, and
a surgeon at St. George's Hospital had tested the treatment in May 1870.
Clarke may have read the medical journal, which also printed letters from
other surgeons who had tried out the operation, or perhaps he heard of the

procedure from colleagues and was eager to try it out himself on the work-house patients. Whichever was the case, Clarke recorded that he was particularly pleased that the patients' recovery was "remarkably accelerated with the prospect of recurrence of the ulceration greatly diminished," and he confidently declared that the operation "bids fair to be of signal benefit to those who from hardships, fatigue or constitutional causes become the subjects of ulceration."[22] It is a matter for conjecture as to whether Clarke was chiefly motivated by a professional interest in experimenting on his patients, as the procedure was in its infancy when he carried it out. No further references were made to the procedure in the medical report book after 1873. Perhaps Clarke undertook this surgery routinely until he left his post, but his successor did not continue it, although, undoubtedly, workhouse patients with ulcerated legs would have continued to be admitted.

The workload expected of poor law medical officers was high and the range of cases they encountered was extensive, certainly in large urban unions and particularly as posts were usually part-time and the doctors had other commitments. Among their duties, record keeping was an essential requirement but, as Price observes, most were such erratic record keepers that their normal practice appears to have been to avoid paperwork wherever possible.[23] This view is certainly borne out by a PLB circular of 1868, which criticized the way medical officers reported to guardians. The circular revealed that reports were often simply verbal or written on loose papers that became lost or went unnoticed. The PLB assumed that, if medical officers kept records in official medical report books supplied by the guardians, entries would be made "with more deliberation and care than heretofore."[24] Clarke was evidently a diligent exception to the rule, as the Local Government Board (LGB) commended him as one of the few medical officers who presented an annual report.[25] His detailed medical report book from 1870 until 1880 records illuminating details of the illnesses and treatment of workhouse patients, as well as reports of defects in the infirmary. Unfortunately for the historian, this is the only existing medical report book in the Leicester records. Few other medical report books survive that contain such a wealth of information. Disappointingly, Clarke's successor, Dr. Bryan, added few entries to this book. Possibly Bryan used a different report book that has not survived. Unlike Clarke, Bryan was also occasionally criticized for his lax record keeping.

The report book, minutes, and correspondence books show that Clarke demonstrated a progressive professional attitude. For instance, children were vaccinated against smallpox by the medical officer, but outbreaks occurred when the disease was undetected, particularly in vagrants who frequented several workhouses on their travels. In fact, Clarke recommended to the guardians that vagrants should be vaccinated against smallpox, but the guardians ignored his recommendation. Clarke was similarly frustrated when the guardians excluded him from the appointment of nurses and ignored his recommendation that nurses should not be employed unless they had previously had one year's training in a hospital or infirmary.[26]

A caring attitude toward his patients can be detected in Clarke's report book. In addition to their medical care, he was keen to improve their living conditions in the infirmary, as he considered their surroundings to be uncomfortable, dull, and cheerless. He suggested to the guardians that the large wards should be furnished with tables and chairs to provide a day section for patients. He thought that flowers or plants in the windows would have a "pleasing affect [sic] alike on patients and visitors" and that there would be willing donations "were the desirability made known." Clarke arranged Christmas entertainments for the children and imbeciles, which he and his wife attended, and he arranged for gifts of tea and tobacco for the sick inmates. Clarke also presided over a presentation made to Mr. William Dickisson, the workhouse master, for his twenty-six years of service.[27] The newspaper cuttings in the records of these events convey the impression that Clarke's involvement in these special occasions was of great benevolent significance to the inmates.

In addition to the skin-grafting procedures mentioned earlier, Clarke regularly performed eye surgery on workhouse patients with the assistance of a district medical officer, Dr. Frank Fullager. The operations they performed included the removal of an eyeball, the correction of squints, and removal of cataracts. Clarke wrote to the guardians to praise Fullager's assistance and to justify the benefits of the procedures to both the patients and the system:

> Two cases of double squint and one of single squint in the schools were operated on with considerable improvement. An old man . . . also underwent, on two different occasions, the operation for cataract in each eye, the result being that he was enabled to read again and go about as usual. A young man . . . was also operated on with much success for a severe affliction of the eyelids, and has been thereby enabled to earn his living. . . . I believe the Board will join with me in an expression of thanks to Mr. Fullager, not only for the unlimited time he has placed at my disposal in the matters, but also for the hearty cooperation he has shown in this work.[28]

On an earlier occasion though, Clarke had been annoyed when the guardians sent a patient to the Nottingham Eye Infirmary without consulting him. He was even more aggrieved when asked to make up the Nottingham surgeon's prescription for the patient, saying that to do so placed him "in the position of a chemist and druggist."[29] This example aptly illustrates the iniquitous situation whereby nonmedical guardians disregarded the expertise of medical officers, and medical officers struggled to establish their professional authority.

With regard to surgical procedures under poor law medical services, E. Hugh MacKay regards that surgery in 1905 would have been limited to incision and drainage of abscesses and amputations for gangrene. Although open surgery for bladder stones existed, he believes it is doubtful that it was used on the infirm poor.[30] Yet, as early as 1874, Clarke recommended that an inmate, John Stringer, aged fifty-three, who had a stone in his bladder as well as ulcers and dropsy, should to be transferred to the General Infirmary. On that occasion, Clarke stated, "He has considerably improved in health since his admission, but . . . our wards are now as a rule so filled (especially with bad or dirty cases) as to scarcely leave any beds unoccupied more than a day or two." Furthermore, he considered that "considerable professional assistance would be necessary for the operation."[31] He implied that he was capable of undertaking the operation, but the overcrowded and dirty conditions of the infirmary presented risks, quite apart from the lack of time and necessary medical support. Clarke also sent a deformed child to a London orthopedic hospital for a limb amputation, recording that the child was sent back "relieved."[32] He was unlikely to be able to undertake these operations without the professional support and equipment that was available in more specialized hospitals.

These instances show that pauper patients received specialist medical treatment that was unavailable within the poor law medical service but that would undoubtedly have been denied to them if they had not become paupers. The Poor Law Continuation Act of 1851 had legalized the use of voluntary hospitals, as the authorities realized it could be more economical for dangerous or difficult cases to benefit from superior medical skills or equipment.[33] Like many other unions, Leicester subscribed to a variety of institutions for specialized medical treatment and convalescence for its pauper patients. Initially, it subscribed to the Leicester General Infirmary and its fever house. Later subscriptions were made to more distant institutions, such as the Buxton Bath charity and the Margate Sea Bathing Infirmary. Scrofulous children were regularly sent to the latter institution, such as Elizabeth Lucas, aged six, who Clarke recorded returned from the sea bathing infirmary "greatly improved in health and strength, and with all of her abscesses healed." He was also pleased to report that she returned "much fatter and stronger than she had ever been."[34]

Another illustration of Clarke's progressive attitude was his concern at the ill health of the workhouse children, many of whom suffered from ophthalmia and scrofula. He condemned the narrow, unhealthy workhouse playground, which was surrounded by manure pits and a piggery for the lack of clean air and space for exercise, and he urged the guardians to provide a larger, more open playground.[35] To improve the children's health, Clarke persuaded the guardians to employ a militia drill sergeant (albeit in private clothes). He thought that drilling would help to develop the children's chests, thereby improving their respiratory organs. Perhaps to persuade the guardians further, he stated that an additional benefit of drilling would be to encourage in the children a "respectful demeanor and good deportment." Clarke was similarly concerned at the coldness of the children's wards and the "filthy" conditions of the boys' urinals. In one report, he graphically described these conditions to the guardians, emphasizing the extra suffering caused to boys with chilblains as they stood in pools of urine at night because there was no light in the water closet. Aware that he might offend the guardians' sensibilities, he apologized for the explicitness of the details.[36]

After thirteen years attending patients at the workhouse, Clarke was appointed as a surgeon at the Leicester General Infirmary, whereupon he resigned his workhouse post. Although it is apparent that Clarke was a conscientious medical officer, he was evidently ambitious to progress his career beyond workhouse medicine and may well have taken that post to further his public profile and gain experience of medical practice on a group of patients with conditions that differed from those presented by his private patients. Indeed, in his history of the Leicester Infirmary, Ernest Frizelle records that Clarke did not become a member of the infirmary staff until 1880 purely because there was no vacancy.[37] Clarke clearly intended to gain a position at the infirmary, as he was part of a deputation to its board to propose an increase in the honorary medical staff. The board agreed with the proposal and, when a surgeon resigned in 1880, Clarke was elected to the post.

Dr. Clement Frederick Bryan

Dr. Clarke's replacement was Dr. Clement Frederick Bryan, also from Leicester and also a student at Guy's Hospital, which he entered at the age of sixteen. He became one of the youngest practitioners in England, being in full practice at the age of twenty-two. He was aged twenty-nine when he became the workhouse medical officer in 1880, and he remained in that post for thirty-four years, until his sudden death in 1914 at the age of sixty-four. Like Clarke, Bryan was also involved in public duties and activities. Both doctors presented public papers and lectures, for example, on the dangers to health caused by a defective sewage system and on the "horrors and dangers" of diphtheria.[38] Bryan was a town councillor for several years and stood as Liberal candidate in 1896. He was instrumental in the establishment of the People's Dispensary in Leicester in 1889, which enabled the poor to obtain medicine and the attendance of a doctor for a small subscription. He was also honorary surgeon to the Leicester Volunteers, and he was elected president of the Leicester Medical Society in 1894.[39] His death was reported in a local newspaper under the heading, "Sudden end to a useful career," indicating that he was well regarded for his professional and public work. The newspaper described him as "a favourite with his pauper patients" and a "staunch Liberal and friend of the working-classes."[40] The latter tribute was due to his work as a surgeon under the Factory Act, which involved reporting accidents caused by machinery and possible contributory negligence by employers, as well as examining children under sixteen years of age to see whether they were fit to work in factories.

Relationships between both medical officers and the guardians were mainly cordial, although they had different priorities regarding the patients. However, the poor law system ensured that guardians ultimately had power over any decisions made by medical officers. The records show, though, that Bryan became noticeably more strident in his dealings with the guardians in his later years at the workhouse, probably due to his experience and confidence, but he perhaps became more irascible in older age and ill health, as he mentioned that he suffered from colitis. He was usually supported by the LGB, which praised him for being a conscientious doctor and generally took his side in any disputes with the guardians. Bryan certainly did not hesitate to assert his medical professionalism and the value of his expertise, as shown in the quote from a letter that he wrote to the guardians to justify his appeal for an increase in his salary:

> Professional men do not work by time, but should be paid according to their opinions or advice, &c, for which they have to undergo a long and expensive training, which after years of experience becomes much more valuable. I am quite aware that a younger and more inexperienced man might do the work but I am certain that one who has been used to the work and has the courage of his opinion is a very great saving to the Ratepayers and I am quite sure that the Master and other officers will bear me out in this (namely) that in the treatment of tramps alone I am able to detect imposture and malingering which one who had not been used to it could not possibly do as he would be afraid lest he should make a mistake, which I am pleased to say has not been done to my knowledge during the time I have had the honour to be your Medical Officer. Again the quick detection of isolation of infectious and contagious diseases is another great saving. Also the statistics of cures of acute diseases will bear any favourable comparison with other large institutions.[41]

An example of an occasion where Bryan stood his ground against the guardians is shown by his reaction to their suggestion that he try out a hydropathic treatment recommended by another doctor who had claimed to cure scarlet fever in five days by means of hot baths. Bryan told the guardians in no uncertain terms that "having been a medical officer to the workhouse for over sixteen years, and without a single death from scarlet-fever, I cannot allow any interference with my medical treatment of the patients as

I, and I alone, am responsible and best able to judge what treatment is the best for those under my care."[42] The guardians reluctantly let the matter go, as Bryan was supported by the LGB. Indeed, an LGB inspector, Dr. H. Stevens, penciled in this remark on a report on the dispute: "Dr. Clarke is a very experienced man and I think there is a great deal too much 'gas' in the Leicester Board Room. . . . The medical officer holds his own with the guardians. This requires no further attention."[43]

An aspect of the system that could cause disputes between guardians and medical officers was the provision of medical extras, such as meat, bread, milk, eggs, and alcohol. Unlike medicines, which were usually provided by medical officers, medical extras were financed from the poor rates. Poorly paid doctors could be tempted to abuse the system, but doctors recognized that many workhouse patients were malnourished due to a poor and inadequate diet and that food was often more beneficial than medicine. Few disputes were recorded between the Leicester medical officers and guardians over medical extras. Indeed, Clarke thanked the guardians for "so liberally" allowing him to order mutton chops and eggs, which he valued "far more than stimulants for broken down and debilitated constitutions."[44] On one occasion when a poor law district auditor queried the amount of medical extras that Bryan had ordered, Bryan explained the need for this type of treatment for patients:

> The extras are ordered when I think it necessary for the health of an inmate, probably because they require different food (such as in the case of the man who has had an egg daily for years) as he is a rheumatic subject. I have always been very careful in the ordering of extras, but amongst so many aged and those of a debilitated constitution, extras are obliged to be given particularly to those who are unable to masticate or digest the ordinary diet.[45]

The Treatment of Workhouse Patients

Although workhouse patients were regarded as medically uninteresting, the Leicester records demonstrate that its workhouse patients presented a complex range of illnesses. A brief scan of the union's correspondence, minutes, and medical report book reveals a range of different illnesses and conditions that patients presented. The list is by no means exhaustive, but provides a snapshot of the medical care required: "Cancer, chicken pox, debility, diabetes, diarrhea, dysentery, epilepsy, erysipelas, heart disease, imbecility, insanity, itch (scabies), measles, ophthalmia, paralysis, puerperal fever, scarlet fever, senility, smallpox, tuberculosis or consumption, phthisis, scrofula, typhoid, typhus, ulcerated legs, venereal disease, whooping cough."

Besides infirmary patients, workhouse inmates were also treated as outpatients, and accident and emergency cases were sometimes delivered to the workhouse by ambulance. For example, in 1873 Clarke noted that "among the accidents admitted were a case of fractured thigh, two cases of fracture of the upper arm, one of fractured ribs, and two of fracture of the fore-arm."[46] Paupers with infectious conditions were also frequently admitted, which promoted further cases of sickness and disease. Infectious diseases were difficult to control at the workhouse due to inadequate accommodation and insufficient nurses to attend patients, which resulted in cross-infection. For example, measles regularly swept through wards containing young children and patients, and staff alike caught typhoid during periods when this disease was rife.

Nursing and the Leicester Workhouse

Workhouses generally employed insufficient nurses for the high number of patients and were also notorious for using paupers to help nurse sick inmates. The LGB disapproved of this practice but did not prohibit it. The Leicester guardians evidently permitted the use of pauper assistants (referred to as wardsmen in the records) in its infirmary for most of this period. In 1897, when the LGB requested a report on the alleged mistreatment of patients by pauper assistants in the infirmary, Bryan revealed that he had received constant complaints of the wardsmen's rough treatment of patients and argued that it was absolutely necessary for more nurses to be appointed to cope with the large increase of sick inmates, particularly as there were "many more acute cases to treat than formerly, which require much greater care," as it was "impossible for him to certify that the paupers were fit for any other work in the infirmary except for scrubbing, cleaning and taking messages."[47] Bryan also protested against the wardsmen being allowed to attend the typhoid patients. He complained that "when the patients cry out with hunger, they frequently feed them regardless of consequences." Bryan's strong words clearly had an effect upon the guardians, for he reported in October 1898 that the wardsmen's work had "nearly been done away with," and a workhouse inspection report in 1899 confirmed that inmates no longer helped in the infirmary.[48]

Childbirth

Contrary to poor law regulations, and despite a controversy in 1856 when the parish midwife was accused of gross incompetence, Leicester's medical officers attended only difficult childbirth cases, and the guardians employed midwives who were paid five shillings a case. The LGB appeared to be unaware of this practice until 1872, when it noticed that payments had been made to a midwife. The LGB reminded the guardians that it was "the duty of the medical officer to attend all midwifery cases in the workhouse . . . for which he got a special fee."[49] The guardians insisted that the union had always employed midwives to attend women in labor and that medical officers were called in only for difficult cases. They declared that the poor preferred to have a midwife and, furthermore, it was more economical for the union; by using midwives the union was able to secure the services of a "much superior class of medical man," because the guardians believed that the medical profession regarded midwifery as "a laborious and unremunerative part of the profession."[50] The guardians assured the LGB that midwives were not appointed unless they possessed a medical certificate of competency.[51]

There were relatively few deaths related to childbirth at the workhouse, and the majority of women who gave birth in the workhouse were unmarried. The average number of births was around thirty a year and the records show that Clarke attended only three workhouse childbirth cases in 1872 and two in 1873. He noted in his annual report that the lying-in cases had "as usual done well," indicating that he believed the midwife was sufficiently skilled, as there were few complicated cases that required his attendance.[52] No doubt, however, the midwife was instructed to call on the medical officer only for extremely serious cases. The guardians continued with this policy until 1889, when a midwife's competence was questioned following the death of a woman three days after her baby was delivered. Bryan refused to give a death certificate, as he stated that he should have been sent for at the time of the birth. He reported the case to the coroner, and an inquest was held at which the jury concluded that the woman had died "from exhaustion consequent upon the whole of the afterbirth not having been removed at the proper time."[53] The guardians accepted that the midwife, who had been employed by them for seven years, was "very negligent" by not sending for the medical officer, and she was immediately dismissed. After this, the LGB insisted that Bryan approve her replacement and that he should see all women who had been delivered—and that he alone was responsible for their treatment.[54]

Imbecile and Epileptic Patients

Despite the importance of the poor law in the administration of pauper lunatics, or the key role played by medical officers in the identification and treatment of the pauper insane, very little is known about their treatment within the workhouse, although many studies have been made of the history of insanity and institutions for the insane.[55] The workhouse clearly had its place within the mixed economy of care of the insane.[56] Under the Lunacy

Act of 1862, it was the duty of the workhouse medical officer to decide whether a lunatic was a proper person to remain in the workhouse. The medical officer gave directions on the diet, classification, and treatment of any paupers of unsound mind and reported whether he deemed any pauper to be dangerous or fit to be sent to a lunatic asylum. In reality, the criterion for removal of an insane pauper was predominantly managerial rather than medical, since it was less expensive to maintain paupers in the workhouse than in the asylum and, as the guardians frequently emphasized, their main priority was to keep the rates down.[57]

At the Leicester workhouse, patients classed as lunatics and imbeciles were accommodated in the imbecile wards along with inmates who suffered from senile dementia and epilepsy. Imbecile wards were considered to be safer places for epileptic and senile inmates, where they would ostensibly receive more care and attention. This was mainly due to the padded rooms in the imbecile wards, which meant that epileptic patients could be secluded for short periods either due to mental disturbance after a fit or as a safer place during a fit. Seclusion was always recorded and reported to the medical officer and no restraint was used.[58] After a visit to the workhouse in 1899, a Visiting Commissioner in Lunacy remarked that he was "sorry to see as many as fourteen men and twenty-two women in those wards who . . . display no mental disease."[59] Bryan justified this on the grounds that other commissioners had passed the patients as either epileptics or elderly people with "senile dementia," and he had been told not to certify them when they were old, as it made the lunacy statistics look large, although they agreed that the imbecile wards were the best places for them.[60]

However, conditions in these wards were not necessarily safe or suitable for such patients due to insufficient numbers of attendants and unsuitable furniture. For instance, in 1881 a commissioner reported that some of the epileptic patients were bruised as a result of falling during fits onto brick floors, and an elderly male patient was extensively bruised on the face due to falling from his bed at night. The commissioner recommended that a second paid attendant should be appointed and that a sane pauper ought to be present at night to give assistance.[61] Earlier in 1874 Clarke recommended that John Gray, an eighteen-year-old male epileptic, should be transferred to the asylum, as he considered that, although there was no special indication of insanity, Gray's intellect was weak and his frequent daily fits meant that he was not safe in a chair or able to walk across the ward by himself. The fact that Gray's father was willing for his son to be transferred to the asylum and to pay for part of his maintenance may have influenced this decision.[62]

In addition to inappropriate furniture, patients in the imbecile wards could be at risk from other patients' violent behavior. For example, Rosita Morley "repeatedly struck the other inmates besides pulling off a quantity of hair from one of the others and greatly disturbing them at night."

Fortunately for the patients, she was soon transferred to the local borough asylum, where she was diagnosed as suffering from mania. Similarly, Benjamin Lythall, an epileptic patient, struck an attendant on the head with a roller towel, whereupon he was set upon by the imbecile patients in a "violent attempt to master him."[63] The daily management and care of such patients was undertaken by lone, untrained attendants, while the medical officer's role was simply to decide which patients were dangerous lunatics or curable cases, who were then transferred to the asylum. Imbecile patients who were sufficiently able-bodied were kept occupied by providing useful manual labor in the workhouse, such as chopping sticks, carrying coals, and cleaning wards, and those who were disruptive and difficult to manage were usually contained by seclusion in the padded cell and then sent to the asylum.

Patients' Attitudes

According to a commissioner's report in 1900, the workhouse imbeciles were "happy and contented and many expressed gratification at their treatment."[64] Regrettably, there are very few direct records of any of the workhouse patients' opinions of their medical treatment; no doubt, any complaints that the guardians regarded as trivial went unrecorded. The records occasionally reveal patients' attitudes through reports of incidents regarded as disruptive.[65] George Chamberlain, for example, was one patient who created continual problems for the workhouse staff, according to prolonged correspondence conducted between the guardians and the LGB. In 1872 Clarke reported that Chamberlain had been constantly swearing and using abusive language to the ward nurse. The patient was told that he would not be allowed extras in his diet if he continued swearing, to which he replied with a "torrent of the most foul and filthy language ever uttered." Clarke stated that he regretted that Chamberlain was "subversive of all authority." He even suggested that his behavior was so bad that he should be removed to the Borough Gaol. This evidently did not happen as, in 1877, the doctor again reported that Chamberlain's "abominable and foul" language was a "scandal to the establishment" and "demoralising to the inmates."[66]

    Chamberlain was blind and paralyzed, and it appears that his only recourse was the workhouse infirmary, as his family could not cope with him. A pathetic letter was written on his behalf to the LGB, in which he stated that he was a "poor helpless creature" whose disease had been brought on by serving his country in a foreign climate. In addition to objecting to being put in the itch ward, where he was placed because of his profanities, Chamberlain complained that the guardians refused him admission unless he paid over his entire pension of seven shillings for his maintenance.[67]

The guardians asserted that he was not destitute, and they felt justified in refusing him admission because of his conduct and violent character. They disingenuously reported to the LGB that Chamberlain was in a helpless condition and required a separate room and constant attendance night and day, yet, clearly, he was not put in a separate room but in the itch ward, to which he violently objected, thus provoking further disruption.[68] Clarke noted, somewhat disappointedly, that Chamberlain's disabilities meant that the only punishment available was to put him on an ordinary diet, otherwise he was at a loss to know what else they could do with him.[69]

One further example of a patient's attitude toward her treatment is revealed by Bryan's report on the performance of the nurses. A patient, Sarah Ann Blunt, complained that due to her fear of a particular nurse, she had slept in a wet bed. Furthermore, the nurse had left her uncovered while changing the bedclothes, which had caused her to catch a cold. An investigation revealed that Blunt had a difficult labor for her confinement, and the deputy medical officer had applied instruments that caused a rupture requiring two stitches. When Blunt had been given a bed pan, she had been too embarrassed to use it when the nurse was present. Instead, another patient assisted her, but, unfortunately, the contents were spilled onto the bed. Sarah stated that she was too scared of Nurse Louisa Clowes to tell her what had happened, so she slept in the wet bed. The guardians decided that there was no evidence that the nurse was unduly harsh and remarked that, besides, it was "her duty to be firm in the patient's interest." Clowes confirmed that she did sometimes speak sharply to the patients when it was necessary, but stated that this was "not out of temper." The guardians concluded that it was Blunt's own fault for sleeping in a wet bed and dismissed her claim somewhat patronizingly, adding that "the method of changing the bedclothes employed by Nurse Clowes is only employed by skilled nurses and was therefore no doubt new and strange to Blunt."[70]

The Significance of Medical Officers
to the Quality of Workhouse Medicine

This chapter has provided a snapshot of the range of medical care provided at the Leicester workhouse with the intention of showing that, despite the many deficiencies of the poor law medical service inevitable in a system that embraced deterrence and economy as its central principles, the Leicester workhouse provided a reasonably good medical service in those circumstances. The caliber of its medical officers after 1867 was surprisingly high. Their lengthy periods of service signify a level of satisfaction and commitment on their part, although equally this indicates compliance with the restrictions and iniquities of the system. Even so, their long service provided experience, familiarity, and continuity of care for their patients and enabled them to establish a level of professional authority with the guardians. Naturally, there were many deficiencies, particularly in the quality and adequacy of the infirmary accommodation, the amount of time medical officers spent at their patients' bedsides, and the insufficient numbers of nurses. Nevertheless, the workhouse medical service provided treatment and care that would otherwise have been unavailable to paupers.

The microstudy on which this chapter is based concluded that the medicine practiced at the Leicester workhouse exceeded expectations and confounded the traditional image of workhouse medicine. Medical procedures were undertaken that went far beyond basic medical care, and progressive attitudes toward the medical treatment of workhouse patients were held by at least two of its medical officers. That attitude was pertinently encapsulated by Bryan in a statement he made to the LGB: "The sick poor . . . ought to have the best of treatment and I do not think anything ought to stand in the way of their receiving such treatment."[71]

Notes

1. This chapter is based on a paper delivered at the History of Medicine Unit, University of Birmingham, on November 17, 2007. The paper was based on doctoral research by Angela Negrine (funded by AHRC), "Medicine and Poverty: A Study of the Poor Law Medical Services of the Leicester Union, 1867–1914" (PhD diss. University of Leicester, 2008).

2. Irvine Loudon, *Medical Care and the General Practitioner, 1750–1850* (Oxford: Clarendon, 1986), 227.

3. Margaret Anne Crowther, "Paupers or Patients? Obstacles to Professionalization in the Poor Law Medical Service before 1914." *Journal of the History of Medicine and Allied Sciences* 39 (1984): 47–48.

4. Anne Digby, *Making a Medical Living: Doctors and Patients in the English Market for Medicine, 1720–1911* (Cambridge: Cambridge University Press, 1994), 50.

5. Crowther, "Paupers or Patients," 41–42; Kim P. Price, "A Regional, Quantitative and Qualitative Study of the Employment, Disciplining and Discharging of Workhouse Medical Officers of the New Poor Law throughout Nineteenth-Century England and Wales" (PhD diss., Oxford Brookes University, 2008), 59–60.

6. Felix Driver, *Power and Pauperism: The Workhouse System, 1834–1884* (Cambridge: Cambridge University Press, 1993); Steven King, *Poverty and Welfare in England, 1700–1850: A Regional Perspective* (Manchester: Manchester University Press, 2000).

7. Ruth G. Hodgkinson, *The Origins of the National Health Service: The Medical Services of the New Poor Law, 1834–1871* (London: Wellcome Trust Historical Medical Library, 1967); Jeanne L. Brand, *Doctors and the State: The British Medical Profession and Government Action in Public Health, 1870–1912* (Baltimore: Johns Hopkins Press, 1965); Michael W. Flinn, "Medical Services under the New Poor Law," in *The New Poor Law in the Nineteenth Century*, ed. Derek Fraser (London: Macmillan, 1976);

Margaret Anne Crowther, *The Workhouse System, 1834–1929: The History of an English Social Institution* (London: Batsford, 1981).

8. *Times*, November 12, 1880, reported that "Leicester . . . for some time past has enjoyed the unenviable notoriety of being the most unhealthy large town in England."

9. For a full discussion of the treatment of sick children, see Angela Negrine, "The Treatment of Sick Children in the Workhouse by the Leicester Poor Law Union, 1867–1914," *Family and Community History* 13 (2010): 34–44.

10. Nottingham and Birmingham Unions were exceptional in their insistence that workhouse medical officers worked full-time and were prohibited from taking on private practice. Ennis C. Bosworth, "Public Healthcare in Nottingham, 1750–1911" (PhD diss., University of Nottingham 1996), 209, 237; Alistair E. S. Ritch, "Sick, Aged and Infirm: Adults in the New Birmingham Workhouse, 1852–1912" (MPhil diss., University of Birmingham 2010), 46.

11. Kate M. Thompson, "The Leicester Poor Law Union, 1836–1871" (PhD diss., University of Leicester, 1988), 203.

12. Alexander P. Stewart, *Medical and Legal Aspects of Sanitary Reform (1867)* (Leicester: Leicester University Press, 1969), 42.

13. K. Thompson, "Leicester Poor Law Union," 202.

14. National Archives (hereafter NA), MH9/10, Leicester Union Register of Appointments.

15. NA, MH32/67, Report by Dr. Edward Smith on Provincial Workhouses, April 15, 1867.

16. Price, "Quantitative and Qualitative Study," 85–86.

17. Clarke's work for the asylum contributed to his untimely death when, in October 1900, he was shot in the sacrum by a former patient of the asylum while crossing a road. The patient had threatened to harm Clarke after he had certified him for homicidal tendencies. Clarke partially recovered, but died ten months later, aged sixty-four.

18. Julius St. Thomas Clarke, obituary, *Lancet*, August 31, 1901, 624–25.

19. "The Late Dr. J. St. T. Clarke, M.D., M.S., F.R.C.S.," *Leicester Guardian*, August 10, 1901.

20. Record Office for Leicestershire, Leicester, and Rutland (hereafter ROLLR), G/12/94, Medical Officer's Annual Report, 1872.

21. "The Healing of Wounds by Transplantation," *Lancet*, July 9, 1870, 62.

22. ROLLR, G/12/94, Medical Officer's Annual Report, 1872.

23. Price, "Quantitative and Qualitative Study," 148.

24. ROLLR, G/12/57d/12, Poor Law Board Circular to the Guardians of Poor Law Unions, April 20, 1868.

25. Frances B. Smith, *The People's Health, 1830–1910* (London: Croom Helm, 1979), 386.

26. Despite the high turnover of nursing staff, medical officers were commonly excluded from their appointments.

27. ROLLR, G/12/94, newspaper cutting on "Christmas Day at the Workhouse," 1871; undated newspaper cutting, 1880.

28. ROLLR, G/12/94, Medical Officer's Annual Report, 1873.

29. ROLLR, G/12/94, November 15 and December 12, 1871.

30. E. Hugh MacKay, *The Palace on the Hill: Leicester General Hospital Centenary, 1905–2005* (Leicester: Leicester General Hospital, 2006), 23.

31. ROLLR, G/12/94, March 2, 1874.

32. ROLLR, G/12/94, 1871.

33. See Hodgkinson, *National Health Service*, 196–204, 592–602, for more detailed information on the use of voluntary hospitals as auxiliaries to the poor law medical service.

34. ROLLR, G/12/94, July 28, 1872.

35. ROLLR, G/12/57d/19, August 8, 1879. Due to the limited space in the playground the children were taken for a run in the fields once or twice a week.

36. ROLLR, G/12/94, November 30, 1878.

37. Ernest R. Frizelle, *The Life and Times of the Royal Infirmary at Leicester: The Making of a Teaching Hospital, 1766–1980* (Leicester: Leicester Medical Society, 1988), 221.

38. ROLLR, Pamphlet, vol. 62, paper read by Dr. Clark before the Sanitary Sub-Committee, August 27, 1872; *Leicester Guardian*, September 14, 1901; ROLLR, G/12/8a/36, July 16, 1901.

39. "Dr. Bryan," *Wyvern*, October 16, 1896.

40. "Death of Dr. C. F. Bryan—Sudden End to a Useful Career," *Leicester Daily Post*, March 30, 1915, 5.

41. ROLLR, G/12/57d/36, December 30, 1895.

42. ROLLR, G/12/8a/31, February 16, 1897.

43. NA, MH12/6507, penciled comment by Dr. H. Stevens, February 17, 1897.

44. ROLLR, G/12/94, Medical Officer's Annual Report, 1871.

45. ROLLR, G/12/57b/13, September 14, 1911.

46. ROLLR, G/12/94, Medical Officer's Annual Report, 1873.

47. NA, MH12/6508, Report to Local Government Board by Dr. C. F. Bryan, December 13, 1897; January 15, 1898.

48. NA, MH12/6508, Letter to Local Government Board by Dr. C. F. Bryan, October 28, 1898; NA, MH12/6510, Local Government Board Report on Leicester Workhouse, December 14, 1899.

49. ROLLR, G/12/57d/14, February 16. 1872. Under the General Consolidated Order of 1847, a workhouse medical officer was entitled to a fee of between ten and twenty shillings for such an attendance.

50. Digby, *Making a Medical Living*, 269, notes that medical practitioners regarded midwifery with some ambivalence due to the time involved, but they valued the reliable income.

51. ROLLR, G/12/57b/5, February 24, 1872; G/12/57b/5, April 24, 1874. In 1874 the guardians reiterated that since the formation of the union, it had been their practice to employ midwives for all parish cases. They emphasized that all the lower and lower-middle classes were still attended by midwives and that doctors were called in only for difficult and dangerous cases.

52. ROLLR, G/12/94, Medical Officer's Annual Report, 1872.

53. NA, MH12/6497, Letter to Local Government Board from Dr. C. F. Bryan, November 26, 1889.

54. ROLLR, G/12/57d/30, January 21, 1890, 11; March 18, 1890.

55. Peter Bartlett, *The Poor Law of Lunacy: The Administration of Pauper Lunatics in Mid-Nineteenth-Century England* (London: Leicester University Press, 1999);

Crowther, *Workhouse System*, 164; Edgar Miller, "The Role of the Poor Law in the Care of the Insane in the Nineteenth Century," *History and Philosophy of Psychology* 8 (2006): 22. See also Steven Cherry, *Mental Health Care in Modern England: The Norfolk Lunatic Asylum/St. Andrew's Hospital, c. 1810–1998* (Woodbridge: Boydell Press, 2003); Richard Hunter and Ida Macalpine, *Psychiatry for the Poor: 1851 Colney Hatch Asylum; Friern Hospital, 1973: A Medical and Social History* (Folkestone: Dawsons, 1974); Joseph Melling and Bill Forsythe, *The Politics of Madness: The State, Insanity and Society in England, 1845–1914* (London: Routledge, 2006); Joseph Melling and Bill Forsythe, eds., *Insanity, Institutions and Society, 1800–1914: A Social History of Madness in Comparative Perspective* (London: Routledge, 1999); Cathy Smith, "Family, Community and the Victorian Asylum: A Case Study of the Northampton General Lunatic Asylum and Its Pauper Lunatics," *Family and Community History* 9 (2006): 109–24; David Wright, "Getting Out of the Asylum: Understanding the Confinement of the Insane in the Nineteenth Century," *Social History of Medicine* 10 (1997): 137–55; Wright, *Mental Disability in Victorian England: The Earlswood Asylum, 1847–1901* (Oxford: Clarendon, 2001); David Wright and Anne Digby, eds., *From Idiocy to Mental Deficiency: Historical Perspectives on People with Learning Disabilities* (London: Routledge, 1996).

56. Pamela Dale and Joseph Melling, eds., *Mental Illness and Learning Disability since 1850: Finding a Place for Mental Disorder in the United Kingdom* (London: Routledge, 2006), 4.

57. Driver, *Power and Pauperism*, 106; David Wright, "The Discharge of Pauper Lunatics from County Asylums in Mid-Victorian England: The Case of Buckinghamshire, 1853–1872," in *Insanity, Institutions and Society*, ed. Joseph Melling and Bill Forsythe (London: Routledge, 1999), 103, noted that asylum accommodation cost three times as much as workhouse provision and five times as much as outdoor relief.

58. ROLLR, G/12/57d/12, April 20, 1868.

59. ROLLR, G/12/57d/39, January 31, 1899.

60. ROLLR, G/12/57d/39, March 12, 1899.

61. ROLLR, G/12/57d/21, May 2, 1881.

62. NA, MH12/6484, John Gray, January 18, 1873.

63. Rosita Morley, ROLLR, G/12/94, October 11, 1880; Benjamin Lythall, ROLLR, G/12/57d/24, October 22, 1884.

64. ROLLR, G/12/57d/40, April 2, 1900.

65. Lynn Hollen Lees, *The Solidarities of Strangers: The English Poor Laws and the People, 1700–1948* (Cambridge: Cambridge University Press, 1998), 151–76, asserts that the poor were not always passive recipients of welfare, and they did not necessarily subscribe to this image of themselves.

66. ROLLR, G/12/94, January 6, 1872; October 1875.

67. ROLLR, G/12.57d/16, April 2, 1875.

68. ROLLR, G/12/57b/5, April 8, 1875; June 23, 1876.

69. ROLLR, G/12/94, February 3, 1877.

70. ROLLR, G/12/95, February 1903.

71. Ibid.

Chapter Ten

Workhouse Medicine in the British Caribbean, 1834–38

Rita Pemberton

Workhouse Medicine in Caribbean Literature

A considerable portion of the traditional historiography of the British Caribbean colonies is devoted to the plantation complex, with emphasis on its economic, political, and social systems and the sociocultural characteristics of the African population. Only marginal attention has been paid to issues pertaining to health and medicine. This omission has been addressed in the more recent phase of Caribbean historiography, which includes studies on health and medicine.[1] However, despite its importance in the culture of enslavement, prison and its associated medicine do not feature significantly in the literature. With reference to the workhouse, this chapter discusses the role of medicine in the prison system of the British colonies, to name the medical conditions prevalent in prison, to describe the environment in which workhouse medicine was practiced, to view how considerations of health and medicine impacted the operations of workhouses, and to specify the regulations under which the doctors operated. The objective is to identify the role medical services actually played in the prison system of these colonies during the period from 1834 to 1838. This period witnessed two experiences of freedom: full freedom as occurred in Antigua and partial freedom—if such a state is practically possible—as occurred in the remaining colonies, where the apprenticeship system was operative. Hence the chapter also seeks to determine the extent to which the medical culture in the workhouses differed in free Antigua from that which was developed in the partially free societies.

Research for this chapter has had to rely on those limited sources that are currently accessible. The dearth of secondary sources on this theme is perhaps a reflection of the fragmentary nature of the available primary data. As a consequence of imperial concern with the state of the region's prisons during the 1820s and 1830s, sources are more available for this period. The publication of Diana Paton's *No Bond but the Law* provides secondary sources on the history of punishment, but on workhouse medicine specifically the sources are very limited.[2] So far, none of the journals required to be kept by prison doctors in the British Caribbean have been located. As a result, it is not possible to ascertain what medications were offered to treat the afflictions of the inmates of the workhouses, but a discussion of the workhouse environment and the regulations that governed their operations is possible. Heavy reliance has therefore been placed on the limited available sources from which information has to be culled. Thus, the reports of the prisons authorized by the imperial government—in particular, that of 1836 and the report by Captain J. W. Pringle in 1838—and contemporary sources on the individual colonies and published material on the history of punishment in Jamaica have been used as the base line for this chapter.

The Development of
Penal Institutions in the British Caribbean

Prison, in plantation society, was a representation of the contradictions that characterized the colonial Caribbean, where, despite their lifelong sentence of imprisonment, additional provision for imprisonment of enslaved Africans was considered a necessity. Each plantation had its own jail, which symbolized the absolute power planters held over their enslaved charges. It was the accepted notion that failure to comply with planter orders must be punished and that it was the sole responsibility of planters so to do. Brute force characterized punishment on the plantations, as planters sought to ensure compliance with their orders by instilling fear in the minds of the enslaved. Several forms of punishment were used on Caribbean plantations, but with the increased challenge to enslavement, prison assumed greater importance as an antidote for resistance, particularly during the years when the pace toward abolition quickened.

The nineteenth-century emphasis on prisons was reflected in the increased allocation of prison spaces, the perception of prison as a responsibility of the administration, and the expression of greater interest by the imperial government in the conditions of prisons in the colonies. But the renewed emphasis on prisons was also related to the challenge to enslavement offered across the region, most notably by rebellion in Haiti and by marronage as occurred so significantly in Suriname, Guyana, and Jamaica, as well as the growing force of opposition in England, which was perceived as contributing to the instability of the enslaved population. The proabolitionist stance of the imperial government involved legislation that sought to provide direction in the daily lives of the enslaved, much to the chagrin of the planters, but, as with everything else, planters found ways to circumvent these laws.

According to Paton, in the 1820s there occurred a wave of prison development in Jamaica that matched developments in Europe and the United States, but with a major difference of purpose. She argues that the prisons in Jamaica served to incarcerate enslaved people who tried to escape and were caught, who had been sent for punishment on the private order of their masters or mistresses, or who had been convicted of crimes (19). Prisons served a dual purpose. They were punitive, punishing those who had transgressed, and also reformative, seeking to inculcate desirable habits in the inmates. This aspect of the prison program was based on the notion of the utility of Africans as members of the society that was itself based on the perception of their role as workers in the positions ascribed to them in the plantation complex. As Paton asserts, "prison aimed to recreate their inmates as ideal slaves: subordinate, unresisting, accustomed to hard physical work, and willing to perform it" (49).

Both roles required that inmates must work, hence labor formed a central part of prison activity. Thus workhouses, or houses of correction, were established in the prisons and became a part of the penal landscape of nineteenth-century British Caribbean plantation society, a departure from the pattern in England, where workhouses were separate institutions. Workhouses in the Caribbean were intended to provide rigorous reformative discipline, which included increasing rates of production. It was, however, considered important to establish that those being punished were fit enough to endure the various forms of punishment dispensed in prison. Such verification, needed both at the start and during the exercise, required the support of a medical opinion. Thus, within the prison complex, and especially in the workhouses, there was a clearly defined role for doctors.

The earliest development of an organized prison system occurred in Jamaica, where, until 1759, there was only one penal institution outside of the plantation jails. This changed in 1770 when the Jamaican Assembly passed a series of acts empowering parish authorities to build penal institutions. The first parish jails were established in Kingston, after which the house of correction, or workhouse, became the pattern in the island. By 1820 there were sixteen workhouses across the island, and many parishes had their own jails (19). As a result, "the work houses became the heart of the new Jamaican penal system aimed at enslaved people while the gaols generally confined free people imprisoned for debt" (23). Paton argues that the establishment of the workhouses was primarily a response to running away, which was a major problem on the island. Their establishment provided a network of workhouses through which to advertise runaways and facilitate their capture (27). Central to the operations of the workhouses was the treadmill, which became a fixture in every house of correction in the British colonies. Invented by Sir William Cubitt, the prison treadmill was a paddle wheel structure that simulated walking upstairs at a dictated pace while the prisoner held on to a bar. With the aim of inducing habits of industry and reducing idleness among prisoners, the wheel moved at a fast pace, forcing prisoners to keep up or be injured. Treadmills were introduced to Trinidad in 1824, Berbice in the late 1820s, and the Kingston House of Correction in 1828 (88).

After emancipation, the operations of prisons in Jamaica were regulated by the Jamaican Gaols Act of 1834, which was based on the English Gaols Act of 1823 and required each parish to have a jail and a house of correction (90). Houses of correction were built for each parish of the island and operated according to specified rules. This law authorized a regime of hard labor to prisoners, who were classified according to sex and type of crime. Members of staff were to be professionals, who were fully responsible for the operations of the prison. To prevent abuse of power by prison officials, provision was made for regular prison visits by chaplains, surgeons, and magistrates. The law required that punishment for infractions of prison regulations, which led to solitary confinement or the use of irons, was to be reported within twenty-four hours to a visiting justice (92).

The 1834 act led to a spate of prison construction in Jamaica, with new prisons being established in Morant Bay, Vere, St. Dorothy, and St. John. New rules for houses of correction and jails were issued by magistrates. According to Paton, "the most dramatic effect was the installation of treadmills (or 'treadwheels') in prisons across the island between 1834 and 1836" (93). Therefore, it was during this period that the workhouse culture became firmly established on the island. This was also the period of apprenticeship in Jamaica, when the Emancipation Act specified regulations for punishment of apprentices. This was a new and somewhat unpalatable development for planters, who had been so long accustomed to absolute control of their charges. In fact, they had become wedded to the belief that cruel punishment was the only way to enforce the discipline required to maintain plantation operations and profitability. Thus, in the development of the movement to freedom, the workhouses replaced the whip. Ultimately, in 1838 control of the prisons passed fully out of the hands of planters to the governors of the British Caribbean colonies with the passage of the Act for the Better Government of the Prisons in the West Indies (118).[3]

Basing her assessment on the Jamaica experience, Paton sees the development of prisons as a part of the development of creole society, which included a number of other changes in the society in areas such as hospitals, asylums, and schools (28). Collectively, these demonstrated "the strength and organization of the planter class" (29). She further asserts that "the work houses formed part of this means of ensuring that all slaveholders played their part in the maintenance of slavery," providing the assurance that the state had the means to discipline enslaved Africans should a particular enslaver be negligent. Paton sees the prison system as an "intertwining of private and public punishment" (50), as state sovereignty displaced that of planters during apprenticeship (54) and reflected an imperial commitment to the rule of law that was central to apprenticeship (67). She argues that "the threat of runaways was a major reason for the establishment of workhouses" (27).

The pattern of prison development described by Paton in Jamaica is reflected in other British colonial possessions, as they all made adjustments to their legal codes to make specific regulations for the operations of prisons and houses of correction during the years leading up to and after emancipation. In St. Vincent, where increased public security (as planters saw it) was considered necessary in the years leading up to emancipation, treadmills became a part of the prison infrastructure. After the passing of the Act for Building a Cage and the establishment of a police force in the town of Kingstown on September 22, 1821, the first house of correction in the island, the Kingstown House of Correction, became operative in 1825. During the apprenticeship period two additional houses of correction were established on the island, one in Windward at Colonarie in the Charlotte parish and the other in the leeward area at Barrouaille in the St. Patrick parish. The Kingstown treadmill was established in 1827 and, in 1830 it was placed under the jurisdiction of judges and wardens of the island. The keeper of the cage or his assistant was to superintend the administration of punishment of the prisoners sentenced to labor in a prison that was described as "dirty, bloody and smelly" and organized with a rigid system of internal discipline.

Impending emancipation and the onset of the apprenticeship system in particular stimulated further legislation. To ensure that the processes of apprenticeship and emancipation did not deprive the planters of their ability to control plantation society as they were accustomed, police laws and laws for promoting "the industry and good conduct" of freed people were passed. On June 23, 1834, the Act for the Abolition of Slavery in the Island of St. Vincent and Its Dependencies, in Consideration of Compensation, and for Promoting the Industry and Good Conduct of Manumitted Slaves was passed. It included provisions to establish a police force for the Regulation of Apprenticed Labourers and to carry into effect certain provisions of legislation. Under this law, a police post was set up in every district in St. Vincent. It was the specified duty of the police to prevent and repress crime and enforce obedience to the laws. Planters were required to pay nine pence per day for feeding each laborer sentenced to the treadmill. Each workhouse was to have a penal gang of those sentenced to labor, and these gangs were engaged on public works, roads, or any work necessary for the support of prisoners in the settlement or for public advantage.[4] Thus, during the apprenticeship period there was a strongly felt need to make provision for directing freed people into planter-determined paths of activity and behaviors. The passage of laws to effect this desire is reflective of concerns about the continuity of the traditional plantation operation with its main feature, planter control of the workforce.

The Barbados House of Assembly also made legal provision to administer the houses of correction and the operations of treadmills in 1834. The Emancipation Act was amended to make provision for a matron to preside over female prisoners in the houses of correction, to provide rules for the guidance of the supervisor of the treadmill, and to facilitate the provision of a salaried medical attendant to each house of correction.[5] This emphasis on punishment and the provision of clear rules for the operations of penal institutions during the era of freedom are indicators of a commitment to the rule of law underlined by a fear of freedom that might undermine planter control of labor.

It is clear that the issue of runaways was a major problem for the authorities in Jamaica and some other territories that undoubtedly influenced the establishment of workhouses in the colonies, but it does not necessarily explain the extension of the workhouse culture in colonies that were fully and partially free during the years under study. One of the weaknesses of the existing historiography is the tendency to overlook the Antiguan experience and treat this period of Caribbean history uniformly as the age of apprenticeship. Not only is it of value to understand the forces that influenced the decision to forgo apprenticeship in Antigua, but it is also useful to be able to compare free Antigua with the apprenticeship experience in the other territories. This is important in a study of workhouse medicine because it is essential to establish why workhouses were considered necessary in a free society and how their operations differed, if at all, from those in the world of the partially free.

Antigua was the first territory in the British West Indies to experience full freedom after the Antiguan planters voted in favor of immediate emancipation, which, they were convinced, would be far more advantageous to them than an apprenticeship period. Of major concern to them was that an apprenticeship period would increase their operating costs and provide further opportunities for imperial intervention in the island's affairs. Running away was, therefore, not a major problem for planters in Antigua after 1834 and does not explain the spread of the workhouse culture to that island during the first years of freedom. Recent scholarship has shown that the desire to circumvent the presence of stipendiary magistrates, who were allocated to supervise the apprenticeship system on the island was prominent in the minds of the Antiguan planters. It was felt that these officers symbolized, and would facilitate, imperial control of the affairs of Antigua. Thus, the desire to avoid this state of affairs and prevent "meddling by Downing Street" was one of the main considerations that led to the decision to opt for immediate emancipation in Antigua.[6]

In his observations of the impact of emancipation on Antigua, Louis Rothe, high court assessor and judge of probate in St. Croix, stated that emancipation rendered revisions of the island's criminal law necessary. He noted that during the period of enslavement, masters administered punishment to the enslaved as they saw fit, but after emancipation English criminal law became applicable to the free population. However, it was felt that this legal system, with its complex and lengthy processes, would have impeded rather than facilitated the suppression of crime, the main purpose of the law in the colonial context. Hence, according to Rothe, English law was considered inappropriate to the needs of the population of the colony.[7] Emancipation certainly rendered new laws necessary, especially in Antigua, which would provide the model for freedom in the British colonies. That said, was the suitability or unsuitability of British law the main issue?

The organization of a house of correction in Antigua was provided for in the Police Law of June 31, 1834, and a number of subsequent regulatory measures. According to Rothe, "Sentences to this house of correction eventually became far more common for various laws often prescribed hard labor in it for persons who were unable to pay the fines attached to minor offences."[8] As Rothe indicates, suppression of crime, as defined by the planting interests, was an important consideration during the years of freedom. His references to the increased use of the house of correction for trivial purposes indicate the use of the legal support base for increasing criminalization in the society. Rothe's own evidence suggests that the need to fashion a free society with such restrictions as would permit continued planter control during the age of freedom was central to the actions of planters in Antigua.

On June 21, 1839, the Act for Establishing a New System of Police and for Increasing the Power of the Magistracy of this Island in the Appointment of Rural Constables and for Providing and Regulating a House of Correction made provision for the establishment of a house of correction for the whole island in a former prison building located outside St. John. The building was to be expanded with provision for the kind of work that should be required of persons sentenced to hard labor, including "the treadmill, stone-breaking, etc or similar work, 10 hours per day" and for solitary confinement.[9] Hence, in the free society in Antigua there was an expectation of increased crime that stimulated provision for legal controls over the laboring population. Thus, prisons, workhouses, and, by extension, their hospitals were to be essential features of free society. These sentiments were felt as much in Antigua as they were in those territories where the apprenticeship system was operative.

The Workhouse Environment

Workhouses served a twin purpose; they were punitive and corrective. They were intended to improve the performance of workers who were confined to an environment where the pace of work formed a part of the punishment and, at the same time, demonstrated the rate of production that was expected of them. Additionally, the hard labor sentences required inmates to give service to the parish, underscoring their need to contribute to the community. At the same time, these hard labor sentences were just that—hard. Whatever the form of punishment inflicted on the unfortunate inmates, the message most forcefully conveyed was that the salvation of Africans in the Caribbean context, in free or unfree society, would come through hard labor. Special efforts were made to ensure that inmates remained in the institutions. Security measures required that convicts were fettered with leg irons, which weighed nine to fifteen pounds and were chained together to prevent escape.[10]

In Jamaica, workhouse gangs performed work for the public good. This included repairing roads, cleaning burial grounds, removing filth from public spaces, or being hired out to plantations.[11] Inmates were punished for nonperformance of work and breaches of prison discipline by deprivation of a meal, solitary confinement, spells on the treadmill, or flogging as sentenced by a magistrate. Sentences to hard labor usually implied the treadmill, but there were cases when individuals were given specific sentencing to the treadmill. Prisoners were given spells of fifteen minutes for males and ten minutes for females, usually undertaken in the morning and evening, sometimes at midday.[12] Prisoners were given specific instructions on how to ascend and descend the treadmills, and they were also required to keep pace with the mill or be injured and given additional punishment.[13] Those refusing to walk the wheel were tied by their arms to the hand rail.[14] Each workhouse had the services of a prison doctor to verify that each prisoner was well enough to work the mill.[15] In St. Lucia, where the treadmill was set up in 1834, men also worked the mill for fifteen minutes and women for ten minutes. The treadmill driver would prod those refusing to step with a cat and whip them if they continued to do so after the prodding. Inmates worked the treadmills from 7:00 a.m. to 4:30 p.m. in St. Lucia, while in Tobago treadmill labor and exercise occurred between the hours of 6:00 a.m. and 6:00 p.m., with an hour for lunch and two hours for dinner.[16] In Guyana labor on the treadmill and further exercise occurred from 6:00 to 11:00 a.m. and 1:00 to 5:00 p.m.[17]

Writing about their observation of the state of affairs in the prisons of Jamaica during the apprenticeship period, Joseph Sturge and Thomas Harvey recount observing about a dozen men and women heavily chained at the Halfway Tree workhouse (St. Andrew House of Correction), where it was the practice to put them in chains before trial. They found evidence of flogging and treadmill injury. The system, they said, was open to abuse, as the driver of the penal gang, superintendent of the treadmill, and other similar officers were selected from among those who were sentenced to prison for life. The hospital buildings in a number of estates also left a lot to be desired. They described the hospital at Drax Hall as "a wretched and filthy building," surpassed only by the one at Wiltshire Estate, which they considered so "dirty and offensive" that it was the worst they encountered on an estate. They also reported that some patients were locked up in the hospital and neglected.[18] Their evidence suggests that the emphasis of the workhouses was on punishment and the workhouse environment was replete with situations that required medical intervention.

In his report on the prisons of Jamaica, Captain Pringle noted that the prisoners sentenced to the houses of correction were all apprentices sent there by the local and special magistrates. Those sent by the former were being punished for theft, trespass, and assault and by the latter for disputes between masters and apprentices. The males sentenced to hard labor were engaged in road repair, while the females worked within the prison walls breaking stones. Prisoners were usually sentenced by magistrates to the penal gang for seven to fifteen days and those convicted by the quarter sessions for periods from two to twelve months. Owners of runaways committed to the penal house of correction were required to pay six pence per day for food and two pence for medicine, if required. In most of the houses of correction, there were two or three convicts among the inmates who were sentenced for life as "incorrigible runaways" during slavery.[19]

There does not appear to be a rational relationship between the crimes for which the inmates were incarcerated, the length of time they spent in the prison, and the nature of the punishments administered. Interestingly, the provision for medical supervision of the operation suggests that doctors, or some other medical personnel, spent long hours at the prisons guiding the operations of the workhouses. This does not appear to have been the practice, given the state of sanitation of the prisons and the evidence of injured and neglected sick prisoners in the prison hospitals.

All reports support the view that there was generally a lack of personal cleanliness among the inmates in the prisons of the region. Soap was not allowed in the prisons of Jamaica and St. Vincent.[20] But the hair of inmates, both male and female, was cut short, ostensibly for cleanliness, but more as a punishment. Pringle lamented the lack of prison dress in Jamaica, where clothes were provided to inmates only in extreme circumstances, bedding was noticeably absent, and prisoners slept on a raised bench or on the floor. A similar situation also occurred in Antigua, where Pringle reports that prisoners slept on the floor with no bedding, except for the sick, who slept on stretchers with mattresses and blankets in a special room that was used as a hospital.[21]

Given the emphasis on ability to withstand punishment, diet was important in prison and workhouse medicine. While there was some variation in the different colonies, the dietary provisions at the workhouses were similarly restrictive, with some gender differentiation in the allowances. Inmates in Trinidad were allocated one pound of prepared cornmeal with two ounces of salted fish for breakfast and dinner at a weekly cost per prisoner of three shillings and sixpence. The inmates were required to work between the hours of 6:00 or 9:00 a.m. to 1:00 p.m. and then again from 2:00 to 6:00 p.m., with the intervening hours being used for meals and rest. In Guyana (Demerara and Essequibo), prisoners were given weekly allowances of plantains and salt fish with fresh meat twice per week for inmates and salt fish and plantains alone for slaves.[22]

Some prisoners received money instead of food. In some parts of Jamaica prisoners were given between one shilling, threepence, and tenpence per day, and the apprentices received little over half of that allowance. All were expected to use such funds to buy food from hucksters. Where food was provided, prisoners were usually fed ground roots, cornmeal, salt herring, and shad, a river herring. Their daily food allowance was six large plantains for males and five for females or six pounds of yam or cocoas, along with one herring or shad, except those sentenced by the special magistrate to be fed on plantains and water alone.[23] Clearly, the food provided in the workhouses was not intended to strengthen inmates in preparation for the demanding routines of workhouse punishment. The provisions were less than adequate for laboring people and would have left them barely able to survive. In Montserrat, which did not have a treadmill, the most frequent complaint was that the food was not sufficient.[24]

The houses of correction were administered by the custos and local magistrates who established a management committee to govern the appointment and removal of staff and the formulation of operational regulations. As indicated by Sturge and Harvey, convicts serving life sentences were often given responsibilities as boatswains, who opened and locked female cells, for which they were not paid but instead received food, exemption from labor, and a chance of pardon. The prison supervisors were usually planters or failed business men. Some prisons had a matron who was usually the wife of the supervisor or an elderly woman. These practices made room for a range of abuses to occur in the workhouses, in addition to which facilities were inadequate. What passed for toilet facilities was a "tub . . . in the room for necessary purposes, to be used publicly by all: a disgusting and unwholesome practice, particularly in crowded rooms which is sometimes badly ventilated."[25]

The prevailing workhouse environment could hardly be considered reformative. Despite the regulations, emphasis was overly placed on restrictions, abuse, and force, from which inmates had no recourse. This pattern of operation was common to both free Antigua and the territories with apprenticeship; therefore there was no difference in the workhouse environment in free and partly free societies. This was the environment in which workhouse medicine was practiced.

Medical Provisions in the Workhouses

In all the colonies (except Tobago), prison staff included medical personnel.[26] In Trinidad, where the common jail and house of correction were under the jurisdiction of the Royal Audiencia, superintended by the board of Cabildo, and inspected by the board of magistrates, the workhouse staff included a physician, a superintendent of the treadmill, a warder, and nurse. Separate accommodation was provided for the sick and "lunatics" (considered nuisances), and the surgeon visited every day and whenever he was required.[27] In Antigua there was no provision for seriously sick prisoners, who were removed from the prison on the instruction of the doctor. However, provision was made for mentally ill patients, who were given separate accommodation on the lower floor at the opposite end of the jail and were allowed in the yard for exercise. They were supervised by a medical officer who visited them daily and a nurse who cooked for them.[28] Separate hospital accommodation was not provided in St. Vincent, where prisoners, sick and well, were housed together. The medical officer visited the sick prisoners once or twice per week and whenever his services were requested.[29] In all parts of Jamaica, the medical officer was required to attend the workhouse regularly and was generally paid what was considered a liberal salary.[30] It was a legal requirement that, whenever a death occurred in prison, the supervisor should send for the coroner and an inquest held.[31] In St. Lucia separate facilities were provided but, according to Dr. Nuchet, a prison doctor in St. Lucia for fourteen years, "the building called a hospital is really a shed and is not fit for the sick."[32] As this suggests, the hospital facilities provided in Caribbean workhouses were varied. In some instances, no separate accommodation was provided for the sick, while in others separate rooms were allocated as hospital space. Except in the case of mental illness, there was no separation based on the nature of the afflictions or on gender.

Given the prevailing workhouse conditions, it is no surprise that there were certain ailments common to the institutions in the region. Sturge and Harvey described patients suffering with leprosy, sores, and ulcers in Jamaica lying on the floor of prison hospitals.[33] In the Kingstown House of Correction, fever was the most common complaint.[34] In Jamaica several institutions identified bilious and intermittent fever, other fevers, and dropsy as the most frequently occurring complaints.[35] While the Barbados prison officials reported that dysentery, inflammation, and fever were most prevalent, those in St. Lucia identified flux, fever, and ulcers as most common among their inmates.[36] In addition, they assured that the prison mortality rate was not greater than that of the wider society. In Montserrat common fever, described as slight, and rheumatism were the most frequently occurring complaints, while in Guyana bowel complaints and slight fevers accompanying colds were the most common problems afflicting inmates.[37] The Antigua prison, on the other hand, reported few cases of illness among its prisoners. Lest this be taken as an indication that there was a prevailing state of health at that institution, the system of discharging ill prisoners permitted the authorities to avoid the cost of prison hospital care, renounce any responsibility for the sick prisoners, and, at the same time, provide an aura of liberalism at the institution. It is not clear how these discharged patients fared and what ultimately became of them.

Underreporting seems to have been widespread among other prison officials in the region. It is surprising that pains, wounds, and lacerations, consistent with flogging and workhouse injuries, did not feature more prominently among the afflictions listed as common among workhouse prisoners. It is well known that there was a plethora of injuries from the treadmills. In his evidence to the Pringle investigation, Dr. Moor, partner and acting surgeon in St. George Parish House of Correction in Jamaica, attests that when prisoners returned from the treadmill sessions, he found that they were often affected with pains in their legs and arms. He also claimed that he had seen marks on women's breasts, which possibly resulted from hanging on the treadmill.[38] The testimony of James Williams supports this view of prevalent injury in the workhouses from flogging and the treadmills. Referring to his own experience, Williams recounts receiving such a severe flogging that he was "all cut up and bleeding." He received several other undeserved floggings, followed by a workhouse session after which "he never felt well . . . got sick with fever and head ache and pain in the stomach." He also witnessed an elderly African man who was flogged until he coughed up blood, and then, when sent to the hospital, received no attention because "them say him not sick." He cites instances of other prisoners who not only were weak after floggings but received little attention at the hospital. He refers to cases where women from different estates were wounded from floggings and sessions at the mill and states that all the people who were flogged complained of pain in the stomach.[39] Given the extensive recourse that was made to punishment in the workhouses, the resulting injuries should have preoccupied most attending doctors.

The practice of workhouse medicine required doctors to perform a range of tasks. As Dr. Richard Madden indicates, "the medical men can't pay enough attention to the sick negroes . . . because [they] had so much to do."[40] They gave medical opinions in courts and recommended the release of prisoners for ill health.[41] The duties of doctors were also stipulated by the prison regulations. The St. Vincent regulations stated,

> The medical attendant shall visit the prison three times in every week, and oftener if necessary, and shall keep a journal, in which the names of the patients under his care, and the prescriptions ordered by him, shall be entered, and any observations he may deem requisite; which journal shall be kept in the gaol, and signed by him, and produced to any person having authority over the place of confinement, whenever it shall be required.[42]

In all territories doctors attending prison hospitals and workhouses were required to keep a journal, commonly called the surgeon's book, in which they recorded details of every case they attended, including the patient's name, the disease treated, prescriptions, special diet ordered, and the progress and termination of each case. They also kept a list of convalescents who were directed to take air and exercise in the yard.[43]

Doctors were required to issue medical certificates in cases where serious illness necessitated the release of the prisoner from prison or workhouse on the instructions of the governor and to confirm the fitness of the prisoners to receive punishment.[44] These certificates were issued to planters who submitted them to the magistrates to authorize punishment.[45] Medical examination of prisoners prior to punishment was compulsory, and doctors could remove prisoners from treadmill sessions if they considered the prisoner incapable of continuing. The doctor's permission and medical examination were required before pregnant women could be sent to the treadmill. If the treadmill routine proved too onerous for them, the doctor could end the session and order alternative punishment in the penal gang. All prisoners were to be allowed as much air and exercise as was considered necessary for the preservation of their health.[46]

Doctors were also responsible for the diet of workhouse prisoners. The common practice was reflected in the regulations of the St. Vincent prison and workhouse, which stipulated that "prisoners under the care of surgeons and physicians shall be allowed such diet as may be directed in writing for them."[47] Some doctors inspected the food to ascertain that it was wholesome and would occasionally order a change or prescribe wine, soup, or anything else considered necessary for the patient.[48]

Doctors ordered medicine, which was imported from England, wine, and other items considered necessary for the treatment of the sick.[49] Recognizing the role of alcohol in the practice of medicine in the workhouses, the law in Guyana allowed only the quantities of liquor specified in writing and ordered by the doctor on the prison compound. The cost of medicine was borne by the public and stocks were usually stored in the jail.[50] The doctor was usually aided by the assistant matron, who in his absence administered the medicines he prescribed.

The regulations project the image of an organized system of operation based on the notion of the welfare of the sick prisoners. If any attempt was made to fulfill all the requirements stipulated in these regulations, the doctors attending workhouses would have been certainly oversubscribed. Unfortunately, the journals they were required to keep are as yet unavailable, so it is not possible to comment on how well they discharged their responsibilities and the nature of the treatments they applied. The evidence in the existing reports indicates that conditions in the workhouse hospitals were less than desirable; sanitation was poor, food was inadequate, and patients showed signs of neglect.

Prison and Control in the Age of Freedom

The spate of prison expansion that occurred in the British Caribbean in the decade before emancipation continued into the first years of freedom. During this period there was a perceived need to provide additional prison space, with supporting legal and policing systems in all the colonies. While, as asserted by Paton, these provisions reflect metropolitan influences, there were also local considerations that necessitated their presence. It is argued here that, during the first years of freedom, there occurred a convergence of needs: the imperial need to assert greater control over developments in the colonies and the planter need to continue to exert control over the society in the context of freedom. The fact that prison regulations signified an imperial intent for greater control did not preclude the possibility of continued planter control in the colonies. It is posited here that while the provision of prison and workhouse regulations resulted from imperial insistence, continued planter control was made possible by the operating practices at the institutions. Detailed regulations governed the operations of workhouses and the duties of doctors, but the provision of hospital space was not mandated, and there was no legislation to specify what environmental conditions were considered appropriate for the workhouses. There was variance between the intent of the regulations and the actual practice at the institutions, which permitted planters to continue to wield control. Workhouses, which served as the centers of punishment within the prison system, continued their brutal practices, and the assuaging influence of doctors was not evident. Unsanitary conditions prevailed at the prisons and workhouses and their hospitals and, as a result, diseases and afflictions related to poor sanitation and brutality prevailed. The role identified for doctors seemed to be somewhat idealized, given the realities of the colonies in that era. Moreover, workhouse operations were consistent in both fully and partially free colonies and the medicine practiced there buttressed, rather than relieved, the cruel impositions of prison and workhouse operations of the day on the inmates.

Notes

1. See, for example, Juanita de Barros, Stephen Palmer, and David Wright, eds., *Health and Medicine in the Circum-Caribbean, 1800–1968* (New York: Routledge, 2009).

2. Diana Paton, *No Bond but the Law: Punishment, Race and Gender in Jamaica State Formation, 1780–1870* (Durham: Duke University Press, 2004). Hereafter cited in text.

3. Diana Paton, "The Penalties of Freedom: Punishment in Post-emancipation Jamaica," in *Crime and Punishment in Latin America: Law and Society since Late Colonial Times*, ed. Ricardo D. Salvatore, Carlos Aguirre, and Gilbert M. Joseph (Durham: Duke University Press, 2001), 275–77.

4. Roderick A. McDonald, ed., *Between Slavery and Freedom: Special Magistrate John Anderson's Journal of St. Vincent during the Apprenticeship* (Kingston, Jamaica: University of the West Indies Press, 2001), 71, 137–38, app. 6, pp. 249–53, 18, 23–26, 252–54.

5. Robert H. Schomburgk, *The History of Barbados Comprising a Geographical and Statistical Description of the Island: A Sketch of the Historical Events since the Settlement and an Account of Its Geology and Natural Productions* (London: Cass, 1971), 470.

6. Nsaka Septuf-Ntepua-Sesepkekiu, "Freedom and the Problem of Labour in Antigua, 1834–1838" (MPhil. diss., University of Cambridge, 2007), 38.

7. Louis Rothe, *A Description of the Island of Antigua with Particular Reference to Emancipation's Results, 1846*, trans. Neville A. T. Hall (Mona, Jamaica: University of the West Indies, 1996), 24.

8. Ibid., 22.

9. Ibid., 21.

10. National Archives, Kew, London (hereafter NA), Colonial Office Records (hereafter CO), 318/136, Report of Captain J. W. Pringle on Prisons in the West Indies, Jamaica, 1838, 5–6.

11. Paton, *No Bond*, 40.

12. NA, CO, Report of Captain J. W. Pringle on Prisons in the West Indies, Jamaica, 1838, 318/136, 8.

13. NA, CO, 137/210, Papers Relevant to the Abolition of Slavery in the British Colonies, 57.

14. Ibid., 32.

15. Paton, *No Bond*, 112.

16. NA, CO, 318/136, Pringle on Prisons, pt. 2, St. Lucia, 1838; NA, CO, 318/136; Pringle on Prisons, pt. 2, Tobago, 1838, 94–95.

17. NA, CO, 318/136, Pringle on Prisons, pt. 2, Guyana, 1838, 96.

18. Joseph Sturge and Thomas Harvey, *The West Indies in 1837* (London: Cass, 1837), 168–70, 176, 190, 203–7, 218, 229, 303.

19. NA, CO, 318/136, Pringle on Prisons, Jamaica, 1838, 4, 8, 7.

20. McDonald, *Between Slavery and Freedom*, app. 10, 264–66.

21. NA, CO, 318/136, pt. 2, Antigua, 20.

22. NA, CO, 318/136, Correspondence Relative to the State of the West Indies, Trinidad, 95; Guyana, 96.

23. CO137/210 Correspondence Relative to the State of Gaols in the West Indies, Jamaica, 46.

24. NA, CO, 318/136, pt. 2, Jamaica; Montserrat, 32.

25. Ibid., Montserrat, 6.

26. NA, CO, 318/136. Correspondence Relative to the State of Gaols in the West Indies, Tobago, 94–95. The total staff at the Tobago prison and treadmill consisted of one jailer.

27. NA, CO, 318/136, Correspondence, Trinidad, 95, 96.

28. NA, CO, 318/136, pt. 2, Antigua, 86.

29. McDonald, *Between Slavery and Freedom*, app. 9, p. 265.

30. NA, CO, 137/210. Some were paid between thirty and two hundred pounds. CO, 318/136, Jamaica, 9.

31. Ibid., 47.

32. NA, CO, 318/136, appendix to Pringle on Prisons, 1838, 58.

33. Sturge and Harvey, *West Indies*, 253, 283, 296, 298.

34. McDonald, *Between Slavery and Freedom*, app. 9, p. 265.

35. NA, CO, 318/136, Pringle on Prisons, Jamaica, 1838, 21.

36. NA, CO, 318/136, 48; no. 26, "Return of the Gaols, and of the Number of Prisoners Confined Therein."

37. NA, CO, 318/136, appendix to Pringle on Prisons, 1838, 58, 32, 9, 58; Guyana, 83.

38. NA, CO, 318/136, appendix to Pringle on Prisons, 1838, 48.

39. Diana Paton, ed., *A Narrative of Events, since the First of August, 1834 by James Williams, an Apprenticed Labourer in Jamaica* (Durham: Duke University Press, 2001), 12, 6, 8, 15, 17.

40. *Report of the Select Committee on Negro Apprenticeship in the Colonies Together with Minutes of Evidence*, Parliamentary Papers, 1836, 15 (560), Evidence of Dr. Madden, August 13, 1836.

41. Sturge and Harvey, *West Indies*, 304.

42. McDonald, *Between Slavery and Freedom*, app. 10, clause 19, p. 269.

43. NA, CO, 318/136, 38.

44. McDonald, *Between Slavery and Freedom*, app. 9, p. 265.

45. *Report of Select Committee*, 1836, Evidence of Dr. Madden.

46. NA, CO, 318/136, appendix to Pringle on Prisons, 1838, 58, 31, 48, 17.

47. McDonald, *Between Slavery and Freedom*, app. 10, clause 11, p. 268.

48. NA, CO, 318/136, appendix to Pringle on Prisons, 1838, 58.

49. Ibid., 47.

50. Ibid., 38.

Chapter Eleven

Poverty, Medicine, and the Workhouse in the Eighteenth and Nineteenth Centuries

An Afterword

STEVEN KING

Thinking about Medical Care in the Workhouse

The literature on poverty and medicine has developed considerably since Anne Crowther, Ruth Hodgkinson, Michael Flinn, Joan Lane, and Geoffrey Oxley were building the field.[1] New work—on doctoring contracts, subscriptions by parishes to extraparochial medical institutions, infirmary building programs, the extent of sickness and ill health among the poor, the nature of medical relief under the Old Poor Law, medical negligence, and the medical marketplace—has begun to test ingrained historiographical notions that the nature of medical relief was better under the Old Poor Law than the New and to establish the centrality of sickness to the pauperization process.[2] It has also begun to highlight the essential complexity of medical care for the poor, with considerable regional and intraregional variation overlain by a remarkable expansion in the range of "medical things" that the poor law, Old and New, came to pay for. The sick poor as actors and agents have been given a voice in the flowering of literature on pauper narratives to match that long available for scholars considering the experiences of the insane.[3] And London has moved from a veritable black hole in welfare history to the focus of a renewed appreciation of care and relief for the out-parish, lunatic, venereal, widowed, unemployed, and institutional poor under the Old and New Poor Laws.[4] Medical welfare has been a particularly fruitful field for historians of London, with contributions from Jeremy Boulton on nursing, David Green on medical relief post-1834, and Elaine Murphy on the treatment of the insane. Such work, allied with the London-centric focus of the pre-1834 section of this volume, provides a distinctive agenda for research in the provinces.[5]

Nonetheless, significant gaps in our knowledge on the nature and role of medical care offered in the workhouse remain. Under the Old Poor Law, problems over the very definition of what a workhouse was coalesce with poor record survival so that relatively little is known, outside of interesting ad hoc examples and the large London workhouses analyzed in this volume by Jeremy Boulton, Romola Davenport, Leonard Schwarz, and Kevin Siena, about who workhouse inmates were, how often they were sick, what they were sick with, how they were treated in a medical sense, and how treatment in the workhouse fitted into life cycles of relief and ill health.[6] Even acknowledging that in 1803 only 12–15 percent of the poor were relieved in provincial workhouses, the force of Richard Smith's observation—that a poor grasp of who ended up in workhouses, why, and for how long is a significant hindrance in attempts to understand the meaning of trends in pension expenditure and medical relief—remains very pertinent.[7]

Somewhat paradoxically, the situation has not been much better for the New Poor Law, at least outside of David Green's new analysis of London.[8] Felix Driver has traced the chronology of key changes to the medical fabric of workhouses in different regions, while the study of workhouse medical scandals (such as that in Bridgwater analyzed in chapter 8) has also begun to throw light on generalized standards of medical care, the attitudes of guardians to medical relief, and, in some cases, the detailed treatment regimes employed in workhouse infirmaries.[9] Elizabeth Hurren's work on the crusade against outdoor relief and its corollary of an attack on medical relief, and on the traffic in the bodies of the poor, has done much to expose the dark side of medical relief in the later New Poor Law.[10] Yet, microstudies of the detailed records of poor law unions remain notable by their absence, and some of the most exciting work—on Leicester by Angela Negrine, or Graham Mooney on mid-Victorian London, for instance—has only recently come to fruition.[11] As Keir Waddington has suggested in his discussion of the financing of medicine in the Whitechapel Union, there are formidable challenges to moving beyond the generalities of New Poor Law medical relief offered by Crowther, Hodgkinson, and Flinn. Solving them requires a systematic and coordinated research program.[12] A model is the overlapping work of Leonard Smith, Akihito Suzuki, Joseph Melling, and Cathy Smith, all of whom have been looking at how and why pauper lunatics moved between family and community care, into and through workhouses, on to asylums and prisons, and back again.[13] As Peter Bartlett reminds us, even in the 1890s at least 25 percent of all the lunatic poor were still resident in the workhouse, with poor law unions seeking to provide care "of a standard not dissimilar to that in the County asylum."[14] Smith, in his contribution to this volume, disputes such a rosy view but confirms the importance of the work-house in lunatic care. English welfare historians also have much to learn from their Irish counterparts about using disputes within the workhouse as a lens through which to focus attention on pauper experiences and interpretations of issues such as clothing, diet, and medical care.[15]

In part, one reason for difficulty in understanding the treatment of the sick poor is the fundamental disjuncture between medical and welfare historians in their approaches. Medical historians have considerably advanced our understanding of institutions, such as endowed (teaching) hospitals, the voluntary hospitals, and (to a lesser extent) the dispensary system.[16] There has also been a boom in the study of individual asylums and regional asylum systems.[17] In practice, however, and notwithstanding some eye-watering figures on the number of discrete cases treated by the voluntary hospitals in particular, only the smallest proportion of paupers and the minutest proportion of all sickness episodes experienced by those paupers are likely to have been encompassed by treatment in such institutions.[18] Medical historians, as Sylvia Pinches observes, have been rather less concerned with the more numerous and more extensive medical aid charities set up by private endowment or public subscription.[19] And if they have constructed a strong analytic superstructure for understanding the nature and content of the medical market, the sick poor and the institutions and policies provided by parishes and unions to care for them are almost completely absent from their frame of reference. This gap has not been filled by British welfare historians, who have been only tangentially concerned with the mixed economy of health care for the poor.[20] Indeed, some have wondered whether it is worth studying the sick poor as a discrete group at all.[21] Unsurprisingly, then, an understanding of the exact medical role of the workhouse remains elusive.

The rest of this chapter attempts, broadly, to establish the state of our knowledge on sickness and medical relief for the poor in general and the place of workhouse medicine in particular. It ranges widely over questions such as the structure of the inmate population, the nature of institutional care, the place of that care in the wider medical market, and attitudes toward particular subsets of the sick poor. The chapter suggests avenues for future research, some of which emerge out of contributions by others in this volume. It is important to start, however, with a brief discussion of terms of reference.

Definitional Matters

An increasingly strong appreciation of the visual and physical imprint of workhouses, particularly for London, has not found balance in work on the manuscript sources.[22] Indeed, and especially for the provinces and Wales under the Old Poor Law, defining what a workhouse was and reconstructing what happened there remains problematic. The nature of the problem can be illustrated with brief reference to Northamptonshire. While towns like Kettering were relatively consistent in identifying buildings as a "workhouse" and in maintaining consistent records, other towns and parishes in the county were not.[23] In Welton, which experimented with a "workhouse" on five separate occasions between 1729 and 1834, the vestry made reference variously to "the poorshouse," "the almshouses," "Mr Sheltons [the farmer of the poor] house," "house of industry," and (in a doctor's contract from 1804) "the old people's hospital."[24] Such variations in terminology are repeated for other Northamptonshire parishes and elsewhere. As Jonathan Reinarz and Leonard Schwarz point out in their introductory chapter, the terminology used to define the "workhouse" was partly organic. Different labels may reflect genuine and—as Kevin Siena shows for the St. Margaret's Westminster workhouse in chapter 1—rapid changes in the purpose or physical constellation of workhouse buildings. On the other hand, they may simply have reflected what Susannah Ottaway has labeled in chapter 2 a "lumping tendency," under which very different institutions were casually given the name "workhouse."

How the shifting linguistic register to describe Old Poor Law institutions reflected poor law ideology, the nature and scale of institutional care for the poor and sick poor, and the relationship between indoor and outdoor medical relief, thus remains a complex question. An answer is made more problematic, though it is no less an important task, by the fact that in a place like Welton more or less the same set of buildings were named and renamed in this way. When the parish sold off its property in the 1830s, the "workhouse" comprised four ramshackle houses clustered together, and in the underlying vestry and overseers' records it is usually impossible to discern what "workhouse care" actually entailed.[25] Defining what a workhouse was and locating the institutional population and their medical care is thus problematic, a problem intensified where parishes came together in private or Gilbert incorporations (of the sort discussed in Susannah Ottaway's chapter) or where they shared workhouse provision.

Nor should we believe that definitional issues are cleared up by the New Poor Law. The fact that many poor law unions ended up with overlapping and competing institutional provision at their creation is well known.[26] The broad chronology of workhouse building and improvement is also clear, although, even for the New Poor Law, the concentration of detailed empirical research on the London workhouses is marked.[27] However, the development of the fabric, particularly medical fabric, of the New Poor Law creates new definitional problems. A plan of the Bolton Union workhouse drawn up in March 1898, for instance, shows the engine shed, school, and cottage homes, as well as the workhouse. It does not, however, record the recently completed infirmary or nursing homes located on an adjacent site, leaving only the lock wards and a fever ward in the workhouse itself. In fact, the infirmary had become something very different to the workhouse and was taking large numbers of nonworkhouse patients. What, then, was the relationship between poverty, the workhouse, and medicine in this case? Bolton Union had also maintained separate institutional provision for the blind and other disabled people for more than twenty years by the late 1890s, further complicating the problem of how to define what a workhouse was and what medical function it was supposed to perform.[28] Angela Negrine traces similar issues with regard to the Leicester Union in her contribution to this volume.

To some extent, these problems are as intractable as they are common. Nonetheless, it *is* surprising how little both welfare and medical historians have analyzed relatively plentiful documents—maps of workhouse sites, standing heritage, plans of workhouse buildings, debates about the location and financing of workhouses, rate books, tenders, loan and mortgage documents, and accounts of disturbances—as a way of gleaning how in a medical sense workhouse space might have been used. Such exercises would both yield important findings in their own right and confront some of the definitional problems outlined earlier. In the meantime, accepting the convenient fiction that we can define what and where a workhouse was leads to other questions, one of the most prominent of which is who workhouse inmates and patients were.

Who Were the Workhouse Inmates and Patients?

The broad and widely accepted generalization that workhouses under the Old Poor Law were receptacles for the most costly paupers, those without kin and those with the most entrenched causes of poverty (advanced old age, single women with children, orphans, etc.) is not unproblematic. There is evidence that such institutions experienced high "churn factors" and might sometimes have housed significant numbers of working-age paupers.[29] There were also differences between individual workhouses in the proportion of inmates who were admitted sick or became so. Susannah Ottaway, in this volume and elsewhere, has argued persuasively that the workhouse in eighteenth-century Terling came to focus its activity on the aged, sick, and infirm, despite the widespread acceptance that the aged in particular had natural rights to noninstitutional treatment.[30] Tim Hitchcock suggests that more than half those admitted to the workhouse in St. Luke's Chelsea were in some form "sick" by the mid-eighteenth century. While this figure may have been on the high side compared to other workhouses and other counties, his general findings on the importance of sickness as a factor causing workhouse admission are echoed by Eric Thomas for Berkshire, Ethel Mary Hampson for Cambridgeshire, and Robert Hastings for North Yorkshire.[31]

By contrast, the workhouse in early eighteenth-century St. Martin's had less than 30 percent of its admissions in the strictly sick category, although, as Jeremy Boulton, Romola Davenport, and Leonard Schwarz argue in their contribution, this figure included a high proportion of fever cases such that the workhouse may have played a disproportionate role in protecting the surrounding community from infectious disease. Kevin Siena suggests that, whatever the proportion of sick inmates, the workhouse played a key role as medical institution of last resort in the lives of the poor. Yet patchy evidence from rural and provincial urban workhouses with their very small capacities suggests the workhouse was an adaptable space in which the importance of the sick pauper fluctuated considerably. In Lutterworth, Leicestershire, for instance, the workhouse (capacity twenty-two in 1784) rarely took in the sick poor but broke this rule in the aftermath of smallpox and other epidemics when recovering individuals and malnourished families appear to have been admitted in some numbers.[32]

The picture of workhouse inmates and the importance of sickness as a cause of admission is a little clearer post-1834. Despite the ideological bias of the New Poor Law toward ensuring institutionalized relief, numerous empirical studies have confirmed early generalizations that outdoor relief remained the norm and that "medical need" was often appropriated as a reason for paying outdoor relief of this sort.[33] While the exact composition of workhouse populations varied according to area, chronology, and local economy, census work by Nigel Goose, Andrew Hinde, and others has confirmed Jean Robin's 1990 observation that New Poor Law workhouses became institutions in which children, women, the sick, insane, and above all the most aged were confined.[34] Moreover, there was a distinct trend over time in these and other unions for the importance of "sickness" as a cause of admission and a status of inmates to grow. Just as Kevin Siena sees a "medicalization" of the eighteenth-century workhouse in St. Margaret's Westminster, so a similar medicalization of the New Poor Law might also be observed.

None of this means that medical standards were high, that medical officers were sufficient in number and sufficiently free from the influence of guardians, or that many cases of medical negligence cannot be found. Indeed, Graham Mooney has cast serious doubt on the value of diagnostic and treatment expertise in nineteenth-century London workhouses, something that melds seamlessly into observations by the editors of this volume (and by Samantha Shave) that in the first decades of the New Poor Law many of the workhouse medical staff had limited experience.[35] It is to say, however, that the institutional population of the later New Poor Law in particular was significantly more likely than at any previous time to be sick broadly defined and their poverty to be understood and treated as a soluble medical problem.

Yet if empirical studies have told us more about the workhouse population (and obliquely about the likely character of the sick population in the workhouse), several problems persist in understanding of the medical role of the workhouse. The first is that detailed information on what was actually wrong with workhouse inmates in terms of the range and intensity of diseases is surprisingly thin, even for richly documented places such as Birmingham, explored in this volume by Jonathan Reinarz and Alistair Ritch. Where admission and discharge books survive, they often tell us little about the nature of illnesses and accidents, something as true for the New Poor Law as the Old.[36] Knowing that a majority or significant minority of the institutional population were likely to be sick is one thing. Moving on from this point is complicated and often dependent on the broad surveys employed by Ottaway, chance survival of treatment books of the sort used by Negrine, or proxy records such as guardians' decisions on what sorts of wards to build and what sort of equipment to buy. Under the Old Poor Law, doctors' bills provide the only truly reliable way to juxtapose illness and treatment, and the opportunity for conducting a systematic study of the hundreds of surviving bills for places like Norfolk, Berkshire, Somerset, and Dorset is clear.

A second problem is one of jurisdiction. Kevin Siena argues in chapter 1 that Old Poor Law workhouses in London had an implicit obligation to take patients who could not access other forms of medical care. Like Boulton, Davenport, and Schwarz, he also argues that workhouses might have played the role of conduits, leveraging paupers into institutions, such as voluntary hospitals, where they could not themselves gain admission. Negrine makes the same observation for Leicester under the New Poor Law. Yet if we stray out of London, it is clear that Old and New Poor Law workhouses *might* refuse to take certain paupers, either absolutely or because alternative provision was to be had elsewhere. Even Old Poor Law parishes often had a separate fever house, specialist (home) nursing, and quarantine areas for smallpox and other contagious diseases. The same is true for venereal diseases. Under the New Poor Law, separate wards for such diseases were initially the order of the day, but, increasingly, building and rebuilding the medical fabric involved different sites and recording systems to those occupied by workhouse inmates. In other words, even where workhouse records exist in depth, it is not always clear which subset of the poor and sick poor population they encompass.

A slightly different, but nonetheless overlapping, problem is that the workhouse population tended to be self-selecting. Many thousands of aged paupers became sick or decrepit, but nonetheless resisted the workhouse and the admonitions of officials, who were never given the carceral powers of their German counterparts. The sick poor who ended up in the workhouses of both the Old and New Poor Law were thus a particular subset of all the sick poor, and hence it is difficult to understand what the medical treatment they received meant for them, how representative it was, and under what ideological conditions it was granted. Smith's contention in this volume that nineteenth-century workhouses constituted "holding centers" for the lunatic poor between community and asylum is certainly a caution on this front.

Finally, and one of the themes of the next section of this chapter, there is a danger of seeing the workhouse in isolation. As Bronwyn Croxson has suggested in the context of the Middlesex Hospital, the density and proximity of alternative provision for paupers (and for laboring people before they were driven to pauperism by sickness) could dictate who ended up in the workhouse, what they came with, how long they stayed, and what part workhouse medicine played in their healing. In other words, what really matters for understanding who the workhouse patients were, is the nature, constellation, and accessibility of the mixed economy of health care.[37] In this respect, overarching studies offering the interlinkage of the different elements of the medical market remain sadly lacking, notwithstanding the excellent discussion of the "place" of the St. Margaret's Westminster workhouse offered by Siena in this volume. It is to this theme and to the wider issue of the exact nature of medical care offered by the workhouse that the next section turns.

The Nature and Role of Workhouse Medical Care

Most historians of the Old Poor Law have come to see the scale, variety, and standard of medical relief (however widely or narrowly defined) offered to paupers as relatively good. Reinarz and Ritch make this point well in their chapter for this volume. Early surveys pointed to an increasing range of medical relief in the later eighteenth century and at the willingness of parishes to bear considerable expense in relieving sickness at individual level.[38] For eighteenth-century officials, the question of how to treat sickness represented a moral and practical conundrum rather than simply an economic decision.

Recent microstudies have added nuance and fleshed out the dynamics of particular types of medical care. Jeremy Boulton and Samantha Williams, for instance, have pointed to relatively high levels of nursing care offered in both urban and rural environments in the eighteenth century, while there is evidence that out-parish paupers came to *expect* nursing and midwifery services as part of their customary entitlement.[39] Other elements of medical care have also attracted attention. Whether the rising number of doctors' contracts observed by Williams and Alison Stringer for Bedfordshire and Northamptonshire respectively is an example of good or improving medical care is a moot point.[40] Nonetheless, it is clear that the eighteenth century witnessed a very significant extension of the practice of contracting regular medical care for paupers. The ability to see a doctor was forcefully inserted as a right and parish duty into the lives of the sick poor by the early nineteenth century, part of the wider medicalization of poverty traced by both Siena and Ottaway. In the majority of cases, the implementation of doctors' contracts resulted in a higher overall proportion of resources devoted to medical relief than before.[41]

Of course, the most valuable forms of "medical relief" were the clothing, food, and fuel supplements (as well as the extra cash allowances) associated with being sick. Indeed, there is persuasive evidence that this form of relief in kind for the sick poor increased during the eighteenth century at the same time as provision in kind for other types of paupers all but dried up from the 1790s onward.[42] More widely, the study of pauper narratives clearly indicates that paupers expected sickness and entitlement to be intertwined and that they were sensitive and inventive in their construction and deployment of the rhetoric of sickness to achieve this end.[43] These observations are not to assert that medical care was good; plenty of vestry minutes confirm that the outdoor poor could be badly and even scandalously treated. Nor do they sit at odds with Lynn Hollen Lees's observation that medical relief may have been put under particular pressure as the humanitarian impulse of the late eighteenth century waned under the pressure of the dissolution of interlocking obligations in the early nineteenth century.[44] There is, however, accumulating evidence that sickness was relatively well treated by the eighteenth- and early nineteenth-century parish.

Where the Old Poor Law workhouse fits into this equation is problematic. Boulton, Davenport, and Schwarz have limited evidence of actual medical practice at St. Martin's workhouse, but their proxies—analyzing changes to the workhouse fabric, expenditure trends on external medical solutions, and the number of medical personnel, their salaries, and their rules of engagement—provide an important methodological step forward and suggest a considerable role for the workhouse in health issues in early eighteenth-century London. Focusing on the early nineteenth century, Lynn MacKay argues that almost a third of female admissions to the St. Martin's workhouse in 1817–18 were sick and that the majority of specific workhouse wards listed in the 1817 census of the institution were health related.[45] For another London workhouse, St. Marylebone's, Alysa Levene suggests that a medical function was central and that officials were "progressively-minded . . . especially in the field of medical care."[46] None of this is perhaps surprising if we accept Siena's view that workhouses and hospitals increasingly came to cater to mutually exclusive patient groups. Of course, the representative workhouse under the Old Poor Law was very much smaller than in St. Martin's or St. Marylebone, boasting little by way of dedicated accommodation for the sick and covered (if at all) by staff such as doctors and nurses who were employed mainly to look to the needs of the outdoor poor. About these institutions and their medical care little is known.

This does not mean that the study of the medical dimensions of the Old Poor Law workhouse cannot be taken rather further, as many of the contributions to this volume suggest. Siena's contention that workhouses came to provide basic medical care for the unworldly or the unworthy is particularly compelling. More widely, a survey of workhouses in Northamptonshire suggests that, where parishes had a workhouse, the mean expenditure on drug treatments was some 50 percent higher than parishes that did not, and that the range and depth of medical care deteriorated strongly (and medical or other scandals were more likely to arise) when workhouses were either transferred to or founded by farmers of the poor.[47] Indeed, while it matters where the workhouse was, how it was constituted in terms of buildings, how it was covered by doctors and who was in it, what mattered most for its medical role was who ran it. Overall, however, much of the historiography points to a sense in which the dependent poor under the Old Poor Law obtained a better standard of health care than their independent laboring counterparts.

For most commentators, nothing this positive can be said about the New Poor Law. As Alannah Tomkins (reflecting earlier opinions) reminds us, under the New Poor Law, at least in its initial manifestations, the poor came to "regard medical relief [in the workhouse] at best as undesirable and at worst as repellent."[48] Kim Price's study of the way that medical officers were systematically and periodically undermined by guardians, many of whom felt that they should take the lead in defining sickness as well as shaping its treatment, gives weight to the idea of declining standards in New Poor Law workhouses.[49] That real or invented medical scandals were common is not to be doubted, as Shave argued earlier in this volume. Nor can it be doubted that conditions in general in the immediate post-1834 workhouses tended to be poor.[50] Seeing the positive side of the New Poor Law in medical terms is, however, hampered by both the lack of microstudies and the inability to provide a broad statistical overview, given that most early records make no distinction between the sick and other paupers. Nonetheless, there *were* medically progressive unions, such as Oundle and Brackley in Northamptonshire. In these locations, the survival of interlinking correspondence registers, minutes, and early admissions and discharge books allows us to see an effective medical system—combining relatively high quality clothing, basic but decent food, infirmary wards, and some of the earliest nonpauper nurses in the entire history of the New Poor Law— in microcosm.[51] Such observations link well with the suggestion by Tomkins in this volume that some workhouse inmates actively appreciated the quality of the institutional care they received.

If there is agreement that the early decades of the New Poor Law witnessed (and caused) a decline in the scale and standard of medical care, there is rather less consensus on how and when this situation was put into reverse. Nonetheless, there *was* change. Whether in reaction to workhouse visiting committees, women guardians, commissions of inquiry after scandals, newspaper reporting, or the changing composition of boards of guardians, the ebb and flow of building the fabric of the New Poor Law came to concentrate disproportionately on medical aspects such as infirmary and fever wards. Reinarz and Ritch trace this process very effectively in their chapter. The framework within which workhouse medicine was executed also changed; Kim Price has traced the battle for the professionalization of poor law medical officers and the assertion of medical authority over political authority in poor law unions, identifying the 1870s as a key decade of change.[52] More widely, as Reinarz and Schwarz argue in their introduction, the New Poor Law came to be inscribed into a more general narrative of professionalization. Workhouse infirmaries also became spaces where medical education and the needs of the poor intersected or competed; many London and Oxbridge students learned their trade on the bodies of the poor, so the workhouse became both a diagnostic and training space.[53] Certainly, medical and health issues took up a lot of the time of workhouse staff.[54] This is unsurprising in the sense that changes to the physical infrastructure of workhouses allowed for the creation of new assessment wards to stand alongside treatment and recuperation wards. And, of course, we know from the work of Carol Helmstadter and Stuart Wildman that there was a progressive (if not linear, or, in its early stages, robust) increase in the number, training, and professionalization of nursing staff in the workhouse.[55]

By the 1890s the scale, depth, and range of medical care in the workhouse might be regarded more optimistically than in the immediate aftermath of 1834. As workhouses came to do less (particularly as certain groups were removed from its ambit) and became more susceptible to statisticalization and comparison, their medical dynamics became more complex. The results were not always positive or sustained. Yet the average floor space devoted to medicine in workhouses increased almost continuously after 1865. Moreover, the range of equipment to be found in workhouse infirmaries was superior to some hospitals, and some of the facilities (particularly sanatoria) available to the dependent poor were rather more advanced than those available to the laboring poor in the same areas. The range of diseases with which workhouses engaged increased after 1880 in particular.[56] As Negrine has shown with her discussion of early skin grafts, medical innovation could also develop within such facilities. Keir Waddington's model of change in the intent, fabric, and scope of the New Poor Law ties medical progress not to the will of the guardians, democratization (though this was important), or central inspection and information, but to the diversification of income flows.[57] Such a model resonates strongly with my own work on Bolton, but, whatever its cause, there is a distinct development of the professional, material, and ideological space of the New Poor Law infirmary in particular during the later nineteenth century.

These observations provide, however, only one-half of the equation in understanding what workhouse medical care was and locating its role. Equally important, as Siena observes in his chapter, is the issue of the wider mixed economy of health care within which such provision sat. While microstudies of New Poor Law unions are, at least in the published domain, notable by their absence, the historiography of alternative, supplementary, and competing elements of the medical market for poor people has grown increasingly dense. Work on infirmaries and dispensaries and their medical, social, ideological, and political significance has proved particularly fruitful.[58] To this literature, we might add a burgeoning historiography on quacks, friendly societies, worker subscription charities, lying-in and other medical charities, specialist institutions (such as lock and eye hospitals or blind institutions), medical self-help and self-dosing, and the individual charitable work of doctors themselves.[59]

Even though spatial and chronological coverage of many of these areas remains patchy, it is possible to discern, certainly from the later eighteenth century, an increasingly dense and interlinked medical market for the poor. By way of example, Walter Brett, the registrar of the Bath Hospital, wrote to the Wiltshire parish of Cricklade on November 9, 1837, to say that

> Ann Noad was discharged the waters not being proper for her case, and the Medical Gentlemen requested that a covered cart with a Bed in it might be sent to remove her. Not having heard from the Overseer, I am again directed to urge the immediate compliance with their former directions. We have now 17 females minuted for admission, and we have not a bed empty to receive one of them. Under the circumstances they hope no further delay will take place.[60]

This letter provides both evidence in relation to Noad herself (showing, for instance, that Cricklade were willing to pay for an expensive sojourn in Bath) and the wider medical market: seventeen other paupers were on the waiting list, suggesting that parishes resorted widely to this treatment. Anne Borsay's work on the Bath hospital confirms its position as a major provider for the poor of a very wide hinterland.[61] In this context, easy and traditional distinctions, such as those between urban and rural areas, can be shown as wanting. Some urban areas had a denuded medical economy of makeshifts, while many rural communities could boast access to a range of medical services for the poor way beyond that which would be justified on a strictly per capita basis. As Negrine shows in chapter 9, what mattered for the place of the poor in the medical market was often the strength or absence of particular driving characters rather than simplistic typologies of community types and locations.

Such historiographical advances notwithstanding, three basic problems remain in any attempt to understand this mixed economy. The first is our inability to discern the relative balance of power, influence, and impact among the various elements at different times and in different places. Siena suggests that, for London, the workhouse came to play a decisive role in treating diseases—such as syphilis—which closed off other areas of the mixed economy of health care. Outside London, however, the evidence is less compelling. In Northamptonshire, for instance, the poor law in general and the workhouse in particular came to play a much smaller role in the medical market tapped by the poor by the early and mid-nineteenth century than had been the case before.[62] A second problem is the issue of the agency of poor people in moving between the different elements of the mixed economy of health care. In essence, how many people were, like Ann Noad, clearly directed through different aspects of the medical market by the overseer? Alternatively, how many were like Edward Wilkes, who wrote from his sick bed in the Bristol Infirmary ("No. 2 Mens Ward") on February 2, 1811, to ask if the parish would have

> the Goodness to assist me by the way of Letting me have a few Garment shuch as a shurt & stockings and shoes & Jackett as I ham know in Bristol Infirmary Layup with two Bad leags and have be so for several Months and having no frend I ham under the nesity of trubling you the Gentlemen of the falcuty Desired that I should send to you as I have nothing scarse to hide my Nackedness If the Infirmary Releaves the Poor with medicall and shurgery assistance they will not find Close on less I have the above mention articuls I shall be dismissed from the house to my Parish to the upper Parish Cricklade with a Pass and there for to reseive surgical and other assistance fit for a poor object in my distress.[63]

Wilkes had got himself signed into the hospital, presumably after getting a note from a subscriber; he was in charge of the medical process. This fits keenly with a literature suggesting that, in the closing decades of the Old Poor Law, the sick poor could and did exercise considerable agency over the nature and location of their treatment.[64] What is much less clear is how much agency we see before 1800 and after 1834, and there has been little recent work on the latter period in particular to illuminate this issue outside the chapter by Tomkins in this volume. The final problem is consequent on this observation. That is, one of the key challenges for welfare and medical historians is to locate the treatments offered by the parish in general and the workhouse in particular into the health and relief life cycles of the poor themselves.

The Workhouse and Life Cycles of Ill Health and Medical Care

Understanding where workhouse medical care fitted into a life cycle is contingent, for both the Old and New Poor Laws, on understanding the dynamics of several intertwining issues: the way in which workhouse care related to medical relief offered to the same person outside the workhouse; the relationship between medical care (institutional and otherwise) for the individual and that for the wider family; the mechanism by which medical care and medical relief was rationed; the fate of those turned away; the relationship between workhouse care and background medical standards; and pauper understanding of entitlement to medical relief. Did the workhouse, for instance, deal disproportionately with those in the last extremis of sickness and old age, as Boulton, Davenport, and Schwarz imply in their chapter, or did workhouse care rumble into life for a much wider range of illnesses, acting perhaps as a focus for what we now know as respite care? For the insane, were workhouses an integral part of the mixed economy of care as Smith suggests, or simply a money-saving receptacle? And did workhouses provide long-term care for key groups like the aged, or was tenure in the workhouse brief and of last resort? There has been important progress on fitting the pieces of this jigsaw together. Claudia Edwards and Susannah Ottaway have talked directly and indirectly about age-based rationing of health care in the eighteenth and nineteenth centuries.[65] Historians working on pauper letters have also begun to provide a fractured picture of life-cycle dimensions of health and medical relief. For the Old Poor Law, the work of Boulton and Schwarz in creating pauper biographies promises much in this direction too. The study of scandals and medical neglect cases can provide us with ideal, typical life-cycle examples, while crime records and the narratives of those admitted to refuges, of the sort used by Peter King, also offer a window onto pauper life cycles.[66]

These studies notwithstanding, remarkably little is known specifically about the life cycles and treatment histories of the sick poor. Some things can be inferred from the structure of workhouse populations. It *is* likely, for instance, that the workhouse was the locus for a disproportionate amount of end-of-life care for the aged, something that is also borne out in frequent pleas by union clerks to parish officers for them to take back their dead for burial, given pressure on workhouse burial grounds. Equally likely is that workhouse medical care under both Old and New Poor Laws figured disproportionately in the life cycles of those with the least kin and of children, as Siena suggests in his chapter.[67] Nonetheless, studies of pauper narratives in the eighteenth and nineteenth centuries have begun to show that the poor had ingrained expectations of access to medical relief and care in their own homes and that they accessed, as we have seen, diverse aspects of the mixed economy of health care. It is likely, in other words, that workhouse medicine played a very limited part in most of the life cycle of the dependent poor, except perhaps in London.

Going further than these broad suppositions involves bringing together sources and methodologies from medical and welfare history, geography, and historical demography. Thus, little work has been done on the excellent patient and doctor-case files now available for some later nineteenth-century hospitals and workhouses, despite the fact that, as Lynsey Cullen is beginning to demonstrate, the extraordinary archives of some of the London hospitals provide the entire health and relief histories of patients and their families.[68] More widely, the sorts of interlinkage between family reconstitutions and poor law records conducted by Richard Smith need to be systematically developed.[69] And it is certainly possible to navigate the parish archives to reconstruct for particularly problematic sick families the threads of the mixed economy of health care; to create, in other words, medical biographies or (as Siena styles them) the "backstories." In this context, the nineteenth century remains a strangely neglected period, as illustrated by the almost complete failure to follow up record-linkage models offered by Jean Robin, Pamela Sharpe, Barry Reay, and Di Cooper and Moira Donald.[70] It is certainly difficult to untangle the experiences of "ordinary" poverty and that of medical care and relief from the details available in many nineteenth-century union records. Nonetheless, careful analysis of strategically selected unions, a duplication in other words of the Boulton and Schwarz strategy for seventeenth- and eighteenth-century London or that of Virginia Crossman for Ireland, can potentially tell us much about medical relief and the place of workhouse medicine in the mixed economy of health care in the period post-1834.

The Mad, the Disabled, and the Very Bad

One other way forward is to develop the productive work currently being accomplished on particular groups of "patients," among whom the insane and the venereal stand at the forefront and are explored in this volume by Smith and Siena.[71] To them, we might add the blind and the deaf, along with those disabled by loss of limbs or limb function, especially in wartime.[72] The aged and decrepit poor, drawn low by what they often called the "trials of their age," have also found a voice in the rush to explore pauper narratives.[73] For these elements of the sick poor, four broad overarching observations might be made. First, it is clear that the vast majority of these particular patient groups were offered and desired care through a combination (increasingly a formalized combination) of community, kin, and outdoor relief. This was as true for the New Poor Law as the Old, and Elizabeth Hurren's analysis of the agency of the poor in the face of the attempted withdrawal of traditional forms of medical relief in the later nineteenth century provides strong support to this broad generalization.[74] In other words, what is surprising is not how

much institutional care there was, but how little. Cathy Smith's percep-
tive analysis of the inmates of the Northampton General Lunatic Asylum,
resonating with earlier work on Devon, shows that even for arguably the
most problematic group of patients, the insane, most care most of the
time was offered outside institutions.[75]
  Second, there has been a new focus on the agency of the individual and
their families, communities, and sponsors. Much of the historiographical work, however, has concentrated on the outdoor and out-parish poor.
While Negrine in her chapter refers to the assertion of agency by dispu-
tation for institutional inmates, the question of how far the sick and disabled who did find themselves in a workhouse can be said to have had
agency remains one of the core lacunae in the literature. Only more work
on medical negligence cases, workhouse riots, workhouse visiting, and (for
the New Poor Law) the letters between unions and the central authorities
will reveal more on this issue.
  A third observation is that, judged holistically, a concentration on the
experiences of particular patient groups has generated a largely positive
assessment of the medical relief offered to them, something explored in this
volume by Tomkins. There were, of course, rogue parishes and unions, and
arguably we need to know much more about the sorts of scandals reviewed
by Shave and Reinarz and Ritch as a way of establishing expectation bench-
marks. Nonetheless, Old Poor Law historians have come to accept Joan
Lane's conclusion (itself a development of work by Dorothy George and
Geoffrey Oxley) that pre-1834 officials were willing to go to very considerable lengths to contain, cure, or ameliorate the sickness episodes of particular groups, such as the insane or the venereal.[76] Thus, when John Mitchel,
vicar of Isleworth, wrote to the Oxfordshire parish of Rotherfield Greys
on the subject of Anthony Harris, he pointed to the fact that he "became
deranged in his Intellect some months ago, & it is now no longer safe to
himself & others that he should be permitted to roam at large." Citing a tendency for Harris to wander off, the vicar suggested,

> It will be necessary to place him somewhere in confinement—Indeed it ought
> to have been done long ago—I will undertake through the Medium of some
> Friends to procure his admission into St. Luke's Hospital, provided you are
> disposed to indemnify me for the Expence—There must be a Deposit of Six
> Pounds in the Hands of the Treasurer on his Admission, & 2 Housekeepers
> must enter into a Bond of 100£ to remove him from the Hospital at the
> Expiration of the 12 Months, provided he should be deemed incurable.[77]

Thus began a sojourn in the asylum that was to last until the early 1830s and
cost the small parish of Rotherfield Greys many hundreds of pounds.
  The particular place of care in the workhouse in the generalization
that the Old Poor Law responded positively to the health needs of certain

subgroups of the poor is difficult to fathom, not least because of the poor record survival for many early workhouses. Yet for places that do have a full set of bills submitted to overseers (for example in Mortlake, Surrey), it is clear that the sickest of the sick poor were treated as generously as their outdoor counterparts.[78] To carry this analysis forward to the New Poor Law is rather more problematic, given our lack of understanding of the day-to-day execution of medical relief in union workhouses. However, and as Negrine argues, sick paupers and medical officers came to know what good treatment was and to expect it.[79] Indeed, my own work on Bolton Union suggests that a considerable amount was spent on utilizing the latest technology, on securing temporary specialist treatment for the poor, and on finding out and implementing best medical practice from elsewhere.[80]

Finally, notwithstanding these advances, and for both the Old Poor Law and the New, several weaknesses in the secondary literature remain. One of them centers on the treatment of sick children. The general surveys of Hugh Cunningham, Harry Hendrick, and Frank Crompton have not, particularly for the eighteenth century, told us much about sick children and whether they were treated different from adults or indeed at all.[81] This observation applies particularly to rural areas and the provinces, where a study of the bills submitted for doctoring the poor point to remarkably few children being treated. Another weakness is that our perspectives on the treatment, agency, and institutionalization of groups such as the blind and deaf are disproportionately informed by studies of large urban areas. The experience of these groups in many old provincial towns, the urban areas of the new manufacturing districts, East Anglia, the North, the northern midlands, the rural west, and much of Wales awaits a reconstruction, even though the records in some of these areas are excellent. To these weaknesses we might add the fact that the resurgence of interest in the narratives of poverty written by paupers themselves has largely left institutional populations and the mid- and later nineteenth century behind. The latter observation is surprising in the sense that Elizabeth Hurren's work on the dwarf Margaret Price, writing to the central poor law authorities, suggests the presence of a large number of very revealing narratives.[82] Moreover, even for the most studied of the sick poor, the insane pauper, our grasp of where institutional provision fitted into a life cycle of health needs; what factors influenced families and parishes to seek, maintain, and end institutional care; and what forms of care families themselves offered to the insane remains relatively fragile. In short, there is a pressing need to disaggregate the broad category of the "sick poor" and to carry out detailed, systematic, large-scale, and comparative analysis of the health-care experiences and life cycles of sickness of different subgroups, such as the aged, children, victims of epidemic disease, and so on. Only in this way will it be possible to reconstruct the nature of workhouse medicine, to locate its role in the mixed economy of health care, and to reconstruct official and pauper attitudes toward institutional care.

An Agenda for the Future

Notwithstanding important work on doctor contracts, workhouse scandals, poor law medical officers, and the (particularly nineteenth-century) composition of workhouse populations, our understanding of the character, scale, and scope of workhouse medical care remains surprisingly thin. Equally, how such medical care was cemented in to the local mixed economy of health care and into the life cycles of ill health and medical treatment experienced by the sick poor remains very much a closed book. To some extent, these lacunae in the existing literature reflect genuine problems of definition and source coverage and scale. Sometimes, they reflect an ingrained belief that the sick poor, institutionalized or not, are unworthy of study in their own right. Yet, as this afterword has attempted to show and other chapters in the volume elaborately demonstrate, detailed microstudies can reveal much that carries the debate forward. They also suggest a spectrum of key questions or areas of research for the future, over and above the general need for more microstudies, across the entire New Poor Law period to 1929. Among them, five issues spring directly from the chapters brought together in this volume. First, was the workhouse under the Old and New Poor Laws a central component of the mixed economy of health care, acting, as Siena and Boulton, Davenport, and Schwarz argue, both as a locus for health care and a conduit for paupers to other medical destinations? Did its role vary at times of crisis—during epidemics for example—and according to life-cycle stage? Related to this broad issue, a second avenue for future research is the regionality of the health-care role of the workhouse and the "medicalization" process traced by several contributors to this volume. While the question of rural-urban differences is an obvious one, given the essentially urban focus of the chapters, it is the potentially differing role of the workhouse in the medical lives of the dependent poor between south and north or east and west that provides the most intriguing research agenda.

A third issue centers around the key influences on the nature and quality of health care offered in the workhouse at different dates. Was the nature and scope of health care simply and directly related to the scale and source of income at parish and union level? How were centralized initiatives, such as 1842 General Medical Order, appropriated at the local level? Did long-established staff lead to better medical care and higher expenditure, as Negrine suggests in her chapter? What role did medical journals, professional organizations, and scandal-related inquiries play in setting baseline medical standards? And, as Crossman suggests, did increased spending on medical relief, especially facilities, simply lead to more sick paupers? A related and fourth issue is the susceptibility of workhouse medicine to pressure from above—particularly the politicization of the welfare system traced by Crossman in her chapter and Elizabeth Hurren elsewhere—and to pauper agency from below. The considerable volumes of official and pauper correspondence extant for both the Old and New Poor Law may provide an important signpost in this respect. Finally, there is a sense in which we simply need to know more about the sickness and medical welfare experiences of paupers across the life cycle. Success in this area in part reflects the chance survival of records such as the treatment books used by Negrine, but there remains a considerable body of sources—patient case records for voluntary hospitals, for instance—that can facilitate a much more detailed appreciation of the role of the workhouse in the sentiments, practices, and expectations of the dependent poor.

Notes

1. Margaret Anne Crowther, *The Workhouse System, 1834–1929: The History of an English Social Institution* (London: Batsford, 1981); Ruth G. Hodgkinson, *The Origins of the National Health Service: The Medical Services of the New Poor Law, 1834–1871* (London: Wellcome Trust Historical Medical Library, 1967); Michael W. Flinn, "Medical Services under the New Poor Law," in *The New Poor Law in the Nineteenth Century*, ed. Derek Fraser (London: Macmillan, 1976), 45–66; Joan Lane, *A Social History of Medicine: Health, Healing and Disease in England, 1750–1950* (London: Routledge, 2001); Geoffrey Oxley, *Poor Relief in England and Wales, 1601–1834* (Newton Abbott: David and Charles, 1974).

2. Exemplified most clearly in the survey by Margaret Anne Crowther, "Health Care and Poor Relief in Provincial England," in *Health Care and Poor Relief in 18th and 19th Century Northern Europe*, ed. Ole P. Grell, Andrew Cunningham, and Robert Jütte (Aldershot, UK: Ashgate, 2002), 203–19. For contributions about the centrality of sickness, see to Andreas Gestrich, Elizabeth Hurren, and Steven King, eds., *Poverty and Sickness in Modern Europe: Narratives of the Sick Poor* (London: Continuum, 2012).

3. See Steven King, "'Stop This Overwhelming Torment of Destiny': Negotiating Financial Aid at Times of Sickness under the English Old Poor Law, 1800–1840," *Bulletin of the History of Medicine* 79, no. 2 (2005): 228–60; Peter Bartlett, "The Asylum, the Workhouse and the Voice of the Insane Poor in 19th-Century England," *International Journal of Law and Psychiatry* 21 (1998): 421–32.

4. See, for instance, Kevin Siena, *Venereal Disease, Hospitals and the Urban Poor: London's "Foul Wards," 1600–1800* (Rochester: University of Rochester Press, 2004).

5. Jeremy Boulton, "Welfare Systems and the Parish Nurse in Early Modern London, 1650–1725," *Family and Community History* 10 (2007): 127–51; David Green, "Medical Relief and the New Poor Law in London," in Grell, Cunningham, and Jütte, *Health Care and Poor Relief*, 220–45; Elaine Murphy, "The New Poor Law Guardians and the Administration of Insanity in East-London, 1834–1844," *Bulletin of the History*

of Medicine 77 (2003): 45–74; Murphy, "Workhouse Care of the Insane, 1845–1890," in *Mental Illness and Learning Disability since 1850*, ed. Pamela Dale and Joseph Melling (London: Routledge, 2006), 24–45.

6. Though see Mary Fissell, *Patients, Power and the Poor in Eighteenth-Century Bristol* (Cambridge: Cambridge University Press, 1991); and Tim Hitchcock, "The English Workhouse: A Study in Institutional Poor Relief in Selected Counties, 1696–1750" (DPhil diss., Oxford University, 1985); Tim Hitchcock, "Paupers and Preachers: The SPCK and the Parochial Workhouse Movement," in *Stilling the Grumbling Hive: The Response to Social and Economic Problems in England, 1689–1750*, ed. Lee Davison et al. (Stroud: Sutton, 1992), 145–66.

7. *Abstract of Answers and Returns under the Act for Procuring Returns Relative to Expense and Maintenance of the Poor in England*, Parliamentary Papers, 1803–4 (13), 378; Richard Smith, "Ageing and Well-Being in Early Modern England: Pension Trends and Gender Preferences under the English Old Poor Law, c. 1650–1800," in *Old Age from Antiquity to Post-Modernity*, ed. Paul Johnson and Pat Thane (London: Routledge, 1998), 64–95, on 73–77.

8. David R. Green, *Pauper Capital: London and the Poor Law, 1790–1870* (Farnham, UK: Ashgate, 2010).

9. Felix Driver, *Power and Pauperism: The Workhouse System, 1834–1884* (Cambridge: Cambridge University Press, 1993); Kim P. Price, "A Regional, Quantitative and Qualitative Study of the Employment, Disciplining and Discharging of Workhouse Medical Officers of the New Poor Law throughout Nineteenth-Century England and Wales" (PhD diss., Oxford Brookes University, 2008).

10. Elizabeth T. Hurren, *Protesting about Pauperism: Poverty, Politics and Poor Relief in Late-Victorian England, 1870–1900* (Woodbridge: Boydell, 2007); Hurren, *Dying for Victorian Medicine: English Anatomy and Its Trade in the Dead Poor, c. 1834–1929* (Basingstoke, UK: Palgrave Macmillan, 2012).

11. Angela Negrine, "Medicine and Poverty: A Study of the Poor Law Medical Services of the Leicester Union, 1867–1914" (PhD diss., University of Leicester, 2008); Graham Mooney, "Diagnostic Spaces: Workhouse, Hospital and Home in Mid-Victorian London," *Social Science History* 33 (2009): 357–90.

12. Keir Waddington, "Paying for the Sick Poor: Financing Medicine under the Victorian Poor Law; The Case of Whitechapel Union, 1850–1900," in *Financing Medicine: The British Experience since 1750*, ed. Martin Gorsky and Sally Sheard (Aldershot, UK: Ashgate, 2006), 95–111.

13. Leonard Smith, *Lunatic Hospitals in Georgian England, 1750–1830* (London: Routledge, 2007); Akihito Suzuki, "The Household and the Care of Lunatics in Eighteenth Century London," in *The Locus of Care: Families, Communities Institutions and the Provision of Welfare since Antiquity*, ed. Peregrine Horden and Richard Smith (London: Routledge, 1998), 153–75; Bill Forsythe, Joseph Melling, and Richard Adair, "The New Poor Law and the County Pauper Lunatic Asylum: The Devon Experience, 1834–1884," *Social History of Medicine* 9, no. 3 (1996): 335–55; Cathy Smith, "Family, Community and the Victorian Asylum: A Case Study of the Northampton General Lunatic Asylum and Its Pauper Lunatics," *Family and Community History* 9 (2006): 109–24.

14. Bartlett, "Asylum," 423–24.

15. Alice Clark, "Wild Workhouse Girls and the Liberal Imperial State in Mid-Nineteenth Century Ireland," *Journal of Social History* 37 (2005): 389–409; Virginia Crossman, "The New Ross Workhouse Riot of 1877: Nationalism, Class and the Irish Poor Laws," *Past and Present* 179 (2003): 135–58.

16. As a small selection of relevant material, see Keir Waddington, *Charity and the London Hospitals, 1850–98* (Woodbridge: Boydell, 2000); Steven Cherry, "The Hospitals and Population Growth: The Voluntary General Hospitals, Mortality and Local Populations in the English Provinces in the Eighteenth and Nineteenth Centuries," pts. 1 and 2, *Population Studies* 34, nos. 1–2 (1980): 59–75 and 251–65; Irvine Loudon, *Medical Care and the General Practitioner, 1750–1850* (Oxford: Clarendon, 1986); John V. Pickstone, *Medicine and Industrial Society: A History of Hospital Development in Manchester and Its Region, 1752–1946* (Manchester: Manchester University Press, 1985); Irvine Loudon, "The Origins and Growth of the Dispensary Movement in England," *Bulletin of the History of Medicine* 16 (1981): 322–42. See also the particularly important Jonathan Reinarz, "Mechanizing Medicine: Medical Innovations and the Birmingham Voluntary Hospitals in the Nineteenth Century," in *Devices and Designs: Medical Technologies in Historical Perspective*, ed. Julie Anderson and Carsten Timmermann (Basingstoke, UK: Palgrave Macmillan, 2006), 37–60.

17. In addition to note 16, see Joseph Melling and Bill Forsythe, *The Politics of Madness: The State, Insanity and Society in England, 1845–1914* (London: Routledge, 2006); Steven Cherry, *Mental Health Care in Modern England: The Norfolk Lunatic Asylum/St. Andrew's Hospital, c. 1810–1998* (Woodbridge: Boydell, 2003); Andrew Scull, *The Most Solitary of Afflictions: Madness and Society in Britain, 1700–1900* (New Haven: Yale University Press, 1993).

18. See Alannah Tomkins, "'The Excellent Example of the Working Class': Medical Welfare, Contributory Funding and the North Staffordshire Infirmary from 1815," *Social History of Medicine* 21 (2008): 13–30, for a review of attempts to limit hospital access for the laboring classes even in an institution where they had an effective right to treatment by virtue of contribution.

19. Sylvia Pinches, "Women as Objects and Agents of Charity in Eighteenth-Century Birmingham," in *Women and Urban Life in Eighteenth-Century England: On the Town*, ed. Roey Sweet and Penelope Lane (Aldershot, UK: Ashgate, 2003), 65–86.

20. Though, see Samantha Williams, "Practitioners' Income and Provision for the Poor: Parish Doctors in the Late Eighteenth and Early Nineteenth Centuries," *Social History of Medicine* 18 (2005): 1–28.

21. Fissell, *Patients*, 98.

22. Gavin Lucas, "The Archaeology of the Workhouse: The Changing Uses of Workhouse Buildings at St. Mary's, Southampton," in *The Familiar Past? Archaeologies of Later Historical Britain*, ed. Sarah Tarlow and Susie West (London: Routledge, 1999), 125–39; Kathryn Morrison, *The Workhouse: A Study of Poor Law Buildings in England* (Swindon: English Heritage, 1999); Christine Jackson, "Functionality, Commemoration and Civic Competition: A Study of Early Seventeenth-Century Workhouse Design in Reading and Newbury," *Architectural History* 47 (2004): 77–112.

23. Sarah Peyton, ed., *Kettering Vestry Minutes, 1797–1853* (Northampton: Northamptonshire Record Society, 1933).

24. Northamptonshire Record Office, 356P/7, Welton Vestry Minutes.

25. Ibid.

26. Eric Midwinter, *Victorian Social Reform* (London: Longman, 1968), 23–55.

27. See Green, *Pauper Capital.*

28. Steven King, *Women, Welfare and Local Politics, 1880–1920: "We Might Be Trusted"* (Brighton: Sussex Academic Press, 2005), 46–51.

29. Samantha Shave, "The Dependent Poor? (Re)constructing Individuals' Lives 'on the Parish' in Rural Dorset, 1800–1832," *Rural History* 20 (2009): 67–98; Peyton, *Kettering Vestry Minutes*; Alan Neate, *The St. Marylebone Workhouse and Institution, 1730–1965* (London: London Record Society, 2003).

30. Susannah Ottaway, *The Decline of Life: Old Age in Eighteenth-Century England* (Cambridge: Cambridge University Press, 2004), 250–51.

31. Hitchcock, "English Workhouse," 194–202; Eric Thomas, "The Old Poor Law and Medicine," *Medical History* 24 (1980): 10; Ethel Mary Hampson, *The Treatment of Poverty in Cambridgeshire, 1597–1834* (Cambridge: Cambridge University Press, 1934), 77–84; Robert Hastings, *Poverty and the Poor Laws in the North Riding of Yorkshire* (York: Borthwick Institute, 1982).

32. Leicestershire Record Office, DE 2559 37–69, DE 1463/6, Parish Accounts.

33. Summarized in S. King, *Welfare and Local Politics,* 29–55.

34. Nigel Goose, "Workhouse Populations in the Mid-Nineteenth Century: The Case of Hertfordshire," *Local Population Studies* 62 (1999): 52–69; Goose, "Poverty, Old Age and Gender in Nineteenth-Century England: The Case of Hertfordshire," *Continuity and Change* 20 (2005): 351–84; Andrew Hinde and Fiona Turnbull, "The Population of Two Hampshire Workhouses, 1851–1861," *Local Population Studies* 61 (1998): 38–53; Rosemary Hall, "The Vanishing Unemployed, Hidden Disabled, and Embezzling Master: Researching Coventry Workhouse Registers," *Local Historian* 38 (2008): 111–21; Jean Robin, "The Relief of Poverty in Mid-Nineteenth-Century Colyton," *Rural History* 1 (1990): 193–218.

35. Mooney, "Diagnostic Spaces," 361–64.

36. David Jackson, "The Medway Union Workhouse, 1876–1881: A Study Based on the Admission and Discharge Registers and the Census Enumerators Books," *Local Population Studies* 75 (2005): 11–32.

37. Bronwyn Croxson, "The Price of Charity to the Middlesex Hospital, 1750–1830," in Gorsky and Sheard, *Financing Medicine,* 23–39.

38. Lane, *Social History*; Hilary Marland, *Medicine and Society in Wakefield and Huddersfield: 1780–1870* (Cambridge: Cambridge University Press, 1987).

39. Boulton, "Welfare Systems"; Samantha Williams, "Caring for the Sick Poor: Poor Law Nurses in Bedfordshire, c. 1770–1834," in *Women, Work and Wages in England, 1600–1850,* ed. Penelope Lane, Neil Raven, and Keith Snell (Woodbridge: Boydell, 2004), 141–69.

40. Alison Stringer, "Depth and Diversity in Parochial Healthcare: Northamptonshire, 1750–1830," *Family and Community History* 9 (2006): 43–54; Tomkins, "Excellent Example," 13–14, has argued that the implementation of doctoring contracts constrained pauper choice.

41. Steven King, *Poverty, Sickness and Death in England, 1750–1850* (London: Continuum, forthcoming).

42. Ibid., 76–83.

43. Steven King, "Regional Patterns in the Experiences and Treatment of the Sick Poor, 1800–40: Rights, Obligations and Duties in the Rhetoric of Paupers," *Family and Community History* 10 (2007): 61–75.

44. Lynn Hollen Lees, *The Solidarities of Strangers: The English Poor Laws and the People 1700–1949* (Cambridge: Cambridge University Press, 1998), 36.

45. Lynn MacKay, "A Culture of Poverty? The St. Martin's in the Fields Workhouse, 1817," *Journal of Interdisciplinary History* 26, no. 2 (1995): 221.

46. Alysa Levene, "Children, Childhood and the Workhouse: St. Marylebone, 1769–1781," *London Journal* 33 (2008): 43.

47. S. King, *Poverty, Sickness and Death*, 93–103.

48. Tomkins, "Excellent Example," 14.

49. Price, "Quantitative and Qualitative Study."

50. John Washington, "Poverty, Health and Social Welfare: The History of the Halifax Union Workhouse and the St. John's Hospital, 1834–1972," *Transactions of the Halifax Antiquarian Society* 5 (1997): 83–87.

51. S. King, *Poverty, Sickness and Death*, 263–71.

52. Price, "Quantitative and Qualitative Study."

53. Hurren, *Dying for Victorian Medicine.*

54. David Cox, "The Diary of Edward Lawrence, Master of Wellington Workhouse, 1890–1," in *Shropshire Historical Documents: A Miscellany*, ed. Sylvia Watts (Keele: Keele Centre for Local History, 2000), 149–201.

55. Carol Helmstadter, "The Passing of the Night Watch: Night Nursing Reform in the London Teaching Hospitals, 1856–90," *Canadian Bulletin of Medical History* 11 (1994): 23–69; Helmstadter, "Early Nursing Reform in Nineteenth-Century London: A Doctor-Driven Phenomenon," *Medical History* 46 (2002): 325–50; Stuart Wildman, "Changes in Hospital Nursing in the West Midlands, 1841–1901," in *Medicine and Society in the Midlands, 1750–1950*, ed. Jonathan Reinarz (Birmingham: Midland History, 2007), 98, 104.

56. Mooney, "Diagnostic Spaces."

57. Waddington, "Sick Poor."

58. For an excellent case study, see Jonathan Reinarz, *The Birth of a Provincial Hospital: The Early Years of the General Hospital, Birmingham, 1765–1790* (Stratford-upon-Avon: Dugdale Society, 2003).

59. This is a considerable literature. See, for instance, Roy Porter, *Quacks: Fakers and Charlatans in English Medicine* (Stroud: Tempus, 2000); Simon Seligman, "The Royal Maternity Charity," *Medical History* 24 (1980): 403–18; Bronwyn Croxson, "The Foundation and Evolution of the Middlesex Hospital's Lying-In Service, 1745–86," *Social History of Medicine* 14 (2001): 27–57; Gregory Phillips, *The Blind in British Society: Charity, State and Community, c. 1780–1930* (Aldershot, UK: Ashgate, 2004); Steven King and Alan Weaver, "Lives in Many Hands: Medical Practice in Rural Lancashire, 1700–1820," *Medical History* 45 (2000): 1–47.

60. Walter Brett, quoted in Beryl Hurley, *Cricklade Absent Poor and Warrants for Reputed Fathers, 1787–1837* (Devizes: Wiltshire Family History Society, 2005), 12 (underlining in original).

61. Anne Borsay, *Medicine and Charity in Georgian Bath: A Social History of the General Infirmary, c. 1739–1830* (Aldershot, UK: Ashgate, 1999).

62. S. King, *Poverty, Sickness and Death*, 146–52.

63. Edward Wilkes, quoted in Hurley, *Cricklade Absent Poor*, 14.

64. S. King, "Stop This Overwhelming Torment."

65. Claudia Edwards, "Age-Based Rationing of Medical Care in Nineteenth-Century England," *Continuity and Change* 14 (1999): 227–65; Ottaway, *Decline of Life*.

66. Peter King, *Narratives of the Poor in Eighteenth-Century Britain, vol. 4, Institutional Responses: The Refuge for the Destitute* (London, Pickering and Chatto, 2006).

67. Levene, "Children," 41–59.

68. Lynsey Cullen, "Patient Case Records of the Royal Free Hospital, London" (PhD diss., Oxford Brookes University, 2011).

69. R. Smith, "Ageing and Well-Being."

70. Jean Robin, *The Way We Lived Then* (Aldershot, UK: Ashgate, 2000); Pamela Sharpe, *Population and Society in an East Devon Parish: Reproducing Colyton, 1540–1840* (Exeter: Exeter University Press, 2002); Barry Reay, *Microhistories: Demography, Society, and Culture in Rural England, 1800–1930* (Cambridge: Cambridge University Press, 1996); Di Cooper and Moira Donald, "Households and Hidden Kin in Early Nineteenth-Century England: Four Case Studies in Suburban Exeter, 1821–1861," *Continuity and Change* 10 (1995): 223–78.

71. As well as material mentioned elsewhere in this chapter, see most recently Robert Ellis, "The Asylum, the Poor Law and the Growth of County Asylums in Nineteenth-Century Yorkshire," *Northern History* 45 (2008): 279–93.

72. Phillips, *Blind in British Society*; Anne Borsay, *Disability and Social Policy in Britain since 1750: A History of Exclusion* (Basingstoke, UK: Palgrave Macmillan, 2005); Pamela Dale and Joseph Melling, eds., *Mental Illness and Learning Disability since 1850: Finding a Place for Mental Disorder in the United Kingdom* (London: Routledge, 2006).

73. Jane Pearson, "'Labor and Sorrow': The Living Conditions of the Elderly Residents of Bocking, Essex, 1793–1807," in *Power and Poverty: Old Age in the Pre-industrial Past*, ed. Susannah Ottaway, Lynn Botelho, and Katharine Kittredge (Westport: Greenwood, 2002), 125–42.

74. Elizabeth Hurren and Steven King, "Begging for a Burial: Death and the Poor Law in Eighteenth- and Nineteenth-Century England," *Social History* 30 (2005): 321–41.

75. C. Smith, "Victorian Asylum"; Bill Forsythe, Joseph Melling, and Richard Adair, "Families, Communities and the Legal Regulation of Lunacy in Victorian England: Assessments of Crime, Violence and Welfare in Admissions to the Devon Asylum, 1845–1914," in *Outside the Walls of the Asylum: The History of Care in the Community*, ed. Peter Bartlett and David Wright (London: Athlone, 1999), 153–80.

76. See particularly Siena, *Venereal Disease*.

77. Oxfordshire Record Office, MSS. D.D. Par. Rotherfield Greys, c.11/2.

78. Mortlake Public Library, Poor Law Papers.

79. Negrine, "Medicine and Poverty."

80. S. King, *Welfare and Local Politics*, 115–41.

81. Hugh Cunningham, *The Invention of Childhood* (London: BBC Books, 2006); Harry Hendrick, *Children: New Perspectives on Child Welfare in England, 1872–1989* (London: Routledge, 1994); Frank Crompton, *Workhouse Children: Infant and Child Paupers under the Worcestershire Poor Law, 1780–1871* (Stroud: Sutton, 1997).

82. Hurren and King, "Begging for a Burial."

Selected Bibliography

Anderson, Philip. "The Leeds Workhouse under the Old Poor Law: 1726–1834." *Publications of the Thoresby Society* 56, no. 2 (1980): 75–113.

Anderson, Rev. William. "Workhouse Hospitals in the West of Ireland." In *Transactions of the National Association for the Promotion of Social Science, Belfast Meeting, 1867*, edited by George W. Hastings, 513–19. London: Green, Reader, and Dyer, 1868.

Andrew, Donna. *Philanthropy and Police: London Charity in the Eighteenth Century.* Princeton: Princeton University Press, 1989.

Anstruther, Ian. *The Scandal of the Andover Workhouse.* Stroud: Sutton, 1984.

Avery, David. "Charity Begins at Home: Edmonton Workhouse Committee, 1732–37." Occasional Papers, n.s., 14, Edmonton Hundred Historical Society, 1967.

Bamford, Samuel. *The Autobiography of Samuel Bamford.* Vol. 1, *Early Days.* London: Cass, 1967.

Barker-Read, Mary. "The Treatment of the Aged Poor in Five Selected West Kent Parishes from Settlement to Speenhamland (1662–1797)." PhD diss., Open University, 1988.

Bartlett, Peter. "The Asylum, the Workhouse and the Voice of the Insane Poor in 19th-Century England." *International Journal of Law and Psychiatry* 21 (1998): 421–32.

——. *The Poor Law of Lunacy: the Administration of Pauper Lunatics in Mid-Nineteenth-Century England.* London: Leicester University Press, 1999.

Blackden, Stephanie. "The Board of Supervision and the Scottish Parochial Medical Service." *Medical History* 30, no. 2 (1986): 145–72.

——. "The Poor Law and Health: A Survey of Medical Aid in Glasgow, 1845–1900." In *The Search for Wealth and Stability: Essays in Economic and Social History Presented to M. W. Flinn*, edited by Thomas Christopher Smout, 243–62. London: Macmillan, 1979.

Bochel, Catherine, and Hugh M. Bochel. *The UK Social Policy Process.* Basingstoke, UK: Palgrave Macmillan, 2004.

Bohstedt, John. *The Politics of Provisions: Food Riots, Moral Economy, and Market Transition in England, c. 1550–1850.* Farnham, UK: Ashgate, 2010.

Botelho, Lynn. *Old Age and the English Poor Law.* Rochester: Boydell and Brewer, 2004.

Boulton, Jeremy. "Welfare Systems and the Parish Nurse in Early Modern London, 1650–1725." *Family and Community History* 10 (2007): 127–51.

Boulton, Jeremy, and John Black. "'Those That Die by Reason of Their Madness': Dying Insane in London, 1629–1830." *History of Psychiatry* 23, no. 1 (2012): 27–39.

Boulton, Jeremy, and Leonard Schwarz. "'The Comforts of a Private Fireside'? The Workhouse, the Elderly and the Poor Law in Georgian Westminster: St. Martin-in-the-Fields, 1725–1824," in *Accommodating Poverty: The Households of the Poor in England, c. 1650–1850*, edited by Joanne McEwan and Pamela Sharpe, 221–45. Basingstoke, UK: Palgrave Macmillan, 2011.

———. "The Parish Workhouse, the Parish and Parochial Medical Provision in Eighteenth-Century London." Working paper available at: http://research.ncl.ac.uk/pauperlives/workhousemedicalisation.pdf.

———. "Yet Another Inquiry into the Trustworthiness of Eighteenth-Century London's Bills of Mortality." *Local Population Studies* 85 (2010): 28–45.

Boyer, George R., and Timothy P. Schmidle. "Poverty among the Elderly in Late Victorian England." *Economic History Review* 62 (2009): 249–78.

Brand, Jeanne L. *Doctors and the State: The British Medical Profession and Government Action in Public Health, 1870–1912.* Baltimore: Johns Hopkins Press, 1965.

Brundage, Anthony. *The English Poor Laws, 1700–1930.* Basingstoke, UK: Palgrave Macmillan, 2002.

Buchanan, Colin A. "John Bowen and the Bridgwater Scandal." *Proceedings of the Somerset Archaeological and Natural History Society* 131 (1987): 181–201.

Burnett, John, David Mayall, and David Vincent, eds. *The Autobiography of the Working Class: An Annotated Critical Bibliography.* 3 vols. Brighton: Harvester, 1987.

Bynum, William F. *Science and the Practice of Medicine in the Nineteenth Century.* Cambridge: Cambridge University Press, 1994.

Cassell, Ronald D. *The Irish Dispensary System and the Poor Law, 1836–1872.* Woodbridge: Boydell, 1997.

Cassell, William A. "The Parish and the Poor in New Brentford, 1720–1834." *Transactions of the London and Middlesex Archaeological Society* (1972): 174–95.

Cherry, Steven. "The Hospitals and Population Growth: The Voluntary General Hospitals, Mortality and Local Populations in the English Provinces in the Eighteenth and Nineteenth Centuries." Pts. 1 and 2. *Population Studies* 34, nos. 1 and 2 (1980): 59–75 and 251–65.

———. *Mental Health Care in Modern England: The Norfolk Lunatic Asylum/St. Andrew's Hospital, c. 1810–1998.* Woodbridge: Boydell, 2003.

Clark, Alice. "Wild Workhouse Girls and the Liberal Imperial State in Mid-Nineteenth Century Ireland." *Journal of Social History* 37 (2005): 389–409.

Conrad, Christoph. "Old Age and the Health Care System in the Nineteenth and Twentieth Centuries." In *Old Age from Antiquity to Post-Modernity*, edited by Paul Johnson and Pat Thane, 132–45. London: Routledge, 1998.

Cox, Catherine. "Medical Dispensary Service in Nineteenth-Century Ireland: Access, Transport and Distance." In *Cultures of Care in Irish Medical History, 1750–1970*, edited by Catherine Cox and Maria Luddy, 57–78. Basingstoke, UK: Palgrave Macmillan, 2010.

Cox, David. "The Diary of Edward Lawrence, Master of Wellington Workhouse, 1890–1." In *Shropshire Historical Documents: A Miscellany*, edited by Sylvia Watts, 149–201. Keele: Keele Centre for Local History, 2000.

Crompton, Frank. *Workhouse Children: Infant and Child Paupers under the Worcestershire Poor Law, 1780–1871.* Stroud: Sutton, 1997.

Crossman, Virginia. "The New Ross Workhouse Riot of 1877: Nationalism, Class and the Irish Poor Laws." *Past and Present* 179 (2003): 135–58.

———. *Politics, Pauperism and Power in Late Nineteenth-Century Ireland.* Manchester: Manchester University Press, 2006.

———. *The Poor Law in Ireland, 1838–1948.* Dundalk: Irish Economic and Social History Society, 2006.

Crowther, Margaret Anne. "Health Care and Poor Relief in Provincial England." In *Health Care and Poor Relief in 18th and 19th Century Northern Europe,* edited by Ole P. Grell, Andrew Cunningham, and Robert Jütte, 203–19. Aldershot, UK: Ashgate, 2002.

———. "Paupers or Patients? Obstacles to Professionalization in the Poor Law Medical Service before 1914." *Journal of the History of Medicine and Allied Sciences* 39 (1984): 33–54.

———. *The Workhouse System, 1834–1929: The History of an English Social Institution.* London: Batsford, 1981.

Dale, Pamela, and Joseph Melling, eds. *Mental Illness and Learning Disability since 1850: Finding a Place for Mental Disorder in the United Kingdom.* London: Routledge, 2006.

Davenport, Romola, Leonard Schwarz, and Jeremy Boulton. "The Decline of Adult Smallpox in Eighteenth-Century London." *Economic History Review* 64, no. 4 (2011): 1289–314.

De Barros, Juanita, Stephen Palmer, and David Wright, eds. *Health and Medicine in the Circum-Caribbean, 1800–1968.* New York: Routledge, 2009.

Delany, Paul. *British Autobiography in the Seventeenth Century.* London: Routledge and Kegan Paul, 1969.

Denham, Michael J. "The History of Geriatric Medicine and Hospital Care of the Elderly between 1929 and the 1970s." PhD diss., University College, London, 2004.

Digby, Anne. *From York Lunatic Asylum to Bootham Park Hospital.* York: University of York, Borthwick Papers, 1986.

———. *Making a Medical Living: Doctors and Patients in the English Market for Medicine, 1720–1911.* Cambridge: Cambridge University Press, 1994.

———. *Pauper Palaces.* London: Routledge and Kegan Paul, 1978.

Dobson, Mary J. *Contours of Death and Disease in Early Modern England.* Cambridge: Cambridge University Press, 1997.

Donnelly, Michael. *Managing the Mind: A Study of Medical Psychology in Early Nineteenth-Century Britain.* London: Tavistock, 1983.

Driver, Felix. *Power and Pauperism: The Workhouse System, 1834–1884.* Cambridge: Cambridge University Press, 1993.

Dunkley, Peter. "The 'Hungry Forties' and the New Poor Law: A Case Study." *Historical Journal* 17 (1974): 329–46.

Eden, Sir Frederick Morton. *The State of the Poor.* 3 vols. London: Davis, 1797.

Edwards, Claudia. "Age-Based Rationing of Medical Care in Nineteenth-Century England." *Continuity and Change* 14 (1999): 227–65.

Ellis, Robert. "The Asylum, the Poor Law and the Growth of County Asylums in Nineteenth-Century Yorkshire." *Northern History* 45 (2008): 279–93.

Fissell, Mary. *Patients, Power and the Poor in Eighteenth-Century Bristol.* Cambridge: Cambridge University Press, 1991.

Fleetwood, John F. *The History of Medicine in Ireland.* Dublin: Skelling, 1983.

Flinn, Michael W. "Medical Services under the New Poor Law." In *The New Poor Law in the Nineteenth Century,* edited by Derek Fraser, 45–66. London: Macmillan, 1976.

Forsythe, Bill, Joseph Melling, and Richard Adair. "The New Poor Law and the County Pauper Lunatic Asylum: The Devon Experience, 1834–1884." *Social History of Medicine* 9, no. 3 (1996): 335–55.

Fowler, Simon. *The Workhouse: The People, the Places, the Life behind Doors.* Richmond, Surrey: National Archives, 2007.

Fraser, Derek, ed. *The New Poor Law in the Nineteenth-Century.* London: Macmillan, 1976.

Frizelle, Ernest R. *The Life and Times of the Royal Infirmary at Leicester: The Making of a Teaching Hospital, 1766–1980.* Leicester: Leicester Medical Society, 1988.

Gagnier, Regina. "Social Atoms: Working-Class Autobiography, Subjectivity, and Gender." *Victorian Studies* 30, no. 3 (1987): 335–63.

Geary, Laurence M. *Medicine and Charity in Ireland, 1718–1851.* Dublin: University College Dublin Press, 2004.

———. "'The Most Illiberal and Monopolising Corporation in Existence': The Royal College of Surgeons in Ireland and Professional Appointments to Irish County Infirmaries." In *Borderlands: Essays on Medicine and Literature in Honour of J. B. Lyons,* edited by Davis Coakley and Mary O'Doherty, 106–14. Dublin: Royal College of Surgeons in Ireland, 2002.

———. "The Poor Law Medical Service in Ireland, 1838–1921." In *Poverty and Welfare in Ireland, 1838–1948,* edited by Virginia Crossman and Peter Gray. Dublin: Irish Academic Press, forthcoming.

George, Dorothy. *London Life in the Eighteenth Century.* London: Kegan Paul, 1925.

Gestrich, Andreas, Elizabeth Hurren, and Steven King, eds. *Poverty and Sickness in Modern Europe: Narratives of the Sick Poor.* London: Continuum, 2012.

Gillingwater, Edmund. *An Essay on Parish Workhouses.* Bury Saint Edmunds: J. Rackham, 1786.

Goodwyn, Edwin A. *"A Prison with a Milder Name": The Shipmeadow House of Industry, 1766–1800.* Beccles: Goodwyn, 1987.

Goose, Nigel. "Poverty, Old Age and Gender in Nineteenth-Century England: The Case of Hertfordshire." *Continuity and Change* 20 (2005): 351–84.

———. "Workhouse Populations in the Mid-Nineteenth Century: The Case of Hertfordshire." *Local Population Studies* 62 (1999): 52–69.

Gordon, Ian, Janet Lewis, and Ken Young. "Perspectives on Policy Analysis." In *The Policy Process: A Reader,* edited by Michael Hill, 5–9. London: Harvester Wheatsheaf, 1993.

Green, David R. "Icons of the New System: Workhouse Construction and Relief Practices in London under the Old and New Poor Law." *London Journal* 34 (2009): 264–84.

———. "Medical Relief and the New Poor Law in London." In *Health Care and Poor Relief in 18th and 19th Century Northern Europe,* edited by Ole P. Grell, Andrew Cunningham, and Robert Jütte, 220–45. Aldershot, UK: Ashgate, 2002.

———. *Pauper Capital: London and the Poor Law, 1790–1870.* Farnham, UK: Ashgate, 2010.

Guinanne, Timothy, and Cormac Ó Gráda. "Mortality in the North Dublin Union during the Great Famine." *Economic History Review* 55, no. 3 (2002): 487–506.

Hall, Rosemary, "The Vanishing Unemployed, Hidden Disabled, and Embezzling Master: Researching Coventry Workhouse Registers." *Local Historian* 38 (2008): 111–21.

Hampson, Ethel Mary. *The Treatment of Poverty in Cambridgeshire, 1597–1834.* Cambridge: Cambridge University Press, 1934.

Hanway, Jonas. *The Citizen's Monitor.* London: Dodsley, Sewell, and New, 1780.

Hardy, Sheila. *The House on the Hill: The Samford House of Industry, 1764–1930.* Suffolk: Gipping, 2001.

Harris, Bernard. *The Origins of the British Welfare State: Social Welfare in England and Wales, 1800–1945.* Basingstoke, UK: Palgrave Macmillan, 2004.

Hastings, Robert. *Poverty and the Poor Laws in the North Riding of Yorkshire.* York: Borthwick Institute, 1982.

Haw, George. *From Workhouse to Westminster: The Life Story of Will Crooks MP.* London: Cassell, 1907.

Hearn, George W. *Dudley Road Hospital, 1887–1987.* Birmingham: Postgraduate Centre, Dudley Road Hospital, 1987.

Helmstadter, Carol. "Early Nursing Reform in Nineteenth-Century London: A Doctor-Driven Phenomenon." *Medical History* 46 (2002): 325–50.

———. "The Passing of the Night Watch: Night Nursing Reform in the London Teaching Hospitals, 1856–90." *Canadian Bulletin of Medical History* 11 (1994): 23–69.

Henriques, Ursula. "How Cruel Was the Victorian Poor Law?" *Historical Journal* 11 (1968): 365–71.

Higgenbotham, Peter. *The Workhouse Cookbook.* Stroud: History, 2008.

Higgs, Michelle. *Life in the Victorian and Edwardian Workhouse.* Stroud: Tempus, 2007.

Hinde, Andrew, and Fiona Turnbull. "The Population of Two Hampshire Workhouses, 1851–1861." *Local Population Studies* 61 (1998): 38–53.

Hitchcock, Tim. *Down and Out in Eighteenth-Century London.* London: Hambledon and London, 2007.

———. "The English Workhouse: A Study in Institutional Poor Relief in Selected Counties, 1696–1750." DPhil diss., Oxford University, 1985.

———. "Paupers and Preachers: The SPCK and the Parochial Workhouse Movement." In *Stilling the Grumbling Hive: The Response to Social and Economic Problems in England, 1689–1750,* edited by Lee Davison, Tim Hitchcock, Tim Keirn, and Robert Shoemaker, 145–66. Stroud: Sutton, 1992.

———. "'You Bitches . . . Die and Be Damned': Gender, Authority and the Mob in St. Martin's Roundhouse Disaster of 1742." In *The Streets of London,* edited by Tim Hitchcock and Heather Shore, 69–91. London: Oram, 2003.

Hodgkinson, Ruth G. *The Origins of the National Health Service: The Medical Services of the New Poor Law, 1834–1871.* London: Wellcome Trust Historical Medical Library, 1967.

———. "Poor Law Medical Officers of England, 1834–1871." *Journal of the History of Medicine and Allied Sciences* 11 (1956): 299–338.

———. "Provision for Pauper Lunatics, 1834–1871." *Medical History* 10 (1966): 138–54.

Honeyman, Katrina. *Child Workers in England, 1780–1820: Parish Apprentices and the Making of the Early Industrial Labour Force.* Aldershot, UK: Ashgate, 2007.

Howard, John. *An Account of the Principal Lazarettos in Europe: With Various Papers Relative to the Plague; Together with Further Observations on Some Foreign Prisons and Hospitals; and Additional Remarks on the Present State of Those in Great Britain and Ireland.* Warrington: W. Eyers, 1789.

Humphries, Jane. *Childhood and Child Labour in the British Industrial Revolution.* Cambridge: Cambridge University Press, 2010.

Hunter, Richard, and Ida Macalpine. *Psychiatry for the Poor: 1851 Colney Hatch Asylum; Friern Hospital, 1973: A Medical and Social History.* Folkestone: Dawsons, 1974.

Hurren, Elizabeth T. *Dying for Victorian Medicine: English Anatomy and Its Trade in the Dead Poor, c. 1834–1929.* Basingstoke, UK: Palgrave Macmillan, 2012.

———. *Protesting about Pauperism: Poverty, Politics and Poor Relief in Late-Victorian England, 1870–1900.* Woodbridge: Boydell, 2007.

Hurren, Elizabeth, and Steven King. "Begging for a Burial: Death and the Poor Law in Eighteenth- and Nineteenth-Century England." *Social History* 30 (2005): 321–41.

Jackson, Christine. "Functionality, Commemoration and Civic Competition: A Study of Early Seventeenth-Century Workhouse Design in Reading and Newbury." *Architectural History* 47 (2004): 77–112.

Jackson, David. "The Medway Union Workhouse, 1876–1881: A Study Based on the Admission and Discharge Registers and the Census Enumerators Books." *Local Population Studies* 75 (2005): 11–32.

Jenner, Mark. "Death, Decomposition and Dechristianization? Public Health and Church Burial in Eighteenth-Century England." *English Historical Review* 120, no. 487 (2005): 615–32.

Jones, Kathleen. *A History of Mental Health Services.* London: Routledge and Kegan Paul, 1972.

Kidd, Alan. *State, Society and the Poor in Nineteenth-Century England.* Basingstoke, UK: Palgrave Macmillan, 1999.

King, Peter. *Narratives of the Poor in Eighteenth-Century Britain. Vol. 4, Institutional Responses: The Refuge for the Destitute.* London: Pickering and Chatto, 2006.

King, Steven. *Poverty and Welfare in England, 1700–1850: A Regional Perspective.* Manchester: Manchester University Press, 2000.

———. *Poverty, Sickness and Death in England, 1750–1850.* London: Continuum, forthcoming.

———. "Regional Patterns in the Experiences and Treatment of the Sick Poor, 1800–40: Rights, Obligations and Duties in the Rhetoric of Paupers." *Family and Community History* 10 (2007): 61–75.

———. "'Stop This Overwhelming Torment of Destiny': Negotiating Financial Aid at Times of Sickness under the English Old Poor Law, 1800–1840." *Bulletin of the History of Medicine* 79, no. 2 (2005): 228–60.

———. *Women, Welfare and Local Politics, 1880–1920: "We Might Be Trusted."* Brighton: Sussex Academic Press, 2005.

King, Steven, Thomas Nutt, and Alannah Tomkins, eds. *Narratives of the Poor in Eighteenth-Century Britain.* Vol. 1, *Voices of the Poor: Poor Law Depositions and Letters.* London: Pickering and Chatto, 2006.

King, Steven, and Alan Weaver. "Lives in Many Hands: Medical Practice in Rural Lancashire, 1700–1820." *Medical History* 45 (2000): 1–47.

Lane, Joan. "Medical Education in the Provinces in Eighteenth-Century England." *Bulletin of the Society for the Social History of Medicine* 41 (1987): 28–33.

———. *A Social History of Medicine: Health, Healing and Disease in England, 1750–1950.* London: Routledge, 2001.

Lees, Lynn Hollen. *The Solidarities of Strangers: The English Poor Laws and the People, 1700–1949.* Cambridge: Cambridge University Press, 1998.

Levene, Alysa. "Between Less Eligibility and the NHS: The Changing Place of Poor Law Hospitals in England and Wales, 1929–39." *Twentieth Century British History* 20 (2009): 322–45.

———. *Childcare, Health, and Mortality at the London Foundling Hospital.* Manchester: University of Manchester Press, 2007.

———. "Children, Childhood and the Workhouse: St. Marylebone, 1769–1781." *London Journal* 33 (2008): 41–59.

Levine-Clark, Marjorie. *Beyond the Reproductive Body: The Politics of Women's Health and Work in Early Victorian England.* Columbus: Ohio State University Press, 2004.

———. "Engendering Relief: Women, Ablebodiedness, and the Poor Law in Early Victorian England." *Journal of Women's History* 11, no. 4 (2000): 107–30.

Lomax, Elizabeth. *Small and Special: The Development of Hospitals for Children in Victorian Britain.* London: Wellcome Trust, 1996.

Longmate, Norman. *The Workhouse.* New York: St. Martin's Press, 1974.

Loudon, Irvine. *Medical Care and the General Practitioner, 1750–1850.* Oxford: Clarendon, 1986.

———. "The Origins and Growth of the Dispensary Movement in England." *Bulletin of the History of Medicine* 16 (1981): 322–42.

Love, David. *The Life and Adventures of David Love.* Nottingham: Sutton & Son, 1823.

Lucas, Gavin. "The Archaeology of the Workhouse: The Changing Uses of Workhouse Buildings at St. Mary's, Southampton." In *The Familiar Past? Archaeologies of Later Historical Britain,* edited by Sarah Tarlow and Susie West, 125–39. London: Routledge, 1999.

Luddy, Maria. "'Angels of Mercy': Nuns as Workhouse Nurses, 1861–1898." In *Medicine, Disease and the State in Ireland, 1650–1940,* edited by Greta Jones and Elizabeth Malcolm, 102–17. Cork: Cork University Press, 1999.

MacKay, E. Hugh. *The Palace on the Hill: Leicester General Hospital Centenary, 1905–2005.* Leicester: Leicester General Hospital, 2006.

MacKay, Lynn. "A Culture of Poverty? The St. Martin's in the Fields Workhouse, 1817." *Journal of Interdisciplinary History* 26, no. 2 (1995): 209–31.

———. "Moral Paupers: The Poor Men of St. Martin's, 1815–1819." *Histoire sociale/ Social History* 67 (2001): 115–31.

Mackenzie, Charlotte. *Psychiatry for the Rich: A History of Ticehurst Asylum, 1792–1917.* London: Routledge and Kegan Paul, 1992.

MacKinnon, Mary. "The Use and Misuse of Poor Law Statistics, 1857 to 1912." *Historical Methods* 21 (1988): 5–19.

Marcroft, William. *The Marcroft Family.* London: J. Heywood, 1886.

Marland, Hilary. *Medicine and Society in Wakefield and Huddersfield: 1780–1870.* Cambridge: Cambridge University Press, 1987.

Mascuch, Michael. *Origins of the Individualist Self: Autobiography and Self-Identity in England, 1591–1791.* Stanford: Stanford University Press, 1997.

McCandless, Peter. "'Build! Build!' The Controversy over the Care of the Chronically Insane in England, 1855–70." *Bulletin of the History of Medicine* 53 (1979): 553–74.

———. "Insanity and Society: A Study of the English Lunacy Reform Movement, 1815–1870." PhD diss., University of Wisconsin, 1974.

McCord, Norman. "The Implementation of the 1834 Poor Law Amendment Act on Tyneside." *International Review of Social History* 14 (1969): 90–108.

McKeown, Thomas. *The Role of Medicine: Dream, Mirage or Nemesis.* Oxford: Basil Blackwell, 1979.

Mellett, David J. "Bureaucracy and Mental Illness: The Commissioners in Lunacy, 1845–90." *Medical History* 25 (1981): 221–50.

———. *The Prerogative of Asylumdom: Social, Cultural and Administrative Aspects of the Institutional Treatment of the Insane in Nineteenth-Century Britain.* New York: Garland, 1982.

Melling, Elizabeth, ed., *Kentish Sources.* Vol. 4, *The Poor.* Maidstone: Kent County Council, 1964.

Melling, Joseph, and Bill Forsythe. *The Politics of Madness: The State, Insanity and Society in England, 1845–1914.* London: Routledge, 2006.

Midwinter, Eric. *Victorian Social Reform.* London: Longman, 1968.

Miller, Edgar. "The Role of the Poor Law in the Care of the Insane in the Nineteenth Century." *History and Philosophy of Psychology* 8 (2006): 17–26.

Mooney, Graham. "Diagnostic Spaces: Workhouse, Hospital and Home in Mid-Victorian London." *Social Science History* 33 (2009): 357–90.

Mooney, Graham, Bill Luckin, and Andrea Tanner. "Patient Pathways: Solving the Problem of Institutional Mortality in London during the Later Nineteenth Century." *Social History of Medicine* 12 (1999): 227–69.

Mooney, Graham, and Jonathan Reinarz, eds. *Permeable Walls: Historical Perspectives on Hospital and Asylum Visiting.* Amsterdam: Rodopi, 2009.

Morrison, Kathryn. *The Workhouse: A Study of Poor Law Buildings in England.* Swindon: English Heritage, 1999.

Munkhoff, Richelle. "Searchers of the Dead: Authority, Marginality, and the Interpretation of Plague in England, 1574–1665." *Gender and History* 11, no. 1 (1999): 1–29.

Murphy, Elaine. "The New Poor Law Guardians and the Administration of Insanity in East-London, 1834–1844." *Bulletin of the History of Medicine* 77 (2003): 45–74.

———. "Workhouse Care of the Insane, 1845–1890." In *Mental Illness and Learning Disability since 1850,* edited by Pamela Dale and Joseph Melling, 24–45. London: Routledge, 2006.

Myers, Edward. *A History of Psychiatry in North Staffordshire.* Leek: Churnet Valley Books, 1997.

———. "Lunacy in the Stoke-upon-Trent Workhouse, 1834–1900." *Psychiatric Bulletin* 18 (1994): 492–94.

Nagley, Laurence. "A History of the Summerfield Hospital." *Midland Medical Review* 10 (1975): 10–17.

Neate, Alan. *The St. Marylebone Workhouse and Institution, 1730–1965.* London: London Record Society, 2003.

Negrine, Angela. "Medicine and Poverty: A Study of the Poor Law Medical Services of the Leicester Union, 1867–1914." PhD diss., University of Leicester, 2008.

Newman, Simon, P. *Embodied History: The Lives of the Poor in Early Philadelphia.* Philadelphia: University of Pennsylvania Press, 2003.

O'Mahony, Colman. *Cork's Poor Law Palace: Workhouse Life, 1838–90.* Cork: Rosmathun, 2005.

Ottaway, Susannah. *The Decline of Life: Old Age in Eighteenth-Century England.* Cambridge: Cambridge University Press, 2004.

———. "Medicine and Old Age." In *The Oxford Handbook of the History of Medicine,* edited by Mark Jackson, 338–54. Oxford: Oxford University Press, 2011.

Oxley, Geoffrey. *Poor Relief in England and Wales, 1601–1834.* Newton Abbott: David and Charles, 1974.

Parry-Jones, William L. *The Trade in Lunacy.* London: Routledge & Kegan Paul, 1972.

Paton, Diane. *No Bond but the Law: Punishment, Race and Gender in Jamaica State Formation, 1780–1870.* Durham: Duke University Press, 2004.

———. "The Penalties of Freedom: Punishment in Post-emancipation Jamaica." In *Crime and Punishment in Latin America: Law and Society since Late Colonial Times,* edited by Ricardo D. Salvatore, Carlos Aguirre, and Gilbert M. Joseph, 275–77. Durham: Duke University Press, 2001.

Pearson, Jane. "'Labor and Sorrow': The Living Conditions of the Elderly Residents of Bocking, Essex, 1793–1807." In *Power and Poverty: Old Age in the Pre-industrial Past,* edited by Susannah Ottaway, Lynn Botelho, and Katharine Kittredge, 125–42. Westport, CT: Greenwood, 2002.

Pickstone, John V. *Medicine and Industrial Society: A History of Hospital Development in Manchester and Its Region, 1752–1946.* Manchester, Manchester University Press, 1985.

Pinches, Sylvia. "Women as Objects and Agents of Charity in Eighteenth-Century Birmingham." In *Women and Urban Life in Eighteenth-Century England: On the Town,* edited by Roey Sweet and Penelope Lane, 65–86. Aldershot, UK: Ashgate, 2003.

Porter, Roy. "The Gift Relation: Philanthropy and Provincial Hospitals in Eighteenth-Century England." In *The Hospital in History,* edited by Lindsay Granshaw and Roy Porter, 149–78. London: Routledge, 1989.

———. *Mind Forg'd Manacles: A History of Madness in England from the Restoration to the Regency.* Cambridge: Cambridge University Press, 1987.

Price, Kim. "A Regional, Quantitative and Qualitative Study of the Employment, Disciplining and Discharging of Workhouse Medical Officers of the New Poor Law throughout Nineteenth-Century England and Wales." PhD diss., Oxford Brookes University, 2008.

Railton, Margaret, and Marshall Barr. *Battle Workhouse and Hospital, 1867–2005.* Reading: Berkshire Medical Heritage Centre, 2005.

Reinarz, Jonathan. *The Birth of a Provincial Hospital: The Early Years of the General Hospital, Birmingham, 1765–1790.* Stratford-upon-Avon: Dugdale Society, 2003.

————. *Health Care in Birmingham: The Birmingham Teaching Hospitals, 1779–1939.* Woodbridge: Boydell, 2009.

————. "Investigating the 'Deserving' Poor: Charity and the Voluntary Hospitals in Nineteenth-Century Birmingham." In *Medicine, Charity and Mutual Aid: The Consumption of Health and Welfare in Britain, c. 1550–1950,* edited by Anne Borsay and Peter Shapely, 111–33. Aldershot, UK: Ashgate, 2007.

————. "Mechanizing Medicine: Medical Innovations and the Birmingham Voluntary Hospitals in the Nineteenth Century." In *Devices and Designs: Medical Technologies in Historical Perspective,* edited by Julie Anderson and Carsten Timmermann, 37–60. Basingstoke, UK: Palgrave Macmillan, 2006.

————. "The Transformation of Medical Education in Eighteenth-Century England: International Developments and the West Midlands." *History of Education* 37, no. 4 (2008): 549–66.

Richardson, Ruth. *Death, Dissection and the Destitute.* London: Routledge and Kegan Paul, 1987.

Richardson, Ruth, and Brian Hurwitz. "Joseph Rogers and the Reform of Workhouse Medicine." *British Medical Journal* 299 (1989): 1507–10.

Risse, Gunter. *Mending Bodies, Saving Souls: A History of Hospitals.* Oxford: Oxford University Press, 1999.

Ritch, Alistair E. S. "Sick, Aged and Infirm: Adults in the New Birmingham Workhouse, 1852–1912." MPhil diss., University of Birmingham, 2010.

Roberts, David. "How Cruel Was the Victorian Poor Law?" *Historical Journal* 6 (1963): 97–107.

————. *The Victorian Origins of the Welfare State.* Yale: Yale University Press, 1960.

Robin, Jean. "The Relief of Poverty in Mid-Nineteenth-Century Colyton." *Rural History* 1 (1990): 193–218.

Rogers, James E. Thorold, ed. *Joseph Rogers, MD: Reminiscences of the Workhouse Medical Officer.* London: Unwin, 1889.

Saunders, Janet. "Quarantining the Weak-Minded: Psychiatric Definitions of Degeneracy and the Late-Victorian Workhouse." In *The Anatomy of Madness: Essays in the History of Psychiatry.* Vol. 3, *The Asylum and Its Psychiatry,* edited by William F. Bynum, Roy Porter, and Michael Shepherd, 273–96. London: Routledge, 1988.

Schäfer, Daniel. "'That Senescence Itself Is an Illness': A Transitional Medical Concept of Age and Ageing in the Eighteenth Century." *Medical History* 46 (2002): 525–48.

Scott, James. *Domination and the Arts of Resistance.* New Haven: Yale University Press, 1990.

Scull, Andrew. *The Most Solitary of Afflictions: Madness and Society in Britain, 1700–1900.* New Haven: Yale University Press, 1993.

————. *Museums of Madness: The Social Organisation of Insanity in Nineteenth-Century England.* London: Lane, 1979.

Shave, Samantha. "The Dependent Poor? (Re)constructing Individuals' Lives 'on the Parish' in Rural Dorset, 1800–1832." *Rural History* 20, no. 1 (2009): 67–98.

————. "Poor Law Reform and Policy Innovation in Rural Southern England, c. 1780–1850." PhD diss., University of Southampton, 2010.

Siena, Kevin. "Hospitals for the Excluded or Convalescent Homes? Workhouses, Medicalization and the Poor Law in Long Eighteenth-Century London and Pre-confederation Toronto." *Canadian Bulletin of Medical History* 27, no. 1 (2010): 5–25.

———. "Searchers of the Dead in Long Eighteenth-Century London." In *Worth and Repute: Valuing Gender in Late Medieval and Early Modern Europe*, edited by Kim Kippen and Lori Woods, 123–52. Toronto: Centre for Reformation and Renaissance Studies, 2011.

———. *Venereal Disease, Hospitals and the Urban Poor: London's "Foul Wards," 1600–1800*. Rochester: University of Rochester Press, 2004.

Sigsworth, Eric M. "Gateways to Death? Medicine, Hospitals and Mortality, 1700–1850." In *Science and Society, 1600–1900*, edited by Peter Mathias, 97–110. London: Cambridge University Press, 1972.

Slack, Paul. *From Reformation to Improvement: Public Welfare in Early Modern England*. New York: Oxford University Press, 1999.

Smith, Cathy. "Family, Community and the Victorian Asylum: A Case Study of the Northampton General Lunatic Asylum and Its Pauper Lunatics." *Family and Community History* 9 (2006): 109–24.

Smith, Francis B. *The People's Health, 1830–1910*. London: Croom Helm, 1979.

Smith, James E. "Widowhood and Ageing in Traditional English Society." *Ageing and Society* 4, no. 4 (1984): 429–49.

Smith, Leonard. "The County Asylum in the 'Mixed Economy of Care.'" In *Insanity, Institutions and Society, 1800–1914: A Social History of Madness in Comparative Perspective*, edited by Joseph Melling and Bill Forsythe, 23–47. London: Routledge, 1999.

———. *"Cure, Comfort and Safe Custody": Public Lunatic Asylums in Early Nineteenth-Century England*. London: Leicester University Press, 1999.

———. "Duddeston Hall and the 'Trade in Lunacy,' 1835–65." *Birmingham Historian* 8 (1992): 16–22.

———. "Eighteenth-Century Madhouse Practice: The Prouds of Bilston." *History of Psychiatry* 3 (1992): 45–52.

———. *Lunatic Hospitals in Georgian England, 1750–1830*. London: Routledge, 2007.

———. "The Pauper Lunatic Problem in the West Midlands, 1818–1850." *Midland History* 21 (1996): 101–18.

———. "Sandfield House Lunatic Asylum, Lichfield, 1820–1856." *Staffordshire Studies* 10 (1998): 71–75.

———. "To Cure Those Afflicted with the Disease of Insanity: Thomas Bakewell and Spring Vale Asylum." *History of Psychiatry* 4 (1993): 107–27.

———. "'A Worthy Feeling Gentleman': Samuel Hitch at Gloucester Asylum, 1828–1847." In *150 Years of British Psychiatry*. Vol. 2, *The Aftermath*, edited by Hugh Freeman and German Berrios, 470–99. London: Athlone, 1996.

Smith, Richard. "Ageing and Well-Being in Early Modern England: Pension Trends and Gender Preferences under the English Old Poor Law, c. 1650–1800." In *Old Age from Antiquity to Post-Modernity*, edited by Paul Johnson and Pat Thane, 64–95. London: Routledge, 1998.

Sokoll, Thomas, ed. *Essex Pauper Letters, 1731–1837*. Oxford: Oxford University Press, 2001.

Spicker, Paul. *Policy Analysis for Practice: Applying Social Policy*. Bristol: Policy, 2006.

Stewart, John, and Steven King. "Death in Llantrisant: Henry Williams and the New Poor Law in Wales." *Rural History* 15 (2004): 69–87.

Stringer, Alison. "Depth and Diversity in Parochial Healthcare: Northamptonshire, 1750–1830." *Family and Community History* 9 (2006): 43–54.

Suzuki, Akihito. "The Household and the Care of Lunatics in Eighteenth-Century London." In *The Locus of Care: Families, Communities Institutions and the Provision of Welfare since Antiquity*, edited by Peregrine Horden and Richard Smith, 153–75. London: Routledge, 1998.

Thane, Pat. *Old Age in English History: Past Experiences, Present Issues*. Oxford: Oxford University Press, 2000.

Thomas, Eric. "The Old Poor Law and Medicine." *Medical History* 24 (1980): 1–19.

Thompson, Edward P. *The Making of the English Working Class*. London: Penguin, 1980.

Thompson, Kate M. "The Leicester Poor Law Union, 1836–1871." PhD diss., University of Leicester, 1988.

Thomson, David. "Workhouse to Nursing Home: Residential Care of Elderly People in England since 1840." *Ageing and Society* 3 (1983): 43–70.

Tomkins, Alannah. "'The Excellent Example of the Working Class': Medical Welfare, Contributory Funding and the North Staffordshire Infirmary from 1815." *Social History of Medicine* 21 (2008): 13–30.

———. *The Experience of Urban Poverty, 1723–82: Parish, Charity and Credit*. Manchester: Manchester University Press, 2006.

———. "'Hell with the Lid Off': Re-evaluating the English Workhouse from Working-Class Autobiographies." *Social History of Medicine* (forthcoming).

Townsend, Peter. *The Last Refuge*. London: Routledge and Kegan Paul, 1962.

Troughear, Thomas. *The Best Way of Making Our Charity Truly Beneficial to the Poor; or, The Excellency of Work-Houses in Country Parishes, to Prevent the Evil Effects of Idleness: In a Sermon Preached at Northwood in the Isle of Wight, September the 7th, 1729*. London: Downing, 1730.

Vancouver, John. *An Enquiry into the Causes and Production of Poverty, and the State of the Poor: Together with the Proposed Means for Their Effectual Relief*. London: Edwards, 1796.

Vincent, David. *Bread, Knowledge and Freedom: A Study of Nineteenth-Century Working-Class Autobiography*. London: Methuen, 1982.

Waddington, Keir. *Charity and the London Hospitals, 1850–98*. Woodbridge: Boydell, 2000.

———. "Paying for the Sick Poor: Financing Medicine under the Victorian Poor Law; The Case of Whitechapel Union, 1850–1900." In *Financing Medicine: The British Experience since 1750*, edited by Martin Gorsky and Sally Sheard, 95–111. Aldershot, UK: Ashgate, 2006.

Walter, Tony. *The Revival of Death*. London: Routledge, 1994.

Washington, John. "Poverty, Health and Social Welfare: The History of the Halifax Union Workhouse and the St. John's Hospital, 1834–1972." *Transactions of the Halifax Antiquarian Society* 5 (1997): 83–87.

Webb, Sidney, and Beatrice Webb. *English Local Government: English Poor Law History*. Pt. 1, *The Old Poor Law*. London: Longmans, Green, 1927.

———. *State and the Doctor.* London: Longman, Green, 1910.

Wells, Roger. "Andover Antecedents? Hampshire New Poor-Law Scandals, 1834–1842." *Southern History* 24 (2002): 91–227.

West, Francis Athow, ed. *Memoirs of Jonathan Saville of Halifax.* London: Hamilton, Adams and Co., 1848.

White, Rosemary. *Social Change and the Development of the Nursing Profession.* London: Kimpton, 1978.

Wilde, Joseph. *The Hospital, a Poem in Three Books, Written in the Devon and Exeter Hospital, 1809.* Norwich: Stevenson, Matchett, and Stevenson, 1809.

Wildman, Stuart. "Changes in Hospital Nursing in the West Midlands, 1841–1901." In *Medicine and Society in the Midlands, 1750–1950,* edited by Jonathan Reinarz, 98–114. Birmingham: Midland History, 2007.

Williams, Samantha. "Caring for the Sick Poor: Poor Law Nurses in Bedfordshire, c. 1770–1834." In *Women, Work and Wages in England, 1600–1850,* edited by Penelope Lane, Neil Raven, and Keith Snell, 141–69. Woodbridge: Boydell, 2004.

———. "Practitioners' Income and Provision for the Poor: Parish Doctors in the Late Eighteenth and Early Nineteenth Centuries." *Social History of Medicine* 18 (2005): 1–28.

Wood, Peter. *Poverty and the Workhouse in Victorian Britain.* Stroud: Sutton, 1991.

Woodward, John. *To Do the Sick No Harm: A Study of the British Voluntary Hospital System to 1875.* London: Routledge and Kegan Paul, 1974.

Wright, David. "The Discharge of Pauper Lunatics from County Asylums in Mid-Victorian England: The Case of Buckinghamshire, 1853–1872." In *Insanity, Institutions and Society,* edited by Joseph Melling and Bill Forsythe, 93–113. London: Routledge, 1999.

———. "Getting Out of the Asylum: Understanding the Confinement of the Insane in the Nineteenth Century." *Social History of Medicine* 10 (1997): 137–55.

———. *Mental Disability in Victorian England: The Earlswood Asylum, 1847–1901.* Oxford: Clarendon, 2001.

Wright David, and Anne Digby, eds. *From Idiocy to Mental Deficiency: Historical Perspectives on People with Learning Disabilities.* London: Routledge, 1996.

Wrigley, E. Anthony, and Roger S. Schofield. *The Population History of England, 1541–1871: A Reconstruction.* Cambridge: Cambridge University Press, 1989.

Contributors

JEREMY BOULTON is a professor of urban history at the School of History, Classics, and Archaeology at Newcastle University. He has published widely on many aspects of London's economy, society, and demography between 1550 and 1825. He is currently studying various aspects of welfare and demography in Georgian Westminster. Since 2004 he has, together with Romola Davenport and Leonard Schwarz, been leading the Pauper Lives Project (http://research.ncl.ac.uk/pauperlives), which is based on a detailed reconstruction of the lives of inhabitants of the large parish workhouse of St. Martin in the Fields (1725–1824). This research has been twice funded by the ESRC and also by the Wellcome Trust. Publications from the project have appeared recently in the *History of Psychiatry, Economic History Review, Local Population Studies,* and *Accommodating Poverty: The Housing and Living Arrangements of the English Poor, c. 1600–1850,* edited by Joanne McEwan and Pamela Sharpe (Basingstoke, UK: Palgrave Macmillan, 2011).

VIRGINIA CROSSMAN is a professor of modern Irish history at Oxford Brookes University. She has published widely on the history of government and welfare in Ireland, including, edited with Peter Gray, *Poverty and Welfare in Ireland, 1838–1948* (Dublin: Irish Academic Press, 2011). She is currently working on a monograph titled *The Irish Poor Law: Poverty, Welfare and Community in Ireland, 1850–1914* (Liverpool: Liverpool University Press, forthcoming).

ROMOLA DAVENPORT is a senior research associate at the Cambridge Group for the History of Population and Social Structure at the University of Cambridge. She pursued a career in biology before training as a demographer and is currently investigating the decline of mortality in urban centers of northwestern Europe from 1750 to 1820. Recent publications include, with Leonard Schwarz and Jeremy Boulton, "The Decline of Adult Smallpox in Eighteenth-Century London," *Economic History Review* 64 (2011): 1289–1314.

STEVEN KING is the director of the University of Leicester Centre for Medical Humanities. He publishes widely on topics ranging from industrialization, poverty, and marriage to the nature of the medical marketplace. Recent publications include, edited with Andreas Gestrich and Elizabeth Hurren, *Poverty and Sickness in Modern Europe: Narratives of the Sick Poor, 1780–1938*

(London: Continuum, 2012); "The Healing Tree," in *Invaluable Trees: Cultures of Nature, 1660–1830,* edited by Laura Auricchio, Elizabeth Heckendorn Cook, and Giulia Pacini (Oxford: Voltaire Foundation, 2012), 237–50; and, with Mark Shephard, "Courtship and the Remarrying Man in Late-Victorian England," *Journal of Family History* 37 (2012): 319–40.

ANGELA NEGRINE is an independent scholar who completed a PhD on "Medicine and Poverty: A Study of the Poor Law Medical Services of the Leicester Union, 1867–1914" at the University of Leicester in 2008. She recently published "The Treatment of Sick Children in the Workhouse by the Leicester Poor Law Union, 1867–1914," *Family and Community History* 13 (2010): 34–44.

SUSANNAH OTTAWAY is the David and Marian Adams Bryn-Jones Distinguished Teaching Professor of the Humanities and professor of history at Carleton College, Minnesota, United States. She is the author of *The Decline of Life: Old Age in Eighteenth-Century England* (Cambridge: Cambridge University Press, 2004) and coeditor, with Lynn Botelho, Anne Kugler, and Ingrid Tague, of the eight-volume source collection *Old Age, c. 1600–1800* (London: Pickering and Chatto, 2008–9).

RITA PEMBERTON is a senior lecturer in history at the St. Augustine campus of the University of the West Indies. Her research interests include the history of Caribbean health and environment, agriculture, and, especially, the culture of Tobago. Her most recent publications include "Dirt, Disease and Death: Control, Resistance and Change in the Post Emancipation Caribbean," *História Ciências, Saúde-Manguinhos* 19 (December 2012): 47–58; and "Petticoats, Pathogens and Pollutants: Gender, Law and Sanitation in 19th-Century Trinidad," in *Engendering Caribbean History: Cross Cultural Perspectives,* edited by Verene Shepherd (Kingston, Jamaica: Randle, 2011). She is the coeditor, with Heather Cateau, of *Beyond Tradition: Reinterpreting the Caribbean Historical Experience* (Kingston: Randle, 2006).

JONATHAN REINARZ is a reader and director at the History of Medicine Unit, University of Birmingham, United Kingdom. His recent publications include, edited with Graham Mooney, *Permeable Walls: Institutional Visiting in Historical Perspective* (Amsterdam: Rodopi, 2009); *Healthcare in Birmingham: The Birmingham Teaching Hospitals, 1779–1939* (Woodbridge: Boydell and Brewer, 2009); and, edited with Leonard Schwarz, a special issue of the *Journal for Eighteenth-Century Studies* on "The Enlightenment and the Senses" (35, no. 4, 2012). Forthcoming publications include *Past Scents: Historical Perspectives on Smell* (Champaign: University of Illinois Press, 2013) and an edited collection with Kevin Siena, *A Medical History of Skin: Scratching the Surface* (London: Pickering and Chatto, 2013).

ALISTAIR RITCH is a postgraduate student in the History of Medicine Unit, University of Birmingham, and was previously a consultant physician in geriatric medicine at City Hospital in Birmingham and a senior clinical lecturer at the University of Birmingham, United Kingdom. His MPhil dissertation at the University of Birmingham is on "Sick, Aged and Infirm Adults in the New Birmingham Workhouse, 1852–1912" (available at http://etheses.bham.ac.uk/846). His article "The History of Geriatric Medicine: From Hippocrates to Marjory Warren" is due to be published in 2013 by the *Journal of the Royal College of Physicians of Edinburgh.*

LEONARD SCHWARZ has recently retired as a reader in urban history at the University of Birmingham, where he founded the Birmingham Eighteenth Century Centre. He is the author of *London in the Age of Industrialisation: Entrepreneurs, Labour Force and Living Conditions in the Capital, 1700–1850* (Cambridge: Cambridge University Press, 1992; repr., 2004). Though retired, he continues to research. His main interests are eighteenth- and early nineteenth-century London, on which he has published fairly extensively.

SAMANTHA SHAVE is a research associate in the Faculty of History at the University of Cambridge. Her doctoral thesis, completed at the University of Southampton in 2010, examined the creation, adoption, implementation, and local reworking of both indoor and outdoor poor relief policies in late eighteenth- and early nineteenth-century England. Her publications include "The Dependent Poor? (Re)constructing Individuals' Lives 'on the Parish' in Rural Dorset, 1800–1832," *Rural History* 20, no. 1 (2009): 67–98. A monograph titled *Pauper Policies: Poor Law Practice in England, 1780–1850* is in preparation for Manchester University Press.

KEVIN SIENA is an associate professor of history at Trent University. He is the author of *Venereal Disease, Hospitals and the Urban Poor: London's "Foul Wards,"* *1600–1800* (Rochester: University of Rochester Press, 2004) and editor of *Sins of the Flesh: Responding to Sexual Disease in Early Modern Europe* (Toronto: Centre for Reformation and Renaissance Studies, 2005). He is editing, with Jonathan Reinarz, *A Medical History of Skin: Scratching the Surface* (London: Pickering and Chatto, 2013) and is currently writing a book on class and contagion in eighteenth-century Britain.

LEONARD SMITH is an honorary senior research fellow at the History of Medicine Unit, University of Birmingham, United Kingdom. He has published extensively on the history of psychiatry and mental institutions. His main publications are *"Cure, Comfort and Safe Custody": Public Lunatic Asylums in Early Nineteenth-Century England* (London: University of Leicester Press, 1999) and *Lunatic Hospitals in Georgian England, 1750–1830* (London:

Routledge, 2007). He is currently preparing a history of the development of the lunatic asylum system in the former British West Indies.

ALANNAH TOMKINS is a senior lecturer in history at Keele University, United Kingdom. Her recent publications include "'Who Were His Peers?' The Social and Professional Milieu of the Provincial Surgeon-Apothecary in the Late Eighteenth Century," *Journal of Social History* 44, no. 3 (2011): 915–35; and "'Labouring on a Bed of Sickness': The Material and Rhetorical Deployment of Ill Health in Men's Pauper Letters," in *Poverty and Sickness in Modern Europe: Narratives of the Sick Poor, 1780–1938*, edited by Andreas Gestrich, Elizabeth Hurren, and Steven King (London: Continuum, 2012), 51–68. She is currently writing a book, provisionally titled *Disappointing Doctors: Turbulent Medical Careers in an Age of Professionalization, 1780–1890*.

Index

Printed in the United States
By Bookmasters